# Advanced Studies in Chronic Lymphocytic Leukemia

# Advanced Studies in Chronic Lymphocytic Leukemia

Edited by **Matthew Griffin**

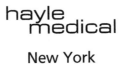

New York

Published by Hayle Medical,
30 West, 37th Street, Suite 612,
New York, NY 10018, USA
www.haylemedical.com

**Advanced Studies in Chronic Lymphocytic Leukemia**
Edited by Matthew Griffin

International Standard Book Number: 978-1-63241-015-3 (Hardback)

Printed in the United States of America.

# Contents

# Preface

The main aim of this book is to educate learners and enhance their research focus by presenting diverse topics covering this vast field. This is an advanced book which compiles significant studies by distinguished experts in the area of analysis. This book addresses successive solutions to the challenges arising in the area of application, along with it; the book provides scope for future developments.

Chronic Lymphocytic Leukemia (CLL) is a disease which has a variable course, and survival rates range from months to decades. It is evident that clinical heterogeneity represents biologic variety with two main subtypes in terms of cellular multiplication, clinical aggressiveness and predictability. As CLL progresses, irregular hematopoiesis leads to pancytopenia and decreased immunoglobulin creation, followed by nonspecific symptoms such as fatigue or malaise. A cure is tough to find in normal cases and postponed treatment (until symptoms develop) is aimed at lengthening life and eliminating symptoms. Experts are playing a crucial role in studying CLL's main source and the role of genetics in the development of this disorder. Research programs are devoted towards comprehending the essential mechanisms underlying CLL with the hope of enhancing treatment options. The book entails a detailed analysis of CLL prognosis and therapy.

It was a great honour to edit this book, though there were challenges, as it involved a lot of communication and networking between me and the editorial team. However, the end result was this all-inclusive book covering diverse themes in the field.

Finally, it is important to acknowledge the efforts of the contributors for their excellent chapters, through which a wide variety of issues have been addressed. I would also like to thank my colleagues for their valuable feedback during the making of this book.

**Editor**

# Part 1

## CLL Prognosis

# Genetics of Chronic Lymphocytic Leukemia: Practical Aspects and Prognostic Significance

N. Put[1], I. Wlodarska[1], P. Vandenberghe[1] and L. Michaux[1,2]
[1]Center for Human Genetics, Catholic University of Leuven, Leuven
[2]Department of Hematology, University Hospital UCL Saint-Luc, Brussels,
Belgium

## 1. Introduction

B-cell chronic lymphocytic leukemia (CLL) is a mature B-cell neoplasm. Affecting mainly the elderly, CLL represents the most common hematological malignancy in Western countries, and 6-7% of non Hodgkin's lymphomas.

The disease course is heterogenous. Clinical staging systems (i.e. Rai and Binet) are used for estimating the tumor burden and prognosis and for making therapeutic decisions in individual patients. However, the evolution, even in the early stages, remains highly variable with at least 50% of cases showing early or late progression. Since the large majority of newly diagnosed cases present with early or intermediate stage, it is important to assess the risk profile within this group.

Several biological variables have been proposed for the prognostic stratification of early stage CLL, including chromosomal abnormalities [as assessed by karyotyping or fluorescent *in situ* hybridization (FISH)], expression of CD38, the proportion of ZAP-70-positive cells, somatic hypermutation of the variable part of the B-cell receptor gene (*IGVH*) and *VH* 3-21 usage. In addition, acquisition of particular chromosomal aberrations could be relevant, i.e. a 17p deletion appearing during the disease course confers resistance to alkylating agents and purine analogs, underscoring the need for defining the genetic patterns of disease evolution.

Here, chromosomal aberrations in CLL will be reviewed. First, the different techniques to detect abnormalities will be described. Second, the CLL-associated (cyto)genetic abnormalities and their relevance for clinical practice will be discussed, with a focus on the role of these aberrations in disease onset, progression, and on their prognostic significance.

## 2. Cytogenetic techniques

Numerous studies have shown that the presence, number, and type of chromosomal aberrations represent an independent predictor of prognosis in CLL (Döhner *et al*, 2000; Juliusson *et al*, 1990; Mayr *et al*, 2006; Van Den Neste *et al*, 2007). Therefore, cytogenetic analysis is now routinely performed in this disease. Different techniques are available to detect chromosomal abnormalities. Conventional cytogenetic analysis (CCA) can be performed, but is hampered by the poor mitotic index of CLL lymphocytes *in vitro*.

Although several mitogens have been used to overcome this problem, alternative approaches allowing analysis of nondividing cells are available, i.e. interphase FISH is widely used and has become the standard technique. In addition multiplex ligation-dependent probe amplification (MLPA) (Coll-Mulet *et al*, 2008; Fabris *et al*, 2011) and more recently analysis by means of different array-platforms (Gunn *et al*, 2008; Hagenkord *et al*, 2010) have been investigated in research and routine setting.

## 2.1 Conventional cytogenetic analysis

CCA or chromosome banding analysis (CBA) examines the patient's chromosomes in a sample of cells. Counting the number of chromosomes and evaluating their structural aberrations (banding patterns) results in the construction of a karyogram and karyotype. The resolution is determined by the number of bands seen in a haploid set of chromosomes (300-850 bands, each band contains approximately 5-10 megabase of DNA) (Shaffer *et al*, 2009). The work-flow of the technical procedure is shown in Fig 1. Peripheral blood is the preferred tissue for CCA in CLL, but bone marrow, lymph node, spleen or effusions can be analyzed as well.

Since CLL is a malignancy of mature B-cells, these cells are often arrested at the $G_0G_1$ phase of the cell cycle and do not divide spontaneously. They accumulate primarily as a result of lack of apoptosis, rather than by accelerated cell division (Chiorazzi, 2007). As a consequence, CLL lymphocytes have a poor mitotic index *in vitro*. Therefore longer culture duration has been introduced, i.e. 72 hours instead of 24-48 hours, and several stimulating agents have been added to the culture medium. Mitogens and agents such as 12-O-tetradecanoylphorbol-13-acetate (TPA), the lectine phyotohemagglutinin (PHA), lipopolysaccharide (LPS) and pokeweed mitogen (PWM), the cytokine interleukin-2 (IL-2) and Epstein-Barr virus, have been used to improve the yield of aberrant metaphases. However, abnormal karyotypes were revealed in only 40–50% of cases (Juliusson *et al*, 1990). These low abnormality detection rates can be attributed to a lack of aberrant metaphases, i.e. proliferation disadvantage of the aberrant B-cell clone, and to the presence of cryptic deletions escaping the low resolution of CCA. Recently, improved culture methods have been introduced, i.e. CD40 ligand (CD40L)-induced cell cycle stimulation, and the immunostimulatory CpG oligonucleotide (DSP30) (Dicker *et al*, 2006; Haferlach *et al*, 2007; Mayr *et al*, 2006; Put *et al*, 2009a; Struski *et al*, 2009).

## 2.1.1 TPA

Before the introduction of DSP30, the phorbol ester TPA was considered to be the stimulating agent of choice to improve the mitotic index of CLL cells. TPA stimulates slowly proliferating immature B-cells by activating protein kinase C. This results in phosphorylation of downstream proteins, maturation of these cells towards a plasmacytoid phenotype and inhibition of apoptosis (Barragan *et al*, 2002). However, the induction of cells in $G_2$ and metaphase is weak (2-10%) (Carlsson *et al*, 1988; Stephenson *et al*, 1991).

In addition, TPA has been shown to induce the IL-2 receptor and CLL colony formation. The addition of the cytokine IL-2 to TPA stimulated CLL cell cultures was reported to directly stimulate CLL proliferation, even in absence of T-lymphocytes (Touw and Lowenberg, 1985). Although the latter findings provide evidence for the addition of IL-2 to TPA cultures, it is not mandatory for successful CCA (Put *et al*, 2009a; Struski *et al*, 2009).

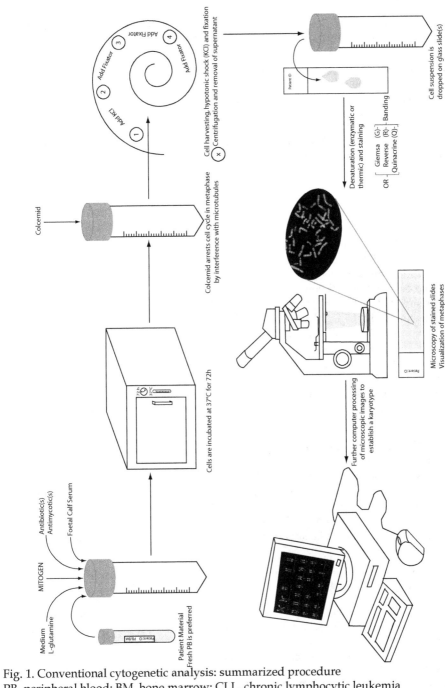

Fig. 1. Conventional cytogenetic analysis: summarized procedure
PB, peripheral blood; BM, bone marrow; CLL, chronic lymphocytic leukemia

### 2.1.2 CD40-ligand (CD40L)

As metaphase induction by TPA is weak and aberration detection is inferior compared with FISH, efforts were made to improve culture methods. In contrast to the environment of lymph node proliferation centers, *in vitro* cultures do not protect the lymphocytes from apoptotic and cytotoxic triggers. The addition of CD40 was able to induce an antiapoptotic profile in CLL cells (Hallaert *et al*, 2008) and therefore it could improve the generation of metaphases. CD40 is an antigen expressed on the surface of normal and malignant B-cells and induces cell cycle progression after activation by its ligand (Buhmann *et al*, 2002). CD40L-induced cell cycle stimulation resulted in a threefold increase in generation of metaphases compared with stimulation with B-cell mitogens such as TPA, LPS and PWM. In addition, the success rate of CCA and aberration detection rate were higher in the CD40L cultures (93% vs. 78% and 89% vs. 22%, respectively) (Buhmann *et al*, 2002). However, this technique is labor-intensive and expensive, and therefore not applicable for routine analysis.

### 2.1.3 DSP30

At the present time, the best CCA results in CLL are obtained with the addition of CpG oligodinucleotides (ODN) and IL-2 to the culture medium. ODN containing a CpG motif, such as DSP30, stimulate cells of the immune system via the Toll-like receptor 9 (TLR9). In humans, the only cell types known to express TLR9 are B-cells and plasmacytoid dendritic cells (Hornung et al., 2002). It has been established that CpG stimulates a broad spectrum of B-cell malignancies, i.e. CLL (Jahrsdorfer *et al*, 2005). CpG induces proliferation in normal B-cells; however, proliferation is weaker and followed by increased apoptosis in CLL cells (Jahrsdorfer *et al*, 2005). The lower proliferative response to CpG-ODN in CLL cells compared with normal B-cells can be overcome by addition of IL-2. Indeed, compared with normal B-cells, CpG causes a stronger induction of the IL-2 receptor α chain (CD25) in CLL, resulting in higher numbers of IL-2 receptors with a stronger affinity. Costimulation with CpG and IL-2 might alter IL-2 signaling in CLL cells in addition to increase cytokine production and surface molecule expression (Decker et al., 2000a).

The use of CpG/IL-2 improves proliferation capacity of CLL cells, and therefore it enables karyotyping in more cases (79-98%). Moreover, the technique yields detection rates of aberrations comparable with interphase FISH (81–83%) (Dicker et al., 2006; Haferlach et al., 2007). Other groups confirmed an improvement of the aberration detection rate in CpG/IL-2 (i.e. an increase of 9-13% of cases with aberrations) compared with TPA stimulated cultures (Put *et al*, 2009a; Struski *et al*, 2009). Moreover, the detection of translocations and del(13q) in particular, has been found to be superior after CpG/IL-2 stimulation compared with TPA (Put *et al*, 2009a).

The influence of CpG/IL-2 on quality of banding and metaphase generation is not clear (Put *et al*, 2009a; Struski *et al*, 2009).

Another question to address is whether abnormalities found after CpG/IL-2 stimulation might be related to activation-induced cytidine deaminase (AID). CpG stimulation of CLL and normal B-cells induces expression of AID, an enzyme that is linked to the development of genetic abnormalities (Capolunghi et al., 2008). However, culturing B-cells of healthy blood donors with CpG/IL-2 did not induce clonal abnormalities, thus validating CpG/IL-2 as a tool for the cytogenetic analysis of CLL (Dicker *et al*, 2006; Put *et al*, 2009a; Wu *et al*, 2008).

In conclusion, CpG/IL-2 should be preferred for routine CCA of CLL. However, as neither conventional cytogenetics nor CLL-specific FISH can detect all aberrations, both techniques should be complementarily applied.

## 2.2 FISH

FISH uses labeled DNA probes directed to selected targets and has a higher resolution than standard cytogenetics (approximately 40 Kb - 1 Mb, depending on the size of the FISH-probes vs. 10 Mb, respectively). Moreover, it can be used on metaphases and on nondividing cells. Sample types that may be used for FISH include in most cases peripheral blood or bone marrow, but also lymph node, spleen or effusions. Either uncultured fresh or frozen cells, cultured fixed cells, or paraffin-embedded tissue sections can be investigated.

The procedure is summarized in Fig 2. Interphase FISH yields high rates of detection of abnormalities, i.e. 80% (Döhner et al, 2000). However, this technique provides only partial information confined to the chromosomal loci examined, whereas CCA gives an overview of all microscopically visible aberrations.

Although FISH is a very sensitive technique, one should consider certain shortcomings. As already mentioned, a limited number of probes is applied. For this reason FISH can underestimate genomic complexity. False-positive and false-negative interpretations occur in 5% of FISH assays (Smoley et al, 2010). Wrong results may be due to i.e. inadequate cut-offs, co-hybridization or poor hybridization of probes, background signals, difficulties in visualizing probe signals in different planes of the nucleus, inadequate probes [in case of microdeletions or microduplications, i.e. ATM or miR-15a/16-1, in which the probe may be too large or not covering the deletion]. Lack of proliferation of the aberrant clone can occur when FISH is performed on cultured material. Furthermore, complex and cryptic translocations may generate special patterns of FISH signals that do not match the normal, expected signal pattern.

In clinical practice, FISH is performed for the regions 17p13 (TP53), 11q13 (ATM), chromosome 12 and 13q14 (RB1 and  miR15.a/16.1). The panel can be extended with probes for the regions 6q21 and 14q32 (IGH). Of interest, particular aberrations detected by FISH (discussed in section 3.1), e.g. loss of 17p13, were identified as major prognostic markers in CLL.

Hence abnormalities detected by FISH may guide patient monitoring and therapeutic decisions. Moreover FISH analysis is recommended for pretreatment evaluation and before subsequent, second- or third-line treatment (Hallek et al, 2008).

## 2.3 MLPA

Since FISH is a quite laborious, time-consuming and expensive technique, MLPA has been developed as an alternative tool. This technique relies on the comparative quantitation of specifically bound probes that are amplified by polymerase chain reaction (PCR) with universal primers. The latter allows simultaneous processing of multiple samples and has proven to be accurate and reliable for identifying deletions, duplications, and amplifications (Coll-Mulet et al, 2008). The procedure is summarized in Fig 3. (Schouten et al, 2002) and an example of MLPA results is shown in Fig 4. In a study comparing FISH and MLPA on 100 samples of untreated early stage (Binet A) CLL patients, a high degree of concordance between both techniques was observed (95%). Seven aberrations were not detected by

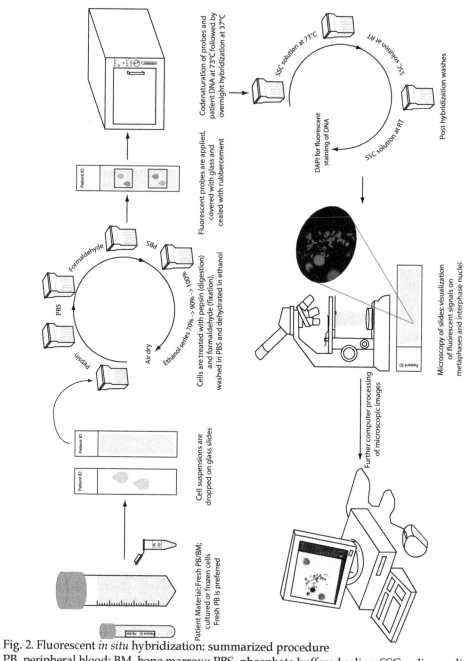

Fig. 2. Fluorescent *in situ* hybridization: summarized procedure
PB, peripheral blood; BM, bone marrow; PBS, phosphate buffered saline; SSC, saline-sodium citrate (SSC) buffer; DAPI, 4',6-diamidino-2-phenylindole

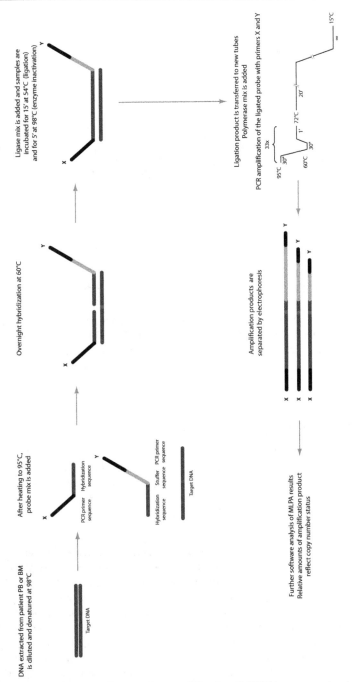

Fig. 3. Multiplex ligation-dependent probe amplification (MLPA): summarized procedure
PB, peripheral blood; BM, bone marrow

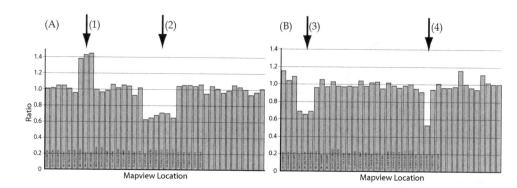

Fig. 4. Example of MLPA analysis performed in two cases of CLL (A and B). Arrows indicate the unbalanced regions: (1) gain of 8q24 and (2) loss of 13q14 in case A, and (3) loss of 6q25 and (4) loss of exon 5 of *TP53* on 17p13 in case B. (Courtesy of M. Jarosova)

MLPA, probably due to the low percentage of leukemic cells (<30%) carrying the aberration (Fabris *et al*, 2011). The sensitivity may even be lower if no B-cell pre-enrichment is performed (i.e. aberrations not detected when the percentage of leukemic cells <50%). Moreover MLPA fails to detect concomitant mono- and biallelic losses at 13q (Fabris *et al*, 2011). However, the availability of multiple probes in MLPA allows the identification of genetic aberrations which are not incorporated in the standard FISH probe panel. In conclusion, MLPA can be used alone or in association with FISH to detect both recurrent and less frequent lesions in CLL.

## 2.4 Comparative genomic hybridization and single nucleotide polymorphism arrays

Very recently (2000s), comparative genomic hybridization arrays (aCGH) and single nucleotide polymorphism (SNP)-arrays have been validated as reliable tools to investigate global genetic abnormalities in CLL with a higher resolution (i.e. 200 basepairs – 10 kilobases), compared with FISH and conventional cytogenetics. Therefore, it allows to detect new, cytogenetically cryptic, recurrent chromosomal changes, such as microdeletions.

However, aCGH has shortcomings as it detects genomic imbalances, but not balanced aberrations. In contrast with aCGH, SNP-arrays have the additional advantage of detecting copy number neutral loss of heterozygosity (cnLOH) or uniparental disomy (UPD). LOH results from the loss of normal function of one allele of a gene in which the other allele has already been inactivated, whereas UPD is a cnLOH in which all copies of an allele are derived from one parent and no copies from the other parent are present. Until now, the application of aCGH and SNP-arrays is restricted to research setting, but may possibly be implemented in routine analysis of CLL in the near future. As many platforms from different companies are available and each platform has its own technical specifications, Fig 5. gives only a brief and general overview of the technique. In the next paragraphs, we will focus in detail on the main results.

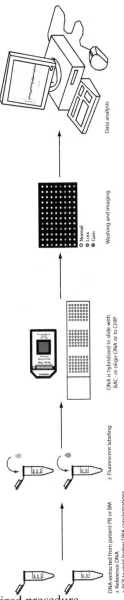

Fig. 5. Array-technology: summarized procedure.
PB, peripheral blood; BM, bone marrow; BAC, bacterial artificial chromosome

## 2.5 Next generation sequencing

Next-generation sequencing (NGS, also known as massively parallel sequencing) technologies have a higher throughput than traditional sequencing methods. It allows millions of sequencing reactions to happen in parallel, using different approaches, either by creating micro-reactors and/or attaching DNA molecules to solid surfaces or beads. Unlike previous methods NGS generates millions of short reads (21-400 base pairs) and does not require amplification as sequencing can be performed from a single DNA molecule. The short reads can be quantified, allowing accurate copy number assessment. Moreover, with approaches that sequence both ends of a DNA molecule (paired end massively parallel sequencing), it has become possible to detect balanced and unbalanced somatic rearrangements (i.e. fusion genes) in a genome-wide fashion. Since each type of NGS has specific artefacts, one should be aware of this phenomenon and new findings should be interpreted with caution (Reis-Filho, 2009). In addition, the high cost of the technique limits its use in (routine) practice.

## 3. Cytogenetic and molecular abnormalities in CLL prognosis

### 3.1 Five prognostically important FISH-categories

A landmark interphase FISH-study of 325 mainly untreated CLL patients identified five prognostically important hierarchical categories: 17p deletion (with or without concomitant lesions), 11q deletion (with no concomitant 17p deletion), 12 trisomy (with neither concomitant 17p- nor 11q deletion), none of these aberrations, and 13q deletion as the sole abnormality (Fig 6. and Fig 7.). Median survival times for patients in these five groups were 32, 79, 114, 111, and 133 months, respectively and the treatment-free survival was 9, 13, 33, 49 and 92 months, respectively (Döhner et al, 2000).

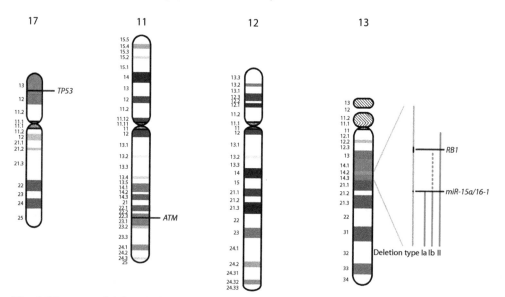

Fig. 6. Idiogram of G-banded chromosomes involved in prognostically important aberrations, at 550-band level.
Commonly deleted regions are indicated in red (caveat: deletions may be larger or smaller).
Del(13q) type Ib can vary in length, as indicated by the dashed line.

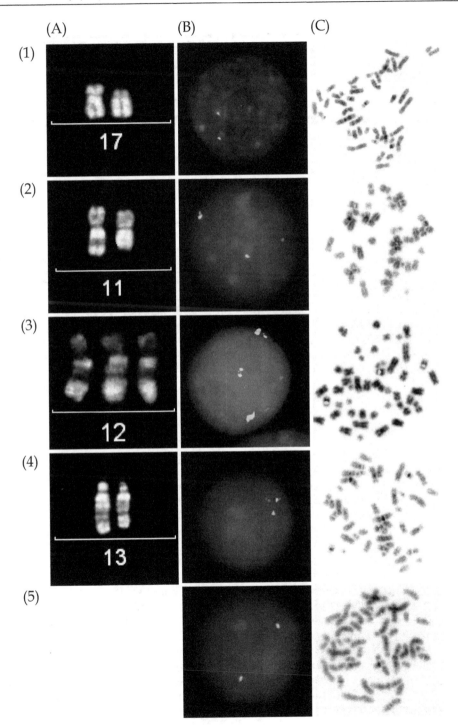

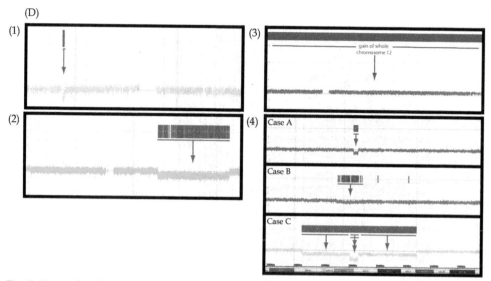

Fig. 7. Examples of the four prognostically important aberrations in CLL, namely del(17p) (1), del(11q) (2), trisomy 12 (3) and del(13q) (4, 5), as observed by CCA (A), interphase FISH (B), metaphase FISH (C) and the Affymetrix 2.7M array platform (D). Applied FISH-probes are specific for *TP53* (red) and centromere 17 (CEP17) (green) (1), for *ATM* (red) and centromere 12 (green) (2+3), for *RB1* (green) and D13S319 (red) (4+5). Note a monoallelic loss of *TP53* (B1, C1, D1 red arrow), monoallelic loss of *ATM* (B2, C2, D2 red arrow), trisomy 12 (B3, C3, D3 blue arrow), a monoallelic (B4, C4, D4 cases A+B+C, single red arrows) and biallelic del(13q) in (B5, C5, D4 case C, double red arrow).

### 3.1.1 17p deletions

Patients with a deletion of 17p have worst outcome. The del(17p) is found in 3-8% of previously untreated patients, although higher incidences up to 45% have been reported in patients with relapsed or refractory CLL, as a consequence of clonal selection (Cramer and Hallek, 2011; Zenz *et al*, 2011). Del(17p) usually encompasses the *TP53* locus at 17p13. A gene-dosage effect of *TP53* has been reported. About 80-90% of the cases harbor a biallelic inactivation of *TP53* (i.e. deletion of one copy and mutation of the remaining copy), but also the monoallelic inactivation of *TP53* is an adverse prognostic marker (Cramer and Hallek, 2011; Zenz *et al*, 2011). The tumor suppressor p53 plays an essential role in inducing apoptosis or cell cycle arrest after DNA damage. Since therapy with purine nucleoside analogues (e.g. fludarabine) and alkylating agents (e.g. chlorambucil) is based on p53-dependent mechanisms, CLL patients with deletion 17p or inactivating mutations of *TP53* are refractory to such chemotherapy (Van Bockstaele *et al*, 2008) and have impaired survival. A threshold of > 20-25% interphase nuclei harboring the del(17p) has been reported to correlate with adverse survival (Catovsky *et al*, 2007; Tam *et al*, 2009). Because of the very poor prognosis, risk-adapted treatment for this subgroup has been developed. Current treatment approaches (in clinical trials) use agents acting independently of p53 (e.g. alemtuzumab, high dose steroids) or allogeneic stem cell transplantation for fit patients (Zenz *et al*, 2011). In the future, optimization of the therapeutic strategies hopefully may improve outcome for this poor prognostic subgroup.

### 3.1.2 11q deletions

Deletions of 11q have been associated with adverse outcome. It is found in about 20% of the patients with CLL (Van Bockstaele *et al*, 2008; Zenz *et al*, 2011). The minimally deleted region (MDR) at 11q22.3-q23.1 harbors the *ATM* (ataxia telangiectasia mutated) gene. ATM is a protein that acts upstream of p53 in the DNA damage response pathway. Mutations of *ATM* have been reported in 12% of patients with CLL and in 30% of patients with del(11q) (Zenz *et al*, 2011). As not all patients with del(11q) have an *ATM* mutation (and vice versa), haplo-insufficiency of ATM or the presence of other tumor suppressor genes in the MDR can be suspected. In the patients with del(11q), the biallelic inactivation of *ATM* leads to a worse clinical outcome (Cramer and Hallek, 2011). Of note, rarely the del(11q) does not encompass *ATM*, but affects the telomerically located *FDX* locus (Heim and Mitelman, 2009). Patients with del(11q) are generally younger, have more B-symptoms and more advanced clinical stages. Furthermore, the del(11q) is typically associated with extensive lymphadenopathy (Cramer and Hallek, 2011; Van Bockstaele *et al*, 2008).

### 3.1.3 Trisomy 12

An intermediate outcome has been described for patients with trisomy 12. While progression free survival (PFS) may be shorter (PFS rate at 3 years of 48-83%), overall survival (OS) is rather favorable (OS rates at 3 years of 86-96%). Trisomy 12 has been associated with atypical morphology or immunophenotype (i.e. stronger surface immunoglobulin and FMC7 expression) (Zenz *et al*, 2011). The aberration is observed in 10-30% of patients (Van Bockstaele *et al*, 2008; Zenz *et al*, 2011). This variation probably reflects differences in patient selection. Partial trisomy 12q was reported in 10-20% of the cases and a minimal common gained region has been confined to 12q13 (Heim and Mitelman, 2009).

The critical genes involved in the trisomy 12 are yet unknown. Small duplications of 12q have been reported and in particular the murine double minute 2 gene (*MDM2*) located at 12q15 has been found amplified in CLL (Merup *et al*, 1997). Overexpression of the MDM2 protein was also observed in CLL and this was significantly more frequent in the advanced rather than the earlier stages (Watanabe *et al*, 1996). The MDM2 SNP309 in B-CLL has been suggested to be an unfavorable prognostic marker; however the results of several recent publications are conflicting (Willander *et al*, 2010). The CLL upregulated gene 1 (*CLLU1*) located at 12q22 was overexpressed exclusively in CLL and its expression was shown to have a strong prognostic significance in patients younger than 70 years, namely higher expression was associated with shorter overall survival (Josefsson *et al*, 2007). However overexpression of *CLLU1* occurs irrespectively of trisomy 12 or other large chromosomal rearrangements (Buhl *et al*, 2006).

Recurrent association of trisomy 12 with *IG*-aberrations, such as t(14;19)(q32;q13), t(14;18)(q32;q21) and del(14)(q24q32), and with trisomy 18 and/or trisomy 19, has been observed in a subset of cases (Heim and Mitelman, 2009). Trisomy 12 with concomitant *TP53* mutations is rare.

### 3.1.4 13q deletions

Although deletions of 13q are often cytogenetically cryptic, they represent the most frequently observed FISH-aberration in CLL, with a prevalence of 40-60% (Van Bockstaele *et al*, 2008). Only when present as a solitary aberration (by FISH), the del(13q) implies a favorable prognosis. Higher percentages (that is > 65% or > 80%) of interphase FISH nuclei showing the del(13q) have been associated with shorter overall survival and time to first treatment (Hernandez *et al*, 2009; Van Dyke *et al*, 2010). The MDR located at 13q14 contains *miR-15a* and *miR-16-1*. These microRNAs are small non-coding RNA genes that regulate gene expression. The *miR-15a/16-1* cluster seems to negatively regulate the expression of multiple genes involved in proliferation and apoptosis (Klein and Dalla-Favera, 2010). Deletion of the MDR-region in mice models suggested that this lesion is sufficient for lymphomagenesis. In some CLL cases without del(13q), downregulation of *miR-15a* and *miR-16-1* has been described, suggesting an epigenetic mechanism suppressing the miR-cluster (Klein and Dalla-Favera, 2010). Mutations in the miR-cluster appear to be very rare (Zenz *et al*, 2011). The del(13q) is most frequently heterozygous (monoallelic, 76% of cases), but can be homozygous (biallelic, 24% of cases). While the former is suggested to be an early event, the latter probably occurs at a later stage. A gene dosage-effect of *miR-15a/16-1* has been reported (Zenz *et al*, 2011). In addition, SNP-arrays showed that the extent of the deletion (Fig 6) is associated with disease characteristics, for example del(13q) type II (long, involving *RB1*, related with disease progression) and del(13q) type I (short, not involving *RB1*, related with disease progression only when associated with other aberrations) (Malek *et al*, 2010; Zenz *et al*, 2011).

### 3.2 Other cytogenetic aberrations

Several other recurrent genomic aberrations have been described in CLL, such as del(6q), del(14)(q24.1q32.33) involving *IGH* (Pospisilova *et al*, 2007), t(1;6)(p35;p25) involving *MUM1/IRF4* (Michaux *et al*, 2005), total or partial trisomy 3, trisomy 8, trisomy 18 and 19 and changes leading to gains of 2p24-25, 3q26-27, and 8q24. These aberrations are rare in CLL (prevalence < 5-10%). Most of the genes involved are not yet identified and their prognostic relevance remains to be investigated (Heim and Mitelman, 2009; Van Bockstaele *et al*, 2008).

### 3.3 Translocations

Translocations have been reported in up to 34-42% of patients with CLL (Mayr *et al*, 2006; Van Den Neste *et al*, 2007). Balanced translocations are relatively rare, but unbalanced non-reciprocal aberrations are frequent and are often observed within complex karyotypes. Although translocations are heterogenous in CLL, many breakpoints are located in regions showing recurrent loss, like 13q14 and 17p13 (Heim and Mitelman, 2009). Chromosomal translocations in general may have a negative impact on response to therapy and survival, especially when unbalanced (Mayr *et al*, 2006; Van Den Neste *et al*, 2007). Balanced translocations, especially those involving immunoglobulin (*IG*) genes, are recurrent, but uncommon (i.e. 5%) (Haferlach *et al*, 2007). Recurrent partners include *BCL2*, *BCL3*, *BCL11A* and *MYC* (Table 2). In published reports (Cavazzini *et al*, 2008; Nowakowski *et al*, 2007), at least part of the cases have unknown partner genes. In most studies, CLL cases with translocations involving *IG* are analyzed as a single group (Cavazzini *et al*, 2008; Juliusson *et al*, 1990). However, the partner gene that becomes overexpressed as a result of the translocation, may be relevant for the outcome. The best described is the *BCL3* gene involved in the t(14;19), often associated with atypical morphology, unmutated *IGVH* genes and inferior prognosis (Cavazzini *et al*, 2008; Chapiro *et al*, 2008; Martin-Subero *et al*, 2007; Nowakowski *et al*, 2007). Similarly, translocations involving *MYC* have been associated with loss (i.e. monosomy) of 17, del(11q) complex karyotype, additional unbalanced translocations and poor prognosis (Put *et al*, 2011). In contrast, translocations involving *BCL2* are associated with mutated *IGVH* genes, trisomy 12, absence of del(11q) and more favorable outcome (Put *et al*, 2009b).

| Translocation[a,b] | Partner Gene | Morphology | IGVH | Associated changes | Prognosis |
|---|---|---|---|---|---|
| t(2;14)(p16;q32) | BCL11a | Atypical | U > M | Trisomy 12 | Uncertain |
| t(8;14)(q24;q32) | MYC | PL /PT | U ≈ M | Monosomy 17p Del(11q) Complex karyotype Unbalanced translocations | Poor |
| t(14;18)(q32;q21) | BCL2 | Typical | M > U | Trisomy 12 Absence of del(11q) | Favorable |
| t(14;19)(q32;q21) | BCL3 | Atypical | U > M | Trisomy 12 | Poor |

PL, prolymphocyte; PT, prolymphocytic transformation; U, unmutated; M, mutated
[a]IG-translocations involve most frequently IGH located on 14q32. Variant translocations involve either IGK on 2p12 or IGL on 22q11
[b] To date, most cases with t(11;14)(q13;q32), involving CCND1, are diagnosed as mantle cell lymphoma; however, rare cases of t(11;14)-positive CLL might exist.

Table 1. Overview of translocations involving immunoglobulin (IG)-genes in CLL

## 3.4 Genomic complexity

Cytogenetic complexity is defined as the presence of three or more clonal chromosomal aberrations. CCA was found to be superior in the detection of complexity, compared with FISH (Haferlach et al, 2007), probably due to the limited number of investigated loci in the latter approach. Complexity is found in a minority of the cases with CLL (10-30%) (Haferlach et al, 2007; Kujawski et al, 2008). A highly significant association was observed between complex aberrant karyotypes and 17p deletions, unmutated IGVH and expression of CD38 (Haferlach et al, 2007). In addition, particular aberrations (i.e. translocations involving MYC) have also been associated with a complex aberrant karyotype (Put et al, unpublished data). Prognostically, patients with complex genomic changes appear to have more aggressive disease. Similarly, genomic complexity detected by SNP-arrays (≥ 3 genetic lesions) has been associated with poor outcome (Kujawski et al, 2008). An impaired apoptotic DNA double-strand break response and multiple genomic deletions, including del(17p), del(11q), and del(13q) type II were identified as independent strong predictors of genomic complexity in CLL. Moreover, a strong independent effect of aberrant p53 function on genomic complexity and a modest effect of decreased ATM function have been observed (Ouillette et al, 2010). Such multiple independent gene defects in CLL may contribute to genomic instability. In addition, telomere dysfunction as a consequence of telomere erosion may also drive genomic instability during the progression of CLL (Lin et al, 2010). Indeed, short telomeres have been associated with a high risk of genomic aberrations and genetic complexity (Roos et al, 2008).

## 3.5 Clonal evolution

Clonal evolution (CE) represents the acquisition of new or additional cytogenetic aberrations during disease course. As a consequence, CCA or FISH should not only be used for initial prognostication of patients with CLL, but also at the time of disease progression or before therapy initiation [FISH is mandatory in this setting for detection of del(17p)]. Initially, CE as evaluated by sequential CCA, was considered infrequent, i.e. in 16% of CLL patients (Oscier et al, 1991). Later studies reported higher frequencies of 25-43% (Fegan et al, 1995; Finn et al, 1998; Haferlach et al, 2007). Interphase FISH studies (Table 2) revealed CE in 27% and 17% after a median follow-up of more than 5 years and 42.3 months, respectively (Shanafelt et al, 2006;

Stilgenbauer *et al*, 2007). Interestingly, CE occurred more frequently among cases with unmutated *IGVH* status (Shanafelt *et al*, 2006; Stilgenbauer *et al*, 2007). However, another study did not find a correlation between CE and unmutated *IGVH*, expression of CD38 and ZAP70 on one hand, but the combination of all three prognostic factors correlated highly significantly with CE and with a shift from lower to higher FISH risk category (Berkova *et al*, 2009). Patients with CE showed progression to more advanced stages, greater need for therapy and a higher hazard ratio for death. Moreover, CE was identified as an independent factor for survival (Stilgenbauer *et al*, 2007). As a consequence, CCA or FISH should not only be used for initial prognostication of patients with CLL, but also at the time of disease progression or before therapy initiation [FISH is mandatory in this setting for detection of del(17p)]

| Reference | CLL Patients (n) | Follow-up (months) | CE: patients (n) | CE: previously treated patients (n) | CE: abnormalities | Other findings |
|---|---|---|---|---|---|---|
| Shanafelt *et al*, 2006 | 108[a] | 67 (23-136) | 18 (11%) | 13 (71%) | del(13q) (72%) > del(17p) (22%) > del(11q) (6%) | CE not confined to unmutated *IGVH* (association ns) Correlation between ZAP70+ and CE CE more frequent after 50 months compared with before 24 months (27% vs. <2%, respectively) |
| Stilgenbauer *et al*, 2007 | 64 | 42 (23-73) | 11 (17%) | 1 (9%) | del(17p) (36%) > del(13q) = del(6q) (27%) > del(11q) (18%) > +8q24 (9%) | CE confined to unmutated *IGVH* CE correlates with progressive clinical stages, greater need for therapy, higher hazard ratio for death CE as independent factor for survival |
| Berkova *et al*, 2009 | 97 | 66 (22-304) | 25 (26%) | 7 (28%) | del(13q) (64%) > del(17p) = del(11q) (16%) > trisomy 12 (4%) | Combination of unmutated *IGVH*, CD38+ and ZAP70+ correlates highly significantly with CE and with a shift from lower to higher FISH risk category |
| Loscertales *et al*, 2010 | 81 | 67 (16-111) | 17 (21%) | 13 (76%) | del(17p) (53%) > del(11q) (35%) | CE not confined to unmutated *IGVH* del(17p) observed in untreated patients |

N, number; CE, clonal evolution; ns, not significant,
[a]Sequential samples were available in 108/159 patients.

Table 2. Overview of clonal evolution investigated by FISH

### 3.6 Molecular karyotyping

The introduction of aCGH and SNP-arrays enables to investigate CLL at a resolution, greatly surpassing this of conventional cytogenetics. Different array-platforms were validated as a powerful, cost-effective tool for clinical risk assessment in CLL (Table 3) (Gunn *et al*, 2008; Hagenkord *et al*, 2010; O'Malley *et al*, 2011). Of note, the sensitivity of these platforms varies and is related to i.e. the resolution of the array. For example, the Affymetrix SNP6.0 array was found to be superior to the 250K array in detecting small aberrations of uncertain significance and equivalent to the 250K array in detecting clinically relevant lesions. Since the cost of the 250K array is lower, it is preferred for routine use. In contrast, the 10K array is not suitable for routine clinical use due to its low resolution (Hagenkord *et al*, 2010).

New recurrent cytogenetic abnormalities were detected by aCGH and SNP-arrays. In Table 3 an overview of selected publications on array-applications in CLL is shown, describing known prognostically important lesions and new molecular cytogenetic findings (Grubor et al, 2009;

Gunn et al, 2008; Gunn et al, 2009; Gunnarsson et al, 2008; Gunnarsson et al, 2010; Gunnarsson et al, 2011; Hagenkord et al, 2010; Kay et al, 2010; Kujawski et al, 2008; Lehmann et al, 2008; O'Malley et al, 2011; Ouillette et al, 2010; Ouillette et al, 2011; Pfeifer et al, 2007; Rinaldi et al, 2011). Other recent studies using array-platforms revealed new insights in the disease: i.e. the genome of CLL appeared to be quite stable over time (Brown et al, 2010); disease progression has been associated with large, but not small copy number alterations (Gunnarsson *et al*, 2010), genomic complexity, 13q deletion in the presence of other aberrations, and 13q deletion type II (that is, deletions involving *RB1*) (Malek *et al*, 2010).

| Reference | Array | Patients (n) | 17 | 11 | 12 | 13 | Other highlighted abnormalities | LOH/CN LOH | Remarks |
|---|---|---|---|---|---|---|---|---|---|
| Pfeifer et al, 2007 | 10K and 50K Affymetrix | 70 | 5.7% | 12.8% | 12.8% | 51.4% | Gain of 2p16 (n=4; *REL, BCL11a*) | 14 patients with 24 large CN LOH > 10 Mb | Recombination hot spots on both sides of *mir15a/16-1*; Slower lymphocyte growth kinetics for monoallelic vs. biallelic del(13q14) |
| Lehmann et al, 2008 | 50K Affymetrix | 56 | 5% | 9% | 7% | 59% | Loss of 6q21 (n=4; *AIM1*) | 4 patients with UPD | Genetic abnormalities of chr 13 (including UPD) are very common events in early stage CLL |
| Ouillette et al, 2008 | 50K Affymetrix | 171 | NA | NA | NA | 48% | NA | 5 patients with CN LOH of 13q14: 4 with extensive LOH but copy loss restricted to a small area at ~D13S319 and 1 without any LOH-associated copy loss (UPD) | Del(13q14) is heterogeneous; Type Ia lesions are uniform with one breakpoint close to the *mir15a/16-1* cluster; Type I lesions correlate with higher *LATS2* RNA levels; *PHLPP* RNA is absent in 50% of del(13q14); 15% CLL have reduced *mir15a/16-1* expression |
| Kujawski et al, 2008 | 50K Affymetrix | 178 | 7-13%[a] | 8-13%[a] | 14-28%[a,b] | 46-28%[a,b] | ≥2, ≥2.5, or ≥3 genomic lesions in 35%, 19%, and 15% of patients, respectively. | 10 patients with UPD | Genomic complexity as an independent risk factor for short TTT in multivariate analysis |
| Gunn et al, 2008 | 44K Agilent | 174 | 4.6% | 11% | 13% | 47% | Gain of 2p (n=5; *NMYC* in 5/5, *REL* and *BCL11a* in 4/5 cases), del(5q) (n=3), del(2q) (n=2), del(8p) (n=2), gain of 8q (n=3), gain of whole-chr 19 (n=1) and 22 (n=3). | NA | Genomic instability (i.e. ≥3 loci not investigated by FISH panels) was observed in 21% of the cases. |
| Gunnarsson et al, 2008 | 32K BAC, 185K Agilent, 250K Affymetrix, and 317K Illumina CA1000 | 10 | 20% | 10% | 20% | 40% | NA | Concordance of large regions; smaller regions escaping detection | All platforms detect large CNAs, however findings are discrepant for small CNAs |
| Gunn et al, 2009 | microarrays BAC array (Combimatrix Molecular Diagnostics) | 187 | NA | NA | NA | NA | Loss of 22q11 (n=28; *ZNF280A, ZNF280B, GGTLC2, and PRAME*) | NA | |
| Gruber et al, 2009 | 85K and 390K NimbleGen (ROMA) | 58 | 5% | 10% | 17% | 40% | Loss of 8p21.2-p12 (n=2; *TRIM35*), 2q37.1 (n=2; *SP100/110/140*), 9p21.3 (n2; *CDKN2A (P16-INK4)*) *and 18q23* (n=2; *NFATC1*) | NA | CNA differences between CD38+ and CD38- cell fractions (3/4 cases) |

Table 3. Overview of selected publications on genomic array-applications in CLL

| Reference | Array | n | 17 | 11 | 12 | 13 | Other aberrations | LOH / UPD | Comments |
|---|---|---|---|---|---|---|---|---|---|
| Kay et al., 2010 | 1M Agilent | 48 | 6.3% | 12.5% | 23% | 52% | Loss of 3q21, 8p11, 10q24, 11q22, 14q24 (all aberrations present in n≥3) | NA | Higher genomic complexity (>15 CNAs or ≥66 Mb length) associated with shorter PFS, poor response to therapy. Loss of p53 function [in pt with del(17p) or del(13q)] was associated with a complex genome |
| Hagenkord et al., 2010 | 10K, 250K and SNP 6.0 Affymetrix | 33 | NA | NA | NA | 55% | Atypical loss of 11q (n=5; not including ATM) and 13q (n=1; not including mir15a/16-1) | 4 patients with UPD: at 17p13 (n=1), 11q22 (n=1), and 13q14 (n=2) | |
| Gunnarsson et al., 2010 | 250K Affymetrix | 203 | 4.4% | 13% | 11% | 54% | Loss of 4p (n=3), 8p (n=5), gain of 8q (n=5), combination of gain of 2p (2p24.3) and loss of 11q (n=5) | All CN regions included a homozygous del(13q) | Genomic complexity (increasing number of CNAs >5 Mb) as a poor-prognostic marker, although a complex genome often included del(17p) and del(11q) |
| Gunnarsson et al., 2011 | 250K Affymetrix | 369+59ᵇ | 4% | 10% | 10.5% | 55% | Acquisition of aberrations of 6q, 9p, 9p and 10q (i.e. clonal evolution) were exclusively associated with UM IGHV | CN LOH on 13q in 3.5%, most with homozygous del(13q) | Genomic complexity (associated with poor prognostic aberrations) and large 13q deletions correlate with inferior outcome. CE correlates with poor prognostic markers and commonly includes the known recurrent aberrations |
| O'Malley et al., 2011 | HemeScan® BAC (Combimatrix Molecular Diagnostics) | 55 | 11% | 9% | 25% | 46% | Loss of 6q (n=3), 8p (n=4), 10q (n=2), 14q32 (n=14), 18q (n=4) and gain of 10q (n=2) | NA | |
| Rinaldi et al., 2011 | SNP 6.0 Affymetrix | 148 | 10% | 10% | 19%ᵈ | 50% | Gains at 2p25.3-p22.3 (n=5; NMYC), 2p22.3 (n=5), 2p16.2-p14 (n=5; REL), 8q23.3-q24.3 (n=7; MYC), losses at 8p23.1-p21.2 (n=7), 8p21.2 (n=7), 17p13.3-p11.2 (n=15), and 17p12-p11.2 (n=22) | NA | Gains at 2p and 8q and TP53 inactivation showed prognostic significance (multivariate analysis, confirmed in a hierarchical model). Gains at 2p determined a higher risk of Richter transformation. Gains at 2p and 8q proposed as relevant novel genomic regions for prognostic stratification |
| Ouillette et al., 2011 | SNP 6.0 Affymetrix | 255 | 10% | 10% | 17% | 51% | Loss at chr 6 (n=7), 8p (n=7), 10q (n=10), 14q (n=9), 18q (n=8), gains at 8q (n=5), 17q (n=6), and 18p (n=6). Recurrent biallelic losses on chr 9 (n=2; P16/CDKN2A) and chr X (n=2). | In the group of CLL with elevated array-based genomic complexity, 3 patients had acquired 17p-UPD | ≥3 subchromosomal aCNA were detected in 20% of the cases. Genomic complexity was identified as an independent and powerful marker for the identification of CLL patients with aggressive disease and short survival |

Table 3 (continued).

17, Del(17p); 11, Del(11q); 12, Trisomy 12; 13, Del(13q); NA, not available; LOH, loss of heterozygosity; CN, copy number neutral; UPD, uniparental disomy; UM, unmutated; M, mutated; IGVH, immunoglobulin heavy chain mutational status; CGH, comparative genomic hybridization; TTT, time to treatment; CNA, copy number alteration; PFS, progression-free survival; CE, clonal evolution;

ᵃUntreated – treated patients, respectively;

ᵇSolitary del(13q) only;

ᶜAt diagnosis + at follow-up, respectively;

ᵈLowest frequency of (partial) gain of 12q

## 3.7 Next generation sequencing

Whole genome sequencing of cases with CLL led to the discovery of several genes, previously unsuspected to be involved in this disease. For example, combining NGS and copy number analysis in 5 patients, < 20 clonal genomic alterations/case and recurrent mutations of NOTCH1, TGM7, BIRC3, and PLEKHG5 were observed (Fabbri et al, 2011). Lesions of MYD88, BIRC3, and PLEKHG5 are all linked to alteration of the NF-κβ pathway. In a screening cohort of 48 CLL cases, NOTCH1 mutations were found in 8.3% of CLL cases at diagnosis and were associated with aggressive disease (i.e. higher frequency of NOTCH1 mutations were associated with Richter transformation and refractoriness to chemotherapy, in 31.0% and 20.8% of the cases, respectively). Moreover NOTCH1 mutation at diagnosis emerged as an independent risk factor for poor survival (Fabbri et al, 2011). Another NGS and exome sequencing study identified four genes that were recurrently mutated, namely NOTCH1, XPO1 predominantly in CLL with unmutated IGVH, and MYD88 and KLHL6 in CLL with mutated IGVH status (Puente et al, 2011). NOTCH1, XPO1 and MYD88 mutations are suspected to be oncogenic changes, contributing to disease progression, based on their patterns of mutation and functional analyses, (Puente et al, 2011). In conclusion, NGS appears to be a highly effective technique in identifying new genetic lesions and future studies are promising to contribute to an improved understanding of disease onset and evolution.

## 4. The origin of cytogenetic abnormalities

Genomic imbalances, such as gains and losses of chromosome segments or whole chromosomes (aneuploidy), are more frequently observed than translocations in CLL. However, in the following paragraphs we will focus mainly on the origin of translocations, in particular translocations involving IG loci, as the underlying mechanisms are quite specific for lymphoid malignancies, i.e. CLL.

### 4.1 The origin of aneuploidy and structural aberrations

Aneuploidy may arise due to defects in segregation of chromosomes during cell division, including multipolar spindles, but also abnormal kinetochore-spindle interactions, premature chromatid separation, centrosome amplification, and abnormal cytokinesis. Defects of centrosome function in particular have been suggested to be involved in a wide variety of human malignancies. Centrosomes have central role in organizing microtubuli and the mitotic spindle. An aberrant number, size, shape of the centrosome, as well as aberrant phosphorylation of centrosome proteins, may missegregate chromosomes, resulting in aneuploid cells. In addition, errors in the separation of sister chromatids could also be a cause of aneuploidy. Finally, checkpoint controls are expected to be abrogated in order to enable unequal chromosome segregation during cell cycle progression (Gollin, 2004; Schwab, 2001).

Structural chromosomal instability results from chromosome breakage and rearrangement due to defects in the cell cycle checkpoints, the DNA damage response and/or loss of telomere integrity (Gollin, 2004). When a chromatid break occurs, an unprotected chromosomal end will probably fuse with either another broken chromatid or its sister chromatid to produce a dicentric chromosome. During the anaphase, the two centromeres are pulled to opposite poles, forming a bridge that breaks, resulting in more unprotected chromosomal ends, thus resulting in breakage-fusion-bridge cycles. Telomere mechanics, defects in DNA damage response and cell cycle checkpoint may play important roles in the development and maintenance of chromosomal instability (Gollin, 2004).

## 4.2 The origin of translocations

Recurrent translocations in CLL often involve *IG* loci. These translocations may follow DNA double strand breaks (DSBs) that are generated during V(D)J recombination (i.e. recombination of Variable, Diversity, and Joining segments of *IG*-genes) and somatic hypermutation (SHM) in developing B-cells and in the context of class switch recombination (CSR) in activated mature B-cells. DSBs in the partner loci may be generated by off-target VDJ recombination, CSR activities or may result from more general factors, such as oxidative metabolism or genotoxic agents. Misrepair of these DSBs can promote oncogenic translocations. When a translocation involves oncogenes or tumor suppressor genes, it can be positively selected in the context of neoplastic transformation. Selection likely plays the main role in the appearance of most clonal translocations in tumors (Gostissa *et al*, 2011).

### 4.2.1 VDJ recombination and RAG-mediated DSB

The complete VDJ recombination involves RAG-mediated cleavage, which generates DSBs, and the DSB repair pathway "classical nonhomologous DNA end-joining" (C-NHEJ). The latter promotes chromosomal integrity and suppresses the formation of translocations. In the absence of C-NHEJ, DSBs still can be joined by alternative end-joining (A-EJ), a process that contributes to oncogenic chromosomal translocations (Gostissa *et al*, 2011; Nussenzweig and Nussenzweig, 2010).

### 4.2.2 SHM, CSR and AID-mediated DSB

Although representing different processes, SHM and CSR are both initiated by AID (Gostissa *et al*, 2011; Perez-Duran *et al*, 2007). SHM generates point mutations, small deletions and insertions in variable region exons. This occurs in the germinal centers (GCs) and allows the selection of B-cells that express higher affinity B-cell receptors. CSR can also occur within the GC, as well as in extrafollicular regions (Gostissa *et al*, 2011).

AID initiates both SHM and CSR in B-cells by deaminating cytosines on the DNA of *IG* genes. The generated lesion can be processed into a mutation (SHM) or a DSB followed by a recombination reaction (CSR) (Perez-Duran *et al*, 2007). CSR requires the generation of AID-initiated DSBs. In contrast, SHM generally does not require DSBs. The latter are only occasionally generated as by-products of AID activity (Gostissa *et al*, 2011). It has been suggested that AID may have a dual role; initiating chromosomal translocations on one hand and generating secondary hits by mutagenesis on the other (Perez-Duran *et al*, 2007). Aberrant SHM and involvement of AID were reported to be involved in mutations of *TP53* (Malcikova et al, 2008), *MYC*, *PAX5* and *RhoH* (Reiniger et al, 2006). Moreover, AID activity has been linked to the generation of DSBs involved in translocations in both *IG* and non-*IG* loci (Gostissa *et al*, 2011). While AID was shown to initiate the formation of translocations and mutations, ATM, p53 and ARF provide surveillance mechanisms to prevent these aberrations (Perez-Duran *et al*, 2007).

AID expression results from interaction with an activated microenvironment. In a study of CLL patients with unmutated *IGVH*, high AID expression was found exclusively in the small subset of cells with ongoing CSR (Palacios *et al*, 2010). In addition, in CLL and small lymphocytic lymphoma, AID expression has been associated with unfavorable clinical course and with adverse biological parameters, i.e. higher proliferation rate, deletion of *ATM* and *TP53* (Leuenberger *et al*, 2010). AID expression has been considered to be predictive for CLL with unmutated *IGVH* status (Palacios *et al*, 2010). However, in other reports the association of AID expression and *IGVH* mutational status is considered controversial (Leuenberger *et al*, 2010).

### 4.2.3 Combined action of RAG and AID

In conclusion, RAG and AID can generate DSBs leading to translocations via VDJ recombination and CSR, respectively. RAG and AID are usually expressed in distinct B-cell developmental compartments. Activity of RAG has been observed in developing bone marrow B-cells, whereas AID activity has been found in peripheral mature B-cells. Breakpoint sequences can provide information regarding the developmental stage at which the translocation occurred (Gostissa *et al*, 2011; Nussenzweig and Nussenzweig, 2010). However, collaboration between RAG and AID in generating translocations has been reported. RAG induced DSBs can persist in the absence of ATM, an essential DNA damage checkpoint regulator, or in absence of the NHEJ factor XRCC4, leading to abnormal or delayed repair of RAG-mediated DSBs. In addition, AID may facilitate off-target DSB formation by RAG. As a consequence RAG and AID-mediated DSBs may coexist and become partners in translocation formation (Nussenzweig and Nussenzweig, 2010). Finally, not all DSBs that are precursors of translocations in lymphomas appear to be initiated by RAG or AID (Gostissa *et al*, 2011). The mechanism(s) involved herein remain largely unknown.

### 4.2.4 Oncogene activation

Most recurrent translocations activate oncogenes, either by generating oncogenic fusion proteins or by deregulating oncogene expression by linking it to strong transcriptional control elements. The *IGH* locus contains two known major transcriptional enhancer regions: the intronic enhancer (iEμ), which promotes optimal VDJ recombination in developing B-cells and the IGH 3' regulatory region (IGH3'RR), which modulates CSR in mature B-cells by long-range (over 100 kb) activation of certain promoters. The IgH3'RR does not gain full enhancer activity until late in B-cell development. It was reported that iEμ has low oncogenic activity, suggesting that VDJ-mediated translocations that retain iEμ near the translocation breakpoint may arise in early B-cell developmental stages but remain oncogenically silent until the IgH3'RR becomes fully active at the mature B-cell stage. Alternatively, the development of mature B-cell tumors from cells carrying VDJ-mediated translocations might reflect the time required for the accumulation of secondary mutations necessary for transformation. Another explanation is that translocations may be generated directly in mature B-cells, either by persisting VDJ breaks arisen at the pro-B-cell stage or by RAG-mediated breaks in peripheral B-cells (Gostissa *et al*, 2011).

## 5. Acknowledgements

N. Put is supported by Fonds voor Wetenschappelijk Onderzoek (FWO) Vlaanderen – Research Foundation Flanders. P. Vandenberghe is a senior clinical investigator of FWO Vlaanderen. We thank E. Van Den Neste and A. Hagemeijer for critical reading of this manuscript.

## 6. References

Barragan, M., Bellosillo, B., Campas, C., Colomer, D., Pons, G. & Gil, J. (2002) Involvement of Protein Kinase C and Phosphatidylinositol 3-Kinase Pathways in the Survival of B-Cell Chronic Lymphocytic Leukemia Cells. *Blood*, Vol.99, No.8, (Apr) 2969-2976

Berkova, A., Zemanova, Z., Trneny, M., Schwarz, J., Karban, J., Cmunt, E., et al. (2009) Clonal Evolution in Chronic Lymphocytic Leukemia Studied by Interphase Fluorescence in-Situ Hybridization. *Neoplasma*, Vol.56, No.5, (Febr) 455-458

Brown, J.R., Hanna, M., Tesar, B., Werner, L., Reynolds, H., Fernandes, S.M., et al. (2010) High Resolution Genomic Analysis in CLL Demonstrates Genomic Stability in Untreated Patients and Novel Markers of Progression in Treated Patients. *ASH Annual Meeting Abstracts*, Vol.116, No.21, (Nov) 2426

Buhl, A.M., Jurlander, J., Jorgensen, F.S., Ottesen, A.M., Cowland, J.B., Gjerdrum, L.M., et al. (2006) Identification of a Gene on Chromosome 12q22 Uniquely Overexpressed in Chronic Lymphocytic Leukemia. *Blood*, Vol.107, No.7, (Apr) 2904-2911

Buhmann, R., Kurzeder, C., Rehklau, J., Westhaus, D., Bursch, S., Hiddemann, W., et al. (2002) CD40L Stimulation Enhances the Ability of Conventional Metaphase Cytogenetics to Detect Chromosome Aberrations in B-Cell Chronic Lymphocytic Leukaemia Cells. *Br J Haematol*, Vol.118, No.4, (Sep) 968-975

Carlsson, M., Totterman, T.H., Matsson, P. & Nilsson, K. (1988) Cell Cycle Progression of B-Chronic Lymphocytic Leukemia Cells Induced to Differentiate by TPA. *Blood*, Vol.71, No.2, (Feb) 415-421

Catovsky, D., Richards, S., Matutes, E., Oscier, D., Dyer, M.J., Bezares, R.F., et al. (2007) Assessment of Fludarabine Plus Cyclophosphamide for Patients with Chronic Lymphocytic Leukaemia (the LRF CLL4 Trial): A Randomised Controlled Trial. *Lancet*, Vol.370, No.9583, (Jul) 230-239

Cavazzini, F., Hernandez, J.A., Gozzetti, A., Russo Rossi, A., De Angeli, C., Tiseo, R., et al. (2008) Chromosome 14q32 Translocations Involving the Immunoglobulin Heavy Chain Locus in Chronic Lymphocytic Leukaemia Identify a Disease Subset with Poor Prognosis. *Br J Haematol*, Vol.142, No.4, (Aug) 529-537

Chapiro, E., Radford-Weiss, I., Bastard, C., Luquet, I., Lefebvre, C., Callet-Bauchu, E., et al. (2008) The Most Frequent t(14;19)(q32;q13)-Positive B-Cell Malignancy Corresponds to an Aggressive Subgroup of Atypical Chronic Lymphocytic Leukemia. *Leukemia*, Vol.22, No. (May) 2123-2127

Chiorazzi, N. (2007) Cell Proliferation and Death: Forgotten Features of Chronic Lymphocytic Leukemia B Cells. *Best Pract Res Clin Haematol*, Vol.20, No.3, (Sep) 399-413

Coll-Mulet, L., Santidrian, A.F., Cosialls, A.M., Iglesias-Serret, D., de Frias, M., Grau, J., et al. (2008) Multiplex Ligation-Dependent Probe Amplification for Detection of

Genomic Alterations in Chronic Lymphocytic Leukaemia. *Br J Haematol*, Vol.142, No.5, (Sep) 793-801

Cramer, P. & Hallek, M. (2011) Prognostic Factors in Chronic Lymphocytic Leukemia-What Do We Need to Know? *Nat Rev Clin Oncol*, Vol.8, No.1, (Jan) 38-47

Dicker, F., Schnittger, S., Haferlach, T., Kern, W. & Schoch, C. (2006) Immunostimulatory Oligonucleotide-Induced Metaphase Cytogenetics Detect Chromosomal Aberrations in 80% of CLL Patients: A Study of 132 CLL Cases with Correlation to Fish, *IGVH* Status, and CD38 Expression. *Blood*, Vol.108, No.9, (November 2006) 3152-3160

Döhner, H., Stilgenbauer, S., Benner, A., Leupolt, E., Krober, A., Bullinger, L., et al. (2000) Genomic Aberrations and Survival in Chronic Lymphocytic Leukemia. *N Engl J Med*, Vol.343, No.26, (Dec) 1910-1916

Fabbri, G., Rasi, S., Rossi, D., Trifonov, V., Khiabanian, H., Ma, J., et al. (2011) Analysis of the Chronic Lymphocytic Leukemia Coding Genome: Role of *NOTCH1* Mutational Activation. *J Exp Med*, Vol.208, No.7, (Jul) 1389-1401

Fabris, S., Scarciolla, O., Morabito, F., Cifarelli, R.A., Dininno, C., Cutrona, G., et al. (2011) Multiplex Ligation-Dependent Probe Amplification and Fluorescence in Situ Hybridization to Detect Chromosomal Abnormalities in Chronic Lymphocytic Leukemia: A Comparative Study. *Genes Chromosomes Cancer*, Vol.50, No.9, (Jun) 726-734

Fegan, C., Robinson, H., Thompson, P., Whittaker, J.A. & White, D. (1995) Karyotypic Evolution in CLL: Identification of a New Sub-Group of Patients with Deletions of 11q and Advanced or Progressive Disease. *Leukemia*, Vol.9, No.12, (Dec) 2003-2008

Finn, W.G., Kay, N.E., Kroft, S.H., Church, S. & Peterson, L.C. (1998) Secondary Abnormalities of Chromosome 6q in B-Cell Chronic Lymphocytic Leukemia: A Sequential Study of Karyotypic Instability in 51 Patients. *Am J Hematol*, Vol.59, No.3, (Nov) 223-229

Gollin, S.M. (2004) Chromosomal Instability. *Curr Opin Oncol*, Vol.16, No.1, (Jan) 25-31

Gostissa, M., Alt, F.W. & Chiarle, R. (2011) Mechanisms That Promote and Suppress Chromosomal Translocations in Lymphocytes. *Annu Rev Immunol*, Vol.29, (Apr) 319-350

Grubor, V., Krasnitz, A., Troge, J.E., Meth, J.L., Lakshmi, B., Kendall, J.T., et al. (2009) Novel Genomic Alterations and Clonal Evolution in Chronic Lymphocytic Leukemia Revealed by Representational Oligonucleotide Microarray Analysis (ROMA). *Blood*, Vol.113, No.6, (Feb) 1294-1303

Gunn, S.R., Bolla, A.R., Barron, L.L., Gorre, M.E., Mohammed, M.S., Bahler, D.W., et al. (2009) Array CGH Analysis of Chronic Lymphocytic Leukemia Reveals Frequent Cryptic Monoallelic and Biallelic Deletions of Chromosome 22q11 That Include the *PRAME* Gene. *Leuk Res*, Vol.33, No.9, (Sep) 1276-1281

Gunn, S.R., Mohammed, M.S., Gorre, M.E., Cotter, P.D., Kim, J., Bahler, D.W., et al. (2008) Whole-Genome Scanning by Array Comparative Genomic Hybridization as a Clinical Tool for Risk Assessment in Chronic Lymphocytic Leukemia. *J Mol Diagn*, Vol.10, No.5, (Sep) 442-451

Gunnarsson, R., Isaksson, A., Mansouri, M., Goransson, H., Jansson, M., Cahill, N., et al. (2010) Large but Not Small Copy-Number Alterations Correlate to High-Risk Genomic Aberrations and Survival in Chronic Lymphocytic Leukemia: A High-

Resolution Genomic Screening of Newly Diagnosed Patients. *Leukemia,* Vol.24, No.1, (Jan) 211-215

Gunnarsson, R., Mansouri, L., Isaksson, A., Goransson, H., Cahill, N., Jansson, M., et al. (2011) Array-Based Genomic Screening at Diagnosis and Follow-up in Chronic Lymphocytic Leukemia. *Haematologica,* Vol.96, No.8, (Aug), 1161-1169

Gunnarsson, R., Staaf, J., Jansson, M., Ottesen, A.M., Goransson, H., Liljedahl, U., et al. (2008) Screening for Copy-Number Alterations and Loss of Heterozygosity in Chronic Lymphocytic Leukemia--a Comparative Study of Four Differently Designed, High Resolution Microarray Platforms. *Genes Chromosomes Cancer,* Vol.47, No.8, (Aug) 697-711

Haferlach, C., Dicker, F., Schnittger, S., Kern, W. & Haferlach, T. (2007) Comprehensive Genetic Characterization of CLL: A Study on 506 Cases Analysed with Chromosome Banding Analysis, Interphase FISH, IGV(H) Status and Immunophenotyping. *Leukemia,* Vol.21, No.12, (December 2007) 2442-2451

Hagenkord, J.M., Monzon, F.A., Kash, S.F., Lilleberg, S., Xie, Q. & Kant, J.A. (2010) Array-Based Karyotyping for Prognostic Assessment in Chronic Lymphocytic Leukemia: Performance Comparison of 10K2.0, 250K Nsp, and SNP6.0 arrays *J Mol Diagn,* Vol.12, No.2, (Mar) 184-196

Hallaert, D.Y., Jaspers, A., van Noesel, C.J., van Oers, M.H., Kater, A.P. & Eldering, E. (2008) c-Abl Kinase Inhibitors Overcome CD40-Mediated Drug Resistance in CLL: Implications for Therapeutic Targeting of Chemoresistant Niches. *Blood,* Vol.112, No.13, (Dec) 5141-5149

Hallek, M., Cheson, B.D., Catovsky, D., Caligaris-Cappio, F., Dighiero, G., Dohner, H., et al. (2008) Guidelines for the Diagnosis and Treatment of Chronic Lymphocytic Leukemia: A Report from the International Workshop on Chronic Lymphocytic Leukemia Updating the National Cancer Institute-Working Group 1996 Guidelines. *Blood,* Vol.111, No.12, (Jun) 5446-5456

Heim, S. & Mitelman, F. (Eds.) (2009) *Cancer Cytogenetics.* Wiley-Blackwell, ISBN 978-0-470-18179-9, Hoboken, N.J. Hoboken, N.J.

Hernandez, J.A., Rodriguez, A.E., Gonzalez, M., Benito, R., Fontanillo, C., Sandoval, V., et al. (2009) A High Number of Losses in 13q14 Chromosome Band Is Associated with a Worse Outcome and Biological Differences in Patients with B-Cell Chronic Lymphoid Leukemia. *Haematologica,* Vol.94, No.3, (Mar) 364-371

Jahrsdorfer, B., Muhlenhoff, L., Blackwell, S.E., Wagner, M., Poeck, H., Hartmann, E., et al. (2005) B-Cell Lymphomas Differ in Their Responsiveness to CpG Oligodeoxynucleotides. *Clin Cancer Res,* Vol.11, No.4, (Feb) 1490-1499

Josefsson, P., Geisler, C.H., Leffers, H., Petersen, J.H., Andersen, M.K., Jurlander, J., et al. (2007) CLLU1 Expression Analysis Adds Prognostic Information to Risk Prediction in Chronic Lymphocytic Leukemia. *Blood,* Vol.109, No.11, (Jun) 4973-4979

Juliusson, G., Oscier, D.G., Fitchett, M., Ross, F.M., Stockdill, G., Mackie, M.J., et al. (1990) Prognostic Subgroups in B-Cell Chronic Lymphocytic Leukemia Defined by Specific Chromosomal Abnormalities. *N Engl J Med,* Vol.323, No.11, (Sep) 720-724

Kay, N.E., Eckel-Passow, J.E., Braggio, E., Vanwier, S., Shanafelt, T.D., Van Dyke, D.L., et al. (2010) Progressive but Previously Untreated CLL Patients with Greater Array CGH Complexity Exhibit a Less Durable Response to Chemoimmunotherapy. *Cancer Genet Cytogenet,* Vol.203, No.2, (Dec) 161-168

Klein, U. & Dalla-Favera, R. (2010) New Insights into the Pathogenesis of Chronic Lymphocytic Leukemia. *Semin Cancer Biol,* Vol.20, No.6, (Dec) 377-383

Kujawski, L., Ouillette, P., Erba, H., Saddler, C., Jakubowiak, A., Kaminski, M., et al. (2008) Genomic Complexity Identifies Patients with Aggressive Chronic Lymphocytic Leukemia. *Blood,* Vol.112, No.5, (Sep) 1993-2003

Lehmann, S., Ogawa, S., Raynaud, S.D., Sanada, M., Nannya, Y., Ticchioni, M., et al. (2008) Molecular Allelokaryotyping of Early-Stage, Untreated Chronic Lymphocytic Leukemia. *Cancer,* Vol.112, No.6, (Mar) 1296-1305

Leuenberger, M., Frigerio, S., Wild, P.J., Noetzli, F., Korol, D., Zimmermann, D.R., et al. (2010) AID Protein Expression in Chronic Lymphocytic Leukemia/Small Lymphocytic Lymphoma Is Associated with Poor Prognosis and Complex Genetic Alterations. *Mod Pathol,* Vol.23, No.2, (Feb) 177-186

Lin, T.T., Letsolo, B.T., Jones, R.E., Rowson, J., Pratt, G., Hewamana, S., et al. (2010) Telomere Dysfunction and Fusion During the Progression of Chronic Lymphocytic Leukemia: Evidence for a Telomere Crisis. *Blood,* Vol.116, No.11, (Sep) 1899-1907

Malcikova, J., Smardova, J., Pekova, S., Cejkova, S., Kotaskova, J., Tichy, B., et al. (2008) Identification of Somatic Hypermutations in the *TP53* Gene in B-Cell Chronic Lymphocytic Leukemia. *Mol Immunol,* Vol.45, No.5, (Mar) 1525-1529

Malek, S., Parkin, B., Collins, R., Shedden, K. & Ouillette, P. (2010) The Prognostic Importance of Various 13q14 Deletions in CLL. *ASH Annual Meeting Abstracts,* Vol.116, No.21, (Nov) 3587

Martin-Subero, J.I., Ibbotson, R., Klapper, W., Michaux, L., Callet-Bauchu, E., Berger, F., et al. (2007) A Comprehensive Genetic and Histopathologic Analysis Identifies Two Subgroups of B-Cell Malignancies Carrying a t(14;19)(q32;q13) or Variant BCL3-Translocation. *Leukemia,* Vol.21, No.7, (Jul) 1532-1544

Mayr, C., Speicher, M.R., Kofler, D.M., Buhmann, R., Strehl, J., Busch, R., et al. (2006) Chromosomal Translocations Are Associated with Poor Prognosis in Chronic Lymphocytic Leukemia. *Blood,* Vol.107, No.2, (Jan) 742-751

Merup, M., Juliusson, G., Wu, X., Jansson, M., Stellan, B., Rasool, O., et al. (1997) Amplification of Multiple Regions of Chromosome 12, Including 12q13-15, in Chronic Lymphocytic Leukaemia. *Eur J Haematol,* Vol.58, No.3, (Mar) 174-180

Michaux, L., Wlodarska, I., Rack, K., Stul, M., Criel, A., Maerevoet, M., et al. (2005) Translocation t(1;6)(p35.3;p25.2): A New Recurrent Aberration in "Unmutated" B-CLL. *Leukemia,* Vol.19, No.1, (Jan) 77-82

Nowakowski, G.S., Smoley, S., Schwager, S., Zent, C.S., Call, T.G., Shanafelt, T.D., et al. (2007) Presence of Immunoglobulin Heavy Chain Gene (*IGH*) Translocations in Chronic Lymphocytic Leukemia Is Related to Poor Prognosis. *ASH Annual Meeting Abstracts,* Vol.110, No.11, (Nov) 2067

Nussenzweig, A. & Nussenzweig, M.C. (2010) Origin of Chromosomal Translocations in Lymphoid Cancer. *Cell,* Vol.141, No.1, (Apr) 27-38

O'Malley, D.P., Giudice, C., Chang, A.S., Chang, D., Barry, T.S., Hibbard, M.K., et al. (2011) Comparison of Array Comparative Genomic Hybridization (aCGH) to FISH and Cytogenetics in Prognostic Evaluation of Chronic Lymphocytic Leukemia. *Int J Lab Hematol,* Vol.33, No.3, (Jun) 238-244

Oscier, D., Fitchett, M., Herbert, T. & Lambert, R. (1991) Karyotypic Evolution in B-Cell Chronic Lymphocytic Leukaemia. *Genes Chromosomes Cancer*, Vol.3, No.1, (Jan) 16-20

Ouillette, P., Collins, R., Shakhan, S., Li, J., Peres, E., Kujawski, L., et al. (2011) Acquired Genomic Copy Number Aberrations and Survival in Chronic Lymphocytic Leukemia. *Blood*, Vol. 118, No.11, (Sep) 3051-3061

Ouillette, P., Fossum, S., Parkin, B., Ding, L., Bockenstedt, P., Al-Zoubi, A., et al. (2010) Aggressive Chronic Lymphocytic Leukemia with Elevated Genomic Complexity Is Associated with Multiple Gene Defects in the Response to DNA Double-Strand Breaks. *Clin Cancer Res*, Vol.16, No.3, (Feb) 835-847

Palacios, F., Moreno, P., Morande, P., Abreu, C., Correa, A., Porro, V., et al. (2010) High Expression of AID and Active Class Switch Recombination Might Account for a More Aggressive Disease in Unmutated CLL Patients: Link with an Activated Microenvironment in Cll Disease. *Blood*, Vol.115, No.22, (Jun) 4488-4496

Perez-Duran, P., de Yebenes, V.G. & Ramiro, A.R. (2007) Oncogenic Events Triggered by AID, the Adverse Effect of Antibody Diversification. *Carcinogenesis*, Vol.28, No.12, (Dec) 2427-2433

Pfeifer, D., Pantic, M., Skatulla, I., Rawluk, J., Kreutz, C., Martens, U.M., et al. (2007) Genome-Wide Analysis of DNA Copy Number Changes and LOH in CLL Using High-Density SNP Arrays. *Blood*, Vol.109, No.3, (Feb) 1202-1210

Pospisilova, H., Baens, M., Michaux, L., Stul, M., Van Hummelen, P., Van Loo, P., et al. (2007) Interstitial Del(14)(q) Involving *IGH*: A Novel Recurrent Aberration in B-NHL. *Leukemia*, Vol.21, No.9, (Sep) 2079-2083

Puente, X.S., Pinyol, M., Quesada, V., Conde, L., Ordonez, G.R., Villamor, N., et al. (2011) Whole-Genome Sequencing Identifies Recurrent Mutations in Chronic Lymphocytic Leukaemia. *Nature*, Vol.475, No.7354, (Jul) 101-105

Put, N., Konings, P., Rack, K., Jamar, M., Van Roy, N., Libouton, J.M., et al. (2009a) Improved Detection of Chromosomal Abnormalities in Chronic Lymphocytic Leukemia by Conventional Cytogenetics Using CpG Oligonucleotide and Interleukin-2 Stimulation: A Belgian Multicentric Study. *Genes Chromosomes Cancer*, Vol.48, No.10, (Oct) 843-853

Put, N., Meeus, P., Chatelain, B., Rack, K., Boeckx, N., Nollet, F., et al. (2009b) Translocation t(14;18) Is Not Associated with Inferior Outcome in Chronic Lymphocytic Leukemia. *Leukemia*, Vol.23, No.6, (Jun) 1201-1204

Reiniger, L., Bodor, C., Bognar, A., Balogh, Z., Csomor, J., Szepesi, A., et al. (2006) Richter's and Prolymphocytic Transformation of Chronic Lymphocytic Leukemia Are Associated with High mRNA Expression of Activation-Induced Cytidine Deaminase and Aberrant Somatic Hypermutation. *Leukemia*, Vol.20, No.6, (Jun) 1089-1095

Put ,N., Van Roosbroeck, K., Konings, P., Meeus, P., Brusselmans, C., Rack, K., Gervais ,C., Nguyen-Khac, F., Chapiro, E., Radford-Weiss, I., Struski, S., Dastugue, N., Gachard, N., Lefebvre, C., Barin ,C., Eclache, V., Fert-Ferrer, S., Laibe, S., Mozziconacci ,MJ., Quilichini ,B., Poirel, HA., Wlodarska, I., Hagemeijer, A., Moreau, Y., Vandenberghe ,P., Michaux, L.; on behalf of the BCGHo and the GFCH. (2011) Chronic lymphocytic leukemia and prolymphocytic  leukemia with MYC translocations: a subgroup with an aggressive disease course.*Ann Hematol*, (Dec). [Epub ahead of print]

Reis-Filho, J.S. (2009) Next-Generation Sequencing. *Breast Cancer Res*, Vol.11 Suppl 3, No.S12, (Dec) 1-7

Rinaldi, A., Mian, M., Kwee, I., Rossi, D., Deambrogi, C., Mensah, A.A., et al. (2011) Genome-Wide DNA Profiling Better Defines the Prognosis of Chronic Lymphocytic Leukaemia. *Br J Haematol*, Vol.154, No.5, (Sep), 590-599

Roos, G., Krober, A., Grabowski, P., Kienle, D., Buhler, A., Dohner, H., et al. (2008) Short Telomeres Are Associated with Genetic Complexity, High-Risk Genomic Aberrations, and Short Survival in Chronic Lymphocytic Leukemia. *Blood*, Vol.111, No.4, (Feb) 2246-2252

Schouten, J.P., McElgunn, C.J., Waaijer, R., Zwijnenburg, D., Diepvens, F. & Pals, G. (2002) Relative Quantification of 40 Nucleic Acid Sequences by Multiplex Ligation-Dependent Probe Amplification. *Nucleic Acids Res*, Vol.30, No.12, (Jun), 1-13

Schwab, M. (Ed.) (2001) *Encyclopedic Reference of Cancer*. Springer, ISBN 978-3-5403-3443-9, Berlin-Heidelberg, New York

Shaffer, L.G., Slovak, M.L. & Campell, L.J. (Eds.) (2009) *ISCN 2009: An International System for Human Cytogenetic Nomenclature*. Karger, ISBN 978-3-8055-8985-7, Basel

Shanafelt, T.D., Witzig, T.E., Fink, S.R., Jenkins, R.B., Paternoster, S.F., Smoley, S.A., et al. (2006) Prospective Evaluation of Clonal Evolution During Long-Term Follow-up of Patients with Untreated Early-Stage Chronic Lymphocytic Leukemia. *J Clin Oncol*, Vol.24, No.28, (Oct) 4634-4641

Smoley, S.A., Van Dyke, D.L., Kay, N.E., Heerema, N.A., Dell' Aquila, M.L., Dal Cin, P., et al. (2010) Standardization of Fluorescence in Situ Hybridization Studies on Chronic Lymphocytic Leukemia (CLL) Blood and Marrow Cells by the CLL Research Consortium. *Cancer Genet Cytogenet*, Vol.203, No.2, (Dec) 141-148

Stephenson, C.F., Desai, Z.R. & Bridges, J.M. (1991) The Proliferative Activity of B-Chronic Lymphocytic Leukaemia Lymphocytes Prior to and after Stimulation with TPA and PHA. *Leuk Res*, Vol.15, No.11, 1005-1012

Stilgenbauer, S., Sander, S., Bullinger, L., Benner, A., Leupolt, E., Winkler, D., et al. (2007) Clonal Evolution in Chronic Lymphocytic Leukemia: Acquisition of High-Risk Genomic Aberrations Associated with Unmutated *VH*, Resistance to Therapy, and Short Survival. *Haematologica*, Vol.92, No.9, (Sep) 1242-1245

Struski, S., Gervais, C., Helias, C., Herbrecht, R., Audhuy, B. & Mauvieux, L. (2009) Stimulation of B-Cell Lymphoproliferations with CpG-Oligonucleotide DSP30 Plus IL-2 Is More Effective Than with TPA to Detect Clonal Abnormalities. *Leukemia*, Vol.23, No.3, (Mar) 617-619

Tam, C.S., Shanafelt, T.D., Wierda, W.G., Abruzzo, L.V., Van Dyke, D.L., O'Brien, S., et al. (2009) De Novo Deletion 17p13.1 Chronic Lymphocytic Leukemia Shows Significant Clinical Heterogeneity: The M. D. Anderson and Mayo Clinic Experience. *Blood*, Vol.114, No.5, (Jul) 957-964

Touw, I. & Lowenberg, B. (1985) Interleukin 2 Stimulates Chronic Lymphocytic Leukemia Colony Formation in Vitro. *Blood*, Vol.66, No.1, (Jul) 237-240

Van Bockstaele, F., Verhasselt, B. & Philippe, J. (2008) Prognostic Markers in Chronic Lymphocytic Leukemia: A Comprehensive Review. *Blood Rev*, Vol.23, No.1, (Jan) 25-47

Van Den Neste, E., Robin, V., Francart, J., Hagemeijer, A., Stul, M., Vandenberghe, P., et al. (2007) Chromosomal Translocations Independently Predict Treatment Failure, Treatment-Free Survival and Overall Survival in B-Cell Chronic Lymphocytic Leukemia Patients Treated with Cladribine. *Leukemia*, Vol.21, No.8, (Aug) 1715-1722

Van Dyke, D.L., Shanafelt, T.D., Call, T.G., Zent, C.S., Smoley, S.A., Rabe, K.G., et al. (2010) A Comprehensive Evaluation of the Prognostic Significance of 13q Deletions in Patients with B-Chronic Lymphocytic Leukaemia. *Br J Haematol*, Vol.148, No.4, (Feb) 544-550

Watanabe, T., Ichikawa, A., Saito, H. & Hotta, T. (1996) Overexpression of the *MDM2* Oncogene in Leukemia and Lymphoma. *Leuk Lymphoma*, Vol.21, No.5-6, (May) 391-397

Willander, K., Ungerback, J., Karlsson, K., Fredrikson, M., Soderkvist, P. & Linderholm, M. (2010) *MDM2* SNP309 Promoter Polymorphism, an Independent Prognostic Factor in Chronic Lymphocytic Leukemia. *Eur J Haematol*, Vol.85, No.3, (Sep) 251-256

Wu, X., Nowakowski, G.S., Smoley, S.A., Arendt, B.A., Peterson, M.A., van Dyke, D., et al. (2008) Cytogenetic Analysis of Normal Human B Cells Following CpG Stimulation: Implications for Interpretation of CpG Induced CLL Metaphase Analysis. *ASH Annual Meeting Abstracts*, Vol.112, No.11, (Nov) 3124

Zenz, T., Mertens, D., Dohner, H. & Stilgenbauer, S. (2011) Importance of Genetics in Chronic Lymphocytic Leukemia. *Blood Rev*, Vol.25, No.3, (May) 131-137

# Prognostic Factors in Chronic Lymphoid Leukemia and Identification of New Clinically Relevant Molecular Markers

José-Ángel Hernández[1], Marcos González[2] and Jesús-María Hernández[2]
[1]Hospital Universitario Infanta Leonor, Madrid,
[2]Hospital Clínico Universitario, Salamanca,
Spain

## 1. Introduction

Chronic lymphocytic leukemia (CLL) is a hematological malignancy with significant clinical heterogeneity, due in part to the genetic alterations that leukemic cells present in each patient (Chiorazzi et al, 2005). CLL has a highly variable clinical course. Traditionally, it has been considered that about one-third of patients will never require treatment, as they will have prolonged survival and they will die from causes unrelated to the disease. In another third of cases, after an indolent phase disease progression occurs. In the remaining third of patients early treatment is required because of the aggressiveness of the disorder. However, due to the routine performance of blood counts in the population, the number of asymptomatic patients is increasing and, conversely, those who require initial treatment account for fewer than 15% of cases (Hernandez et al, 2010). Since the first descriptions of the disease, researchers have attempted to establish prognostic factors with which to make a risk assessment of disease progression and probability of death. The ultimate aim is to try and apply a targeted and early treatment that increases overall survival and quality of life in patients with more aggressive forms, and to determine reliably the cases who do not need further treatment. (Dighiero & Hamblin, 2008).

Historically, there have been two distinct phases in the analysis of prognostic factors in CLL. Until the late 1980s, most prognostic factors were related to clinical presentation, cellular morphology, the pattern of infiltration of the bone marrow and lymphocyte progression over a period of time. Some of these are no longer considered relevant. Since the 1990s several prognostic factors associated with the immunophenotypic profile, cytogenetic features and mutational status of the immunoglobulin heavy chain (IGVH) have been added (Moreno & Montserrat, 2008). However, nomograms and predictors that include common clinical and pathological factors are still valid.

## 2. Prognostic factors in CLL

### 2.1 Clinical characteristics

In most published series, male patients have a more aggressive clinical course and worse survival than women with CLL (Catovsky et al, 1989). More than 30 years ago, Rai and Binet established two staging systems by which patients could be classified into low-, intermediate- and high-risk groups according to the presence or absence of certain clinical features (lymphadenopathy, visceromegalies, anemia and thrombocytopenia) (Binet et al, 1981; Rai et al, 1975). Nowadays, both clinical staging systems are widely used because of their simplicity and applicability. Different stages can be defined: early (Rai 0, Binet A), intermediate (Rai I-II, Binet B) and advanced (Rai III-IV, Binet C). These stages have a median overall survival (OS) of 10-12, 7 and 1.5-4 years, respectively (Tables 1 and 2). The Rai and Binet clinical stages have several limitations: a) they are unable to predict which patients from the initial stages will progress; b) they do not considerer tumor burden; c) they do not take into account the mechanism of cytopenias and d) they do not predict the response to therapy. At present, over 80% of cases are diagnosed in early stage A (0), since very often the diagnosis is made in the context of a routine analysis or of comorbidities that are unrelated to CLL.

| Stage | Clinical features | Overall survival (years) |
|-------|-------------------|--------------------------|
| 0 | Blood and bone marrow lymphocytosis* | 10 |
| I | Lymphocytosis and large lymph nodes | 7 |
| II | Lymphocytosis and splenomegaly and/or hepatomegaly with or without large lymph nodes | 7 |
| III | Lymphocytosis and anemia** (hemoglobin level < 11 g/dL) with or without large lymph nodes, splenomegaly or hepatomegaly | 1,5-4 |
| IV | Lymphocytosis and thrombocytopenia** (platelet count < 100 x 10⁹/L) with or without anemia, large lymph nodes, splenomegaly or hepatomegaly | 1,5-4 |

*Lymphocyte count > 5 x 10⁹/L in peripheral blood and > 30% of nucleated cells in bone marrow aspiration count.**Immune anemias or thrombocytopenias are excluded.

Table 1. Rai clinical stage system.

| Stage | Clinical features | Overall survival (years) |
|-------|-------------------|--------------------------|
| A | Lymphocytosis in peripheral blood and bone marrow* and < 3 lymphoid regions involved**. No anemia, no thrombocytopenia | 12 |
| B | Lymphocytosis in peripheral blood and bone marrow* and ≥ 3 lymphoid regions involved **, with or without splenomegaly and/or hepatomegaly. No anemia, no thrombocytopenia | 7 |
| C | Lymphocytosis * with anemia*** (hemoglobin level < 11 g/dL in male and < 10 g/dL in female) or thrombocytopenia*** (platelet count < 100 x 10⁹/L) | 2-4 |

*Lymphocyte count > 5 x 10⁹/L in peripheral blood and > 30% of nucleated cells in bone marrow aspiration count. **Each cervical, axillary and inguinal area can be unilateral or bilateral. Splenomegaly and hepatomegaly are one lymphoid region (5 areas). ***Immune anemias or thrombocytopenias are excluded.

Table 2. Binet clinical stage system.

## 2.2 Morphological features

Prolymphocytic transformation of CLL carries a worse prognosis, as well as atypical CLL ( > 15% cell morphology is not compatible with the CLL, such as the presence of cleaved nuclei lymphocytes) compared with the typical morphology of CLL. It has recently been reported that patients with more than 30% of nuclear shadows (smudge cells) in the differential count are more likely to have a mutated IGVH pattern and, therefore, a longer time to treatment and better survival (Nowakowski et al, 2007).

The pattern of bone marrow infiltration may be nodular, interstitial, mixed (the most common type) and diffuse. In practice, we have to consider the first three as non-diffuse, because there are prognostic differences between patients with diffuse vs non-diffuse pattern. Patients treated with fludarabine schedules often show a persistent nodular pattern after therapy (nodular partial response), which represents a higher quality response than a partial one. The group at the Hospital Clinic, Barcelona, showed that the presence of a diffuse pattern of bone marrow infiltration is associated with a worse prognosis (Montserrat & Rozman, 1987). However, this prognostic factor was not independently confirmed by others, when new genetic markers were included in the analysis (Geisler et al, 1996).

## 2.3 Markers of proliferation or tumor burden and markers of angiogenesis

A lymphocyte doubling time (LDT) less than 6 months or an increase in lymphocyte count > 50% in 2 months is associated with a worse prognosis because they indicate an increased activity of the disease (Viñolas et al, 1987). In any case, LDT should only be recommended to initiate the treatment of CLL or to establish the prognosis with elevated lymphocyte counts (> 30 x $10^9$/L). Despite their limitations, including the changes that occur during the course of the disease, LDT is a simple and inexpensive method, that is still interpreted in most clinical trials and clinical practice as an indication to start treatment.

Elevation of serum levels of lactate dehydrogenase (LDH), β2 microglobulin (B2M), thymidine kinase (TK) and soluble CD23 also indicate a high tumor burden (Hallek et al, 1996; Sarfati et al, 1996). Of these, LDH, contrary to what is observed in other lymphoproliferative disorders, is of minor relevance, although it is used in clinical practice due to the simplicity of its determination.

Elevated levels of TK are correlated with increased proliferation and predict the progression of CLL. In patients with early-stage CLL, high TK levels are correlated with the expression of CD38, ZAP-70, poor prognostic cytogenetic abnormalities and unmutated IGVH status. Moreover, serum TK levels have an independent value in the differentiation of CLL patients in early stages according to progression-free survival (PFS). Two limitations of the use of TK as a prognostic factor are the variation between laboratories, as well as their levels can be increased in patients with viral infections. However, its prognostic value in early-stage CLL has been fully established.

High levels of serum B2M, a protein that binds to the class I major histocompatibility complex, is one of the most important prognostic factors in some of the reported series. Moreover, their levels are correlated with the expression of CD38 and ZAP-70. Recently, the MD Anderson Cancer Center has proposed a prognostic nomogram that includes age, sex, absolute lymphocyte count, the number of lymphoid areas involved and B2M (Wierda et al,

2007). Furthermore, this group has also confirmed that low levels of B2M are independently associated with better complete responses (CR) rates, disease-free survival (DFS) and OS in patients treated with fludarabine-based schemes, with or without the addition of rituximab. The prognostic value of B2M in patients with impaired renal function is limited. Nevertheless, B2M is currently one of the most important prognostic factors for evaluating patients with advanced-stage CLL.

High levels and/or duplication of soluble CD23 also predicts a worse outcome for patients with CLL, with progression of patients in early stages and decreased survival.

Finally, the rise in the microvascular density and high levels of growth factor (VEGF) are also associated with poor prognosis (Ferrajoli et al, 2001).

## 2.4 Diagnostic imaging

Changes in abdominal computed tomography is a predictor of progression in patients with early-stage CLL, so its inclusion in the initial diagnostic tests can provide clinically relevant information (Muntañola et al, 2007). Even so, there are controversies regarding its value as a prognostic factor.

## 2.5 Immunophenotypic markers expression

### 2.5.1 Expression of CD38

CD38 is expressed in various hematopoietic cells and progenitors, thymus cells, T cells and activated B cells in later stages of differentiation. Determining the expression of CD38 is a useful tool and the results are easily analyzed to determine the prognosis of patients with CLL. However, because it is not a unique antigen of the proliferating cell in CLL it should not be analyzed independently, but along with the CD19 or CD20 and CD5, due to the aforementioned expression in other mononuclear cells. CD38 has been proposed as a prognostic marker in CLL, which has led to CD38 being proposed as a prognostic marker in CLL, indicating a more aggressive disease (Damle et al, 1999; Ghia et al, 2003). However, there is no consensus about the cutoff of positivity. Some authors suggest this to be 7%, although most choose levels above 30%. Different levels of CD38 expression can be observed over the course of the illness, during which its prognostic relevance diminishes. In fact, CD38 expression is not a perfect marker that can be a surrogates for IGVH mutational status, although it is associated with an increased incidence of organomegaly, bad prognosis cytogenetics, high B2M serum level and worse PFS and OS (Hamblin et al, 2002).

### 2.5.2 Expression of ZAP-70

The chain-associated protein zeta 70 (ZAP-70) is an intracellular tyrosine kinase Syk family/ZAP, which is associated with the zeta chain of the T cell receptor (TCR). Its expression is normally restricted to T and NK cells, which initiate the signaling pathways of T cells, resulting in the activation, differentiation and proliferation of effector cell functions in response to TCR stimulation. B cells of CLL may variably express this marker, but its positivity is one of the most powerful prognostic factors for predicting the course of the disease. The expression of ZAP-70 can be performed by various molecular techniques such as western blot, immunohistochemistry, RT-PCR, microarray expression and flow cytometry. One of the weaknesses of its determination by flow cytometry is the lack of reproducibility of the results. Several research groups have attempted to standardize the methodology in recent years (Letestu et al, 2006). It is likely that once it has been determined, along with other clinical and biological markers, it will help clinicians to assess the prognosis in newly diagnosed CLL patients more reliably. Results published by the Barcelona group, with a 20 % cutoff of ZAP-70, determined by flow cytometry (a higher level of expression indicates a worse prognosis) demonstrated significant differences in the OS and PFS of patients with CLL (Crespo et al, 2003). Unlike the case with CD38, ZAP-70 expression seems to be better than IGVH mutational status in predicting the time to receive the first treatment. The concordance between ZAP-70 expression and IGVH mutational status is 75-90% (Rassenti et al, 2004). When the positivity of ZAP70 and CD38 expression are combined, the time to treatment is 30 months, while it is 130 months in cases where both markers are negative.

However, the expression of both CD38 and ZAP-70 has proved controversial in the scientific community regarding its prognostic value for the next reasons: a) different results may be obtained with the same samples in different laboratories (indicating lack of validity and reproducibility of the techniques used), b) there may be temporal variations in the expression of CD38, c) it is difficult to establish the correct cutoff point for the expression of CD38 (<vs> 7% <vs> 30%) and ZAP-70 (the most widely accepted value being 20%), d) a careful separation of T cells for the determination of ZAP-70 by flow cytometry techniques is mandatory, which has meant that, even recently, several experts in this area have tried to systematize the method of determination, and e) a 20-30% discrepancy in the results of ZAP-70 provided by immunophenotyping by flow cytometry and IGVH mutational status has been described.

The CD49d antigen, whose expression is associated with a worse prognosis, has acquired a special significance in recent years (Gattei et al, 2008).

## 2.6 IGVH mutational status

One of the most important genetic parameters to establish the prognosis of patients with CLL is the mutational status of VH genes. Somatic mutations of the VH gene region of the heavy chain of immunoglobulins are present in about half of all CLL cases. In 1999, two research groups reported the importance of this observation as a predictor of disease progression, with survival of 8 years in cases of patients with CLL and unmutated pattern *vs* 24 years in those with mutated status (Damle et al, 1999; Hamblin et al, 1999). Unmutated cases originate from cells in the pregerminal center and clearly have a worse prognosis than mutated CLL cells also arising from the postgerminal center. The definition of non-mutated *vs* mutated pattern resides in a cutoff point, defined arbitrarily as a homology greater than 98% (non-mutated) gene most similar to the germline (Schroeder & Dighiero, 1994).

Patients with CLL and an unmutated status have an unfavorable course and progress more rapidly, as opposed to patients exhibiting a mutated state, whose survival is much better (Figures 1, 2). Unmutated CLL patients have a greater tendency to acquire poor prognostic cytogenetic abnormalities. It has also been observed that, irrespective of mutational status, some VH regions are associated with specific clinical features and different geographical incidences (Ghia et al, 2005). This is the case for IGHV3-21 usage, whose involvement provides a worse prognosis regardless of mutational status and, characteristically, is less prevalent in southern European countries, as confirmed by the results of an Italian group, who even showed that it is less frequent in southern than in northern Italy. This poorer clinical behavior of patients with IGHV3-21 may be explained because of the complementarity determining regions (HCDR3) are shorter and it is possible that the stimulatory influence of some unknown antigen leads to CLL progression. Other genes from the IGHV3 family, the most frequently used subgroup in CLL, are associated with prognosis. Thus, IGHV3-23 is related with a bad prognosis. On the other hand, IGHV3-72 and IGHV3-30 usages indicate good clinical outcomes, including spontaneous regression in anecdotal cases (Dal-Bo et al, 2011). Moreover, the involvement of the IGHV1-69 family, although it does not seem to have a lower survival compared to patients expressing other unmutated genes, and the IGHV4-39 usage occurs mainly in unmutated cases, while the IGHV4-34 and most cases of IGHV3 contain mutated cases. Patients with unmutated state have a poor prognosis if an autologous transplantation is performed, although the graft versus leukemia effect may counteract the therapeutic resistance of these patients if an allogeneic transplant is offered. The rearrangements of IGHV3-48 and IGHV3-53 are also associated with poor prognosis.

IGVH mutational status and cytogenetic abnormalities identified by FISH have a major impact on the survival of patients with CLL, but while cytogenetic changes during the course of the disease are relatively common, IGVH mutational status remains constant over time. One of the limitations of its use is the high cost of testing, due to its laboriousness and the expertise required.

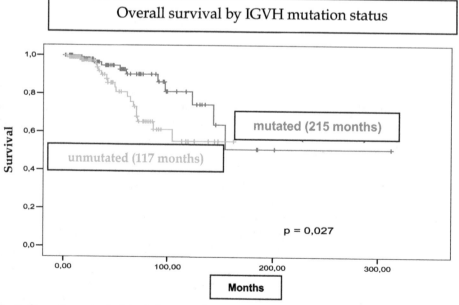

Fig. 1. Overall survival of the Salamanca University series of 226 patients with CLL by IGVH mutation status.

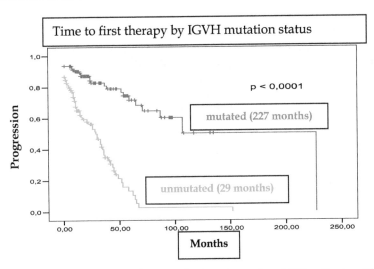

Fig. 2. Time to first therapy of the Salamanca University series of 226 patients with CLL by IGVH mutation status.

## 2.7 Cytogenetics and fluorescence in situ hybridization (FISH)

In 2000, the University of Ulm Group published their results from 325 patients with CLL concerning the relationship of various cytogenetic abnormalities, determined by FISH, with survival (Dohner et al, 2000). Using a panel of eight FISH probes, they analyzed the losses in 6q, 11q, 13q and 17p, the trisomies of 3q26, 8q24 and 12q13 and 14q32 translocations. They found that 82% of patients had chromosomal abnormalities, some of which were of prognostic relevance. In order of frequency, loss of 13q14 was the most frequent (present in 55% of cases), followed by loss of 11q22-23 (18%), trisomy of chromosome 12 (16%), loss of 17p13 (7%) and loss of 6q21 (6%). Only 57 patients (18%) had no abnormalities according to FISH, while 67 and 26 patients had two or more cytogenetic abnormalities, respectively. Median survival of patients with 17p-, 11q-, trisomy 12, normal cytogenetics and 13q- as a single alteration were 32, 79, 114, 111 and 133 months, respectively. In addition, patients with 17p- had the shortest interval before first treatment (9 months), whereas this period was longest in those with 13q- (92 months). In the Cox regression of overall survival time, patients with 17p deletion had a hazard ratio eight times that of other patients, whereas for those with 11q loss the hazard ratio was somewhat less than 3. These results have been reproduced in several series (Figure 3) (Tables 3, 4).

It is of note that some of the cytogenetic changes are related to characteristics of the disease: patients with 11q- tend to be younger and have marked lymphadenopathy, while those with 17p- are resistant to standard treatments, including that with fludarabine. 17p and 11q deletions were independently associated with other prognostic factors, such as IGVH mutation state, and the patients with these deletions had an adverse clinical outcome with progression of CLL and decreased survival (Krober et al, 2006). The British Group recently reported that patients with a more than 20% loss of function of TP53, a gene located on 17p, have a worse prognosis than those with a lower percentage loss (Gonzalez et al, 2011).

On the other hand, although it has customarily been considered that patients with del (13q) have a better prognosis, those with a high number of losses and/or the size of the deletion is greater have a worse prognosis in terms of time to receive the first treatment and survival, as shown recently by four independent groups (Figures 4, 5) (Dal Bo et al, 2011). Our genomic expression profile (GEP) studies have shown that those cases with a high number of losses of 13q have a higher expression of genes related to proliferation and reduced expression of apoptosis-related genes (Hernandez et al, 2009).

The 14q32/IGH translocation is present in 5-7% of CLL cases. Patients with IGH rearrangements can be classified in the intermediate prognosis group, as occurs with 6q deletion CLL patients (Cavazzini et al, 2008).

Clonal evolution may be observed during the course of CLL with the acquisition of new cytogenetic abnormalities (Stilgenbauer et al, 2007). These cytogenetic aberrations occur in 20-45% of patients and are associated with the presence of unmutated state and/or ZAP-70 expression. Therefore, FISH analysis should be done to diagnose CLL, before starting treatment and during relapse.

Finally, it has recently been shown that the presence of chromosomal translocations is associated with poor prognosis in CLL patients and that the length of telomeres is a prognostic factor related to mutation status (Sellmann et al, 2011).

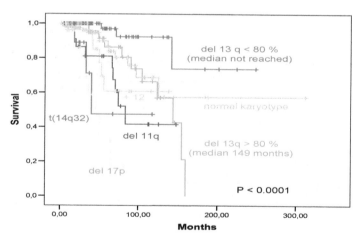

Fig. 3. Overall survival of the Salamanca University series of 350 patients with CLL by FISH group.

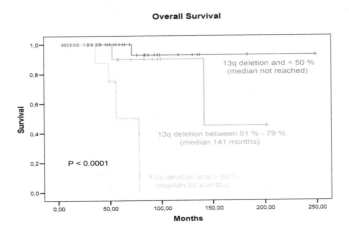

Fig. 4. Overall survival of the Salamanca University series of 109 patients with 13q deletion as unique alteration at diagnosis. A high number of losses in 13q is associated with a worse prognosis.

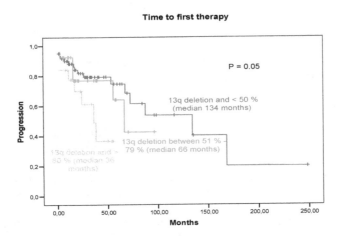

Fig. 5. Time to first therapy of the Salamanca University series of 109 patients with 13q deletion as unique alteration at diagnosis. A high number of losses in 13q is associated with a worse prognosis.

| Study | 13q⁻ | 13q⁻as unique alteration | 11q⁻ | +12 | 17p⁻ | Mutated status | Unmutated status |
|---|---|---|---|---|---|---|---|
| Ulm University | 55 | 36 | 18 | 16 | 7 | 56 | 44 |
| CLL1[1] | 59 | 40 | 10 | 13 | 4 | 41 | 59 |
| CLL4[2] | 53 | 34 | 21 | 11 | 3 | 69 | 31 |
| CLL3[3] | 52 | 27 | 22 | 12 | 3 | 68 | 32 |
| CLL2H[4] | 48 | 14 | 32 | 18 | 27 | 81 | 19 |
| Salamanca University[5] | 46 | 36 | 9 | 12 | 4 | 56 | 44 |

*Results indicate percentages. 1. Patients in Binet A clinical stage without classical indication of therapy. 2. Patients aged < 65 years and Binet B and C clinical stages, included in randomized clinical trial (fludarabine *vs* fludarabine + cyclophosphamide). 3. Patients aged < 60 years and Binet B and C clinical stages, included in a clinical trial of autologous transplantation. 4. Patients refractory to fludarabine included in a clinical trial of subcutaneous alemtuzumab. 5. t(14q32) in 6 % of patients.

Table 3. Incidence of genomic aberrations and IGVH mutational status in several series of the CLL German Study Group and our series from the Salamanca University*

| Variable | Hazard ratio (95% CI*) |
|---|---|
| Deletion 17p | 7.03 (3.23-15.3) |
| IGVH1-69 usage | 2.60 (1.04-6.44) |
| Deletion 11q | 2.52 (1.29-4.90) |
| Normal cytogenetics | 0.47 (0.23-0.97) |
| Deletion 13q as unique aberration | 0.34 (0.18-0.64) |
| Mutated IGVH status | 0.43 (0.20-0.91) |

*CI: confidence interval.

Table 4. Cox regression analysis of overall survival in the series of CLL patients of the CLL patients of the Salamanca University

## 2.8 MicroRNAs

MicroRNAs (miRNA) are a class of RNAs that modulate the expression of post-transcriptional genes. miRNAs are small, non-coding RNAs involved in cancer genesis, apoptosis and the cell metabolism. These molecules show a role in CLL pathogenesis and prognosis (Calin et al, 2005). So, miR-29 has been described as a tumor-suppressing molecule that targets oncogenes like TCL1. This oncogene is overexpressed in CLL and is associated with an unmutated IGVH status, a high level of ZAP-70 expression and high-risk cytogenetics. In CLL patients, TCL1 protein expression is inversely correlated with miR-29 and miR-81 expression. Recently, it has been confirmed that the expression of miR-29 and miR-223 are correlated with poor prognosis. These two miRNAs, ZAP-70 and lipoprotein lipase (LPL) are the four variables comprising a new progressive prognostic score from 0 to 4 with the median TFS decreased from 312 months in the very good prognosis group to 12 months in the poor prognosis group. Also, high and low levels of expression of miR-21 and miR-181b, respectively, have been reported as risk prognostic factors, and miR-15a and miR-

16 expression is related to IGVH mutation status. Finally, a correlation between 17p deletion, TP53 and miR-34a has been reported. It seems likely that miRNA research will be increasingly influential in determining the prognosis of CLL, and some of these molecules may prove to be surrogate markers in this disorder (Ward et al, 2011).

## 2.9 Lipoproteinlipase (LPL) and ADAM 29 gene expression

Recently, several studies have demonstrated the importance of LPL expression, such as that of the principal RNA prognostic marker. A comparative study of RNA-based markers in CLL revealed LPL to be a powerful predictor of clinical outcome. In the initial report the LPL/ADAM29 expression ratio was described as a strong prognosis indicator in CLL, that enabled a better assessment than ZAP-70 in advances stages of CLL (Oppezzo et al, 2005).

## 2.10 Genomic expression profiles

Another area of development is the analysis of gene expression by RNA microarrays, which has led to improved diagnosis and classification of the neoplasms of leukemia patients. Although little information is currently available, the discovery through the analysis of microarray gene expression of a group of genes associated with survival of patients reflects the potential of this technology to detect new markers that may be prognostically relevant. In 2001, it was demonstrated the association between gene expression and mutational pattern and the existence of a homogeneous phenotype related to memory B cells in patients with CLL (Klein et al, 2001; Rosenwald et al, 2001). Subsequently, it was observed that the study of gene expression profiles showed a common molecular signature in patients with CLL, what contributed to the identification of markers of progression or it was different in mutated and unmutated CLL. In addition, genes that are significantly more highly expressed are located in the corresponding aberrant chromosomal regions, indicating the existence of a genetic effect of dose, which may have a pathogenic role in CLL. Significant differences in gene expression according to sex were also found, which suggests that differences in molecular signatures relating to IGVH mutational status may be related to the sex of the patient (Haslinger et al, 2004). Several genes have been implicated in the pathogenesis and prognosis of CLL. Other research lines related to the DNA methylation and the phosphorylation of receptor and adaptor proteins are providing an increasing amount of information about this disease and could have a prognostic role (Prieto-Sanchez et al, 2006). Even so, more work remains to be done in this field (Codony et al, 2009).

## 2.11 Treatment response and prognosis

The quality, depth and length of the response in the CLL treatment are of great prognostic importance. The achievement of a complete or a nodular partial response predicts better DFS and OS. In addition, some therapy schedules, mainly those based on immunochemotherapy (i.e., FCR combination) might overcome the dismal prognosis of patients with CLL and del (11q). On the other hand, negative minimal residual disease (MRD) improves the outcome of CLL patients, in terms of PFS, TTT and OS. Nevertheless, MRD assessment is not recommended in clinical practice, although it might be of great value in the coming years (Cramer & Hallek, 2011).

## 2.12 Comorbidities and prognosis

Performance status, physical fitness and comorbidities are important features in the selection of therapy and thereby in the prognosis of patients with CLL (Zenz et al, 2010). In this context, patients with CLL are divided in three groups: a) Fit or 'Go go' patients, for whom a standard treatment can be administered with the aim of achieving the best response, such as FCR; b) 'Slow go' patients, who should be treated with modified therapies in order to control the disease; c) Unfit or 'No go' patients, who should receive palliative care.

## 2.13 Other prognostic factors

### 2.13.1 Bcl2 and other immunophenotypic markers

Patients who are CD71+ and Bcl2+ have a shorter PFS and OS than those who are CD71- and Bcl2. In a recent paper, the independent prognostic value of bcl-2 was confirmed within ZAP-70 negative patients (Del Poeta et al, 2010). Other immunophenotypic markers, such as soluble CD20, have been investigated as potential prognostic factors in CLL.

### 2.13.2 CD26; CD44

CD26 antigen is strongly upregulated in activated B cells. CD26-positive patients show a shorter time to treatment and this positivity is correlated with ZAP-70 expression or IGVH mutational status (Cro et al, 2009). On the other hand, high levels of soluble CD44 predict the risk of illness progression in patients with early-stage CLL.

### 2.13.3 Circulating endothelial cells (CECs)

In patients with CLL, as occurs in other malignancies, CECs are increased and are correlated with an aggressive clinical outcome. In a recent report, the gene expression profile in patients with higher levels of CECs indicated increased cell survival and proliferation, diminished cell adhesion to the extracellular matrix, and enhanced proangiogenic function. CECs might be considered a biological marker for new targeted antiangiogenic therapies (Rigolin et al, 2010).

### 2.13.4 CLLU1 expression

High CLLU1 expression levels are associated with shorter OS in patients younger than 70 years of age. CLLU1 expression analysis adds prognostic information in risk prediction in CLL patients with the exception of those who have an unmutated IGVH status (Josefsson et al, 2007).

### 2.13.5 Interleukin (IL) 6, IL-8 and IL-10

IL-6 is a strong predictor of shorter survival in CLL patients with advanced disease. Furthermore, high levels of IL-8 are associated with shorter OS (Wierda et al, 2003). Finally, IL-10 levels are elevated in patients with CLL and are correlated with adverse clinical and biological characteristics of the disease and with shorter survival. The role of several IL inhibitors in the treatment of patients with CLL is currently being explored (Fayad et al, 2001) .

### 2.13.6 Matrix metalloproteinase-9 (MMP9)

MMP9 is involved in migration and tissue invasion in patients with CLL. The combined macromolecular cell surface complex formed by CD38, CD49d, CD44 and MMP9 is associated with a dismal prognosis, and, recently, it has been suggested as a novel therapeutic target (Buggins et al, 2011).

### 2.13.7 PEG10 expression

The overexpression of the paternally expressed gene 10 (PEG10) is observed in high-risk CLL patients, defined by high levels of LPL mRNA expression. Recently, PEG10 has been proposed as a new marker in CLL by Austrian and German researchers (Kainz et al, 2007).

### 2.13.8 Telomerase activity and telomere length

Several reports have illustrated the role of telomerase activity and telomere length in cancer prognosis. In CLL, short telomeres and high telomerase activity are associated with poor prognosis (Sellmann et al, 2011). Telomerase inhibitors are being investigated as novel targeted therapies in CLL.

### 2.13.9 TOSO/FCMR expression

Recently, the overexpression of the new gene TOSO (or FC mu receptor [FCMR, FAIM3/TOSO]) has been shown to be associated with the Binet clinical stage, IGVH mutation status, age and time to treatment in CLL. Furthermore, a high level of expression of TOSO is an independent predictor of shorter SLT in CLL (Hancer et al, 2011). However, no correlation has been found between the expression of TOSO and ZAP-70 or CD38. On the other hand, overexpression of FCMR seems to promote chromosomal abnormalities.

### 2.13.10 Tumor necrosis factor (TNF) alpha

MD Anderson Clinical Cancer investigators reported several years ago a correlation between elevated TNF-alpha levels and advanced clinical stage patients, high B2M levels and lower hemoglobin and platelet counts (Ferrajoli et al, 2002).

### 2.13.11 Rel A DNA binding

Researchers from Cardiff University recently demonstrated the importance of the NF-kappa B subunit Rel A in CLL (Hewamana et al, 2009). Rel A DNA binding appears to be strongly associated with advanced Binet stage, time to first therapy and survival. In addition, it seems to have the unique capacity to predict the duration of response to therapy.

## 3. Conclusions

A wide variety of prognostic factors have been studied in CLL, but clinical staging according to Binet or Rai systems, LTD and B2M are the main clinical and biological prognostic markers. Cytogenetics, using FISH (especially using the del (17p) probe), and expression of CD38 and ZAP-70 as surrogate markers for the IgVH mutational status are used routinely worldwide, although CD38 and ZAP-70 are not mandatory in clinical practice. New markers such as LPL, miR29c and TCL7 predict OS in CLL. On the other hand, the evaluation of patient physical fitness and the assessment of the response to therapy are critical elements.

Recently, sequencing the CLL genome and advances in computing and robotics have produced a revolution in general genetics and CLL (Puente et al, 2011). The combination of these methodologies has led to the development of microarray technology, enabling thousands of genes to be analyzed simultaneously. In CLL patients, the gene expression profile indicates that significantly differentiated genes are located in regions with chromosomal aberrations. However, the evidence linking specific genetic alterations using FISH or mutational status to the results of arrays is still not very consistent.

## 4. References

Binet, JL.; Auquier, A.; Dighiero, G., et al. (1981). A new prognostic classification of chronic lymphocytic leukemia derived from a multivariate survival analysis. *Cancer*, Vol.48, No.4, pp. 198-206, ISSN 0008-543X.

Buggins, AG.; Levi, A.; Gohil, S., et al. (2011). Evidence for a macromolecular complex in poor prognosis CLL that contains CD38, CD49d, CD44 and MMP-9. *Br J Haematol*, Vol.154, No.2, pp. 216-222, ISSN 1365-2141.

Calin, GA.; Ferracin, M.; Cimmino, A., et al. (2005). A microRNA signature associated with prognosis and progression in chronic lymphocytic leukemia. *N Engl J Med*, Vol.353, No.17, pp. 1793-1801. ISSN 1533-4406.

Catovsky, D.; Fooks, J. & Richards, S. (1989). Prognostic factors in chronic lymphocytic leukaemia: the importance of age, sex and response to treatment in survival. A report from the MRC CLL 1 trial. MRC Working Party on Leukaemia in Adults. *Br J Haematol*, Vol.72, No.2, pp. 141-149. ISSN 0007-1048.

Cavazzini, F.; Hernández, JA.; Gozzetti, A., et al. (2008). Chromosome 14q32 translocations involving the immunoglobulin heavy chain locus in chronic lymphocytic leukemia identify a disease subset with poor prognosis. *Br J Haematol*, Vol.142, No.4, pp. 529-537. ISSN 1365-2141.

Chiorazzi, N.; Rai, KR. & Ferrarini, M. (2005). Chronic lymphocytic leukemia. *N Engl J Med*, Vol.352, No.8, pp. 804-815. ISSN 1533-4406.

Codony, C.; Crespo, M.; Abrisqueta, P., et al. (2009). Gene expression profiling in chronic lymphocytic leukaemia. *Best Pract Res Clin Haematol*, Vol.22, No.2, pp. 211-22.ISSN 1532-1924.

Cramer, P. & Hallek, M. (2011). Prognostic factors in chronic lymphocytic leukemia-what do we need to know?. *Nat Rev Clin Oncol*, Vol.8, No.1, pp. 38-47. ISSN 1759-4782.

Crespo, M.; Bosch, F.; Villamor, N., et al. (2003). ZAP-70 expression as a surrogate for immunoglobulin-variable-region mutations in chronic lymphocytic leukemia. *N Engl J Med*, Vol.348, No.18, pp. 1764-1775. ISSN 1533-4406.

Cro, L.; Morabito, F.; Zucal, N., et al. (2009). CD26 expression in mature B-cell neoplasia: its possible role as a new prognostic marker in B-CLL. *Hematol Oncol*, Vol.27, No.3, pp. 140-7. ISSN 1099-1069.

Dal Bo, M.; Rossi, FM.; Rossi, D., et al. (2011a). 13q14 deletion size and number of deleted cells both influence prognosis in chronic lymphocytic leukemia. *Genes, Chromosomes Cancer*, Vol.50, No.8, pp. 633-643. ISSN 1098-2264.

Dal-Bo, M; Del Giudice, I; Bomben, R., et al. (2011b). B-cell receptor, clinical course and prognosis in chronic lymphocytic leukaemia: the growing saga of the IGHV3 subgroup gene usage. *Br J Haematol*, Vol.153, No.1, pp. 3-14. ISSN 1365-2141.

Damle, RN.; Wasil, T.; Fais, F., et al. (1999). Ig V gene mutation status and CD38 expression as novel prognostic indicators in chronic lymphocytic leukemia. *Blood*, Vol.94, No.6, pp. 1840-1847. ISSN 0006-4971.

Del Poeta, G.; Del Principe, MI.; Maurillo, L., et al. (2010). Spontaneous apoptosis and proliferation detected by BCL-2 and CD71 proteins are important progression indicators within ZAP-70 negative chronic lymphocytic leukemia. *Leuk Lymphoma*, Vol.51, No.1, pp. 95-106. ISSN 1029-2403.

Dighiero, G. & Hamblin, TJ. (2008). Chronic lymphocytic leukaemia. *Lancet*, Vol.371, No.9617, pp. 1017-1029. ISSN 1474-547X.

Dohner, H.; Stilgenbauer, S.; Benner, A., et al. (2000). Genomic aberrations and survival in chronic lymphocytic leukemia. *N Engl J Med*, Vol.343, No.26, pp. 1910-1916. ISSN 0028-4793.

Fayad, L; Keating, MJ.; Reuben, JM., et al. (2001). Interleukin-6 and interleukin-10 levels in chronic lymphocytic leukemia: correlation with phenotypic characteristics and outcome. *Blood*, Vol.97, No.1, pp. 256-263. ISSN 0006-4971.

Ferrajoli, A; Keating, MJ; Manshouri, T., et al. (2002). The clinical significance of tumor necrosis factor-alpha plasma level in patients having chronic lymphocytic leukemia. *Blood*, Vol.100, No.4, pp. 1215-1219. ISSN 0006-4971.

Ferrajoli, A.; Manshouri, T.; Estrov, Z., et al. (2001). High levels of vascular endothelial growth factor receptor-2 correlate with shortened survival in chronic lymphocytic leukemia. *Clin Cancer Res*, Vol.7, No.4, pp. 795-799. ISSN 1078-0432.

Gattei, V.; Bulian, P.; Del Principe, MI., et al. (2008). Relevance of CD49d protein expression as overall survival and progressive disease prognosticator in chronic lymphocytic leukemia. *Blood*, Vol.111, No.2, pp. 865-873. ISSN 0006-4971.

Geisler, CH.; Hou-Jensen, K.; Jensen, OM., et al. (1996). The bone-marrow infiltration pattern in B-cell chronic lymphocytic leukemia is not an important prognostic factor. Danish CLL Study Group. *Eur J Haematol*, Vol.57, No. 4, pp. 292-300. ISSN: 0902-4441.

Ghia, P.; Guida, G.; Stella, S., et al. (2003). The pattern of CD38 expression defines a distinct subset of chronic lymphocytic leukemia (CLL) patients at risk of disease progression. *Blood*, Vol.101, No.4, pp. 1262-1269. ISSN 0006-4971.

Ghia, P.; Stamatopoulos, K.; Belessi, C., et al. (2005). Geographic patterns and pathogenetic implications of IGHV gene usage in chronic lymphocytic leukemia: the lesson of the IGHV3-21 gene. *Blood*, Vol.105, No. 4, pp. 1678-1685. ISSN 0006-4971.

Gonzalez, D,; Martínez, P., Wade, R., et al. (2011). Mutational status of the TP53 gene as a predictor of response and survival in patients with chronic lymphocytic leukemia: results from the LRF CLL4 trial. *J Clin Oncol*, Vol.29, No.16, pp. 2223-2229. ISSN 1527-7755.

Haferlach, T.; Kohlmann, A.; Schnittger, S., et al. (2005) Global approach to the diagnosis of leukemia using gene expression profiling. *Blood*, Vol.106, No.4, pp. 1189-1198. ISSN 0006-4971.

Hallek, M.; Wanders, L.; Ostwald, M., et al. (1996). Serum beta(2)-microglobulin and serum thymidine kinase are independent predictors of progression-free survival in chronic lymphocytic leukemia and immunocytoma. *Leuk Lymphoma*, Vol.22, No.5-6, pp. 439-447. ISSN 1042-8194.

Hamblin, TJ.; Davis, Z.; Gardiner, A., et al. (1999). Unmutated Ig V(H) genes are associated with a more aggressive form of chronic lymphocytic leukemia. *Blood*, Vol.94, No.6, pp. 1848-1854. ISSN 0006-4971.

Hamblin, TJ.; Orchard, JA.; Ibbotson, RE, et al. (2002). CD38 expression and immunoglobulin variable region mutations are independent prognostic variables in chronic lymphocytic leukemia, but CD38 expression may vary during the course of the disease. *Blood*, Vol. 99, No.3, pp. 1023-1029. ISSN 0006-4971.

Hancer, VS.; Diz-Kucukkaya, R. & Aktan M. (2011). Overexpression of Fc mu receptor (FCMR, TOSO) gene in chronic lymphocytic leukemia patients. *Med Oncol*. 2011 Jan 25. [Epub ahead of print]. ISSN 1559-131X.

Haslinger, C.; Schweifer, N.; Stilgenbauer, S., et al. (2004). Microarray gene expression profiling of B-cell chronic lymphocytic leukemia subgroups defined by genomic aberrations and VH mutation status. *J Clin Oncol*, Vol.22, No.19, pp. 3937-3949. ISSN 0732-183X.

Hernández, JA.; González, M. & Hernández, JM. (2010). Chronic lymphoid leukemia. *Med Clin (Barc)*, Vol.135, No.4, pp. 172-178. ISSN 0025-7753.

Hernández, JA.; Rodríguez, AE.; González, M., et al. (2009). A high number of losses in 13q14 chromosome is associated with a worse outcome and biological differences in patients with B chronic lymphoid leukemia. *Haematologica*, Vol.94, No.3, pp. 364-371. ISSN 1592-8721.

Hernandez, JM.; Mecucci, C.; Criel, A., et al. (1995). Cytogenetic analysis of B cell chronic lymphoid leukemias classified according to morphologic and immunophenotypic (FAB) criteria. *Leukemia*, Vol.9, No.12, pp. 2140-2146. ISSN 0887-6924.

Hewamana, S.; Lin, TT.; Rowntree, C., et al. (2009). Rel a is an independent biomarker of clinical outcome in chronic lymphocytic leukemia. *J Clin Oncol*, Vol.27, No.5, pp. 763-769. ISSN 1527-7755.

Josefsson, P.; Geisler, CH.; Leffers, H., et al. (2007). CLLU1 expression analysis adds prognostic information to risk prediction in chronic lymphocytic leukemia. *Blood*, Vol.109, No.11, pp. 4973-4979. ISSN 0006-4971.

Kainz, B.; Shehata, M.; Bilban, M., et al. (2007). Overexpression of the paternally expressed gene 10 (PEG10) from the imprinted locus on chromosome 7q21 in high-risk B-cell chronic lymphocytic leukemia. *Int J Cancer*, Vol.121, No.9, pp. 1984-1993. ISSN 0020-7136.

Klein, U.; Tu, Y.; Stolovitzky, GA., et al. (2001). Gene expression profiling of B cell chronic lymphocytic leukemia reveals a homogeneous phenotype related to memory B cells. *J Exp Med*, Vol.194, No.11, pp. 1625-1638. ISSN 0022-1007.

Krober, A.; Bloehdorn, J.; Hafner, S., et al. (2006). Additional genetic high-risk features such as 11q deletion, 17p deletion, and V3-21 usage characterize discordance of ZAP-70 and VH mutation status in chronic lymphocytic leukemia. *J Clin Oncol*, Vol.24, No.6, pp. 969-975. ISSN 1527-7755.

Lai, R.; O'Brien, S.; Maushouri, T., et al. (2002). Prognostic value of plasma interleukin-6 levels in patients with chronic lymphocytic leukemia. *Cancer*, Vol.95, No.5, pp. 1071-1075. ISSN 0008-543X.

Letestu, R.; Rawstron, A.; Ghia, P.; et al. (2006). Evaluation of ZAP-70 expression by flow cytometry in chronic lymphocytic leukemia: A multicentric international harmonization process. *Cytometry B Clin Cytom*, Vol.70, No.4, pp. 309-314. ISSN 1552-4949.

Molica, S.; Vitelli, G.; Levato, D., et al. (2003). Increased serum levels of matrix metalloproteinase-9 predict clinical outcome of patients with early B-cell chronic lymphocytic leukaemia. *Eur J Haematol*, Vol.70, No.6, pp. 373-378. ISSN 0902-4441.

Montserrat, E. New prognostic markers in CLL. (2006). *Hematology Am Soc Hematol Educ Program*, pp. 279-284. ISSN 1520-4391.

Montserrat, E. & Rozman, C. (1987). Bone marrow biopsy in chronic lymphocytic leukemia: a review of its prognostic importance. *Blood Cells*, Vol.12, No.2, pp. 315-326. ISSN 0340-4684.

Moreno, C. & Montserrat, E. (2008). New prognostic markers in chronic lymphocytic leukemia. *Blood Rev*, Vol.22, No.4, pp. 211-219. ISSN 0268-960X.

Muntañola, A.; Bosch, F.; Arguis, P., et al. (2007). Abdominal computed tomography predicts progression in patients with Rai stage 0 chronic lymphocytic leukemia. *J Clin Oncol*, Vol.25, No.12, pp. 1576-1580. ISSN 1527-7755.

Nowakowski, GS.; Hoyer, JD.; Shanafelt, TD., et al. (2007). Using smudge cells on routine blood smears to predict clinical outcome in chronic lymphocytic leukemia: a universally available prognostic test. *Mayo Clin Proc*, Vol.82, No.4, pp. 449-453. ISSN 0025-6196.

Oppezzo, P.; Vasconcelos, Y.; Settegrana, C., et al. (2005). The LPL/ADAM29 expression ratio is a novel prognosis indicator in chronic lymphocytic leukemia. *Blood*, Vol.106, No.2, pp. 650-7. ISSN 0006-4971.

Orfao, A.; Gonzalez, M.; San Miguel, JF., et al. (1989). B-cell chronic lymphocytic leukaemia: prognostic value of the immunophenotype and the clinico-haematological features. *Am J Hematol*, Vol.31, No.1, pp. 26-31. ISSN 0361-8609.

Prieto-Sanchez, RM.; Hernandez, JA.; Garcia, JL., et al. (2006). Overexpression of the *VAV* proto-oncogene product is associated with b-cell chronic lymphocytic leukaemia displaying loss on 13q. *Br J Haematol*, Vol.133, No.6, pp. 642-645. ISSN 0007-1048.

Puente, XS.; Pinyol, M.; Quesada, V., et al. (2011). Whole-genome sequencing identifies recurrent mutations in chronic lymphocytic leukemia. *Nature*, Vol.475, No.7354, pp. 101-105. ISSN 1476-4687.

Rai, KR.; Sawitsky, A.; Cronkite, EP., et al. (1975). Clinical staging of chronic lymphocytic leukemia. *Blood*, Vol.46, No.2, pp. 219-234. ISSN 0006-4971.

Rassenti, LZ.; Huynh, L.; Toy, TL., et al. (2004). ZAP-70 compared with immunoglobulin heavy-chain gene mutation status as a predictor of disease progression in chronic lymphocytic leukemia. *N Engl J Med*, Vol.351, No.9, pp. 893-901. ISSN 1533-4406.

Rigolin, GM.; Maffei, R.; Rizzotto, L., et al. (2010). Circulating endothelial cells in patients with chronic lymphocytic leukemia:clinical-prognostic and biologic significance. *Cancer*, Vol.116, No.8, pp. 1926-1937. ISSN 0008-543X.

Rosenwald, A.; Alizadeh, AA.; Widhopf, G., et al. (2001). Relation of gene expression phenotype to immunoglobulin mutation genotype in B cell chronic lymphocytic leukemia. *J Exp Med*, Vol.194: No.11, pp. 1639-1647. ISSN 0022-1007.

Sarfati, M.; Chevret, S.; Chastang, C., et al. (1996). Prognostic importance of serum soluble CD23 level in chronic lymphocytic leukemia. *Blood*, Vol.88, No.11, pp. 4259-4264. ISSN 0006-4971.

Schroeder, HW. Jr. & Dighiero, G. (1994). The pathogenesis of chronic lymphocytic leukemia: analysis of the antibody repertoire. *Immunol Today*, Vol.15, No.6, pp. 288-294. ISSN 0167-5699.

Sellmann, L.; de Beer, D.; Bartels, M., et al. (2011). Telomeres and prognosis in patients with chronic lymphocytic leukaemia. *Int J Hematol*, Vol.93, No.1, pp. 74-82. ISSN 1865-3774.

Stilgenbauer, S.; Sander, S.; Bullinger, L., et al. (2007). Clonal evolution in chronic lymphocytic leukemia: acquisition of high-risk genomic aberrations associated with unmutated VH, resistance to therapy, and short survival. *Haematologica*, Vol.92, No.9, pp. 1242-1245. ISSN 1592-8721.

Viñolas, N.; Reverter, JC.; Urbano-Ispizua, A., et al. (1987). Lymphocyte doubling time in chronic lymphocytic leukemia: an update of its prognostic significance. *Blood Cells*, Vol.12, No.2, pp. 457-470. ISSN 0340-4684.

Ward, BP.; Tsongalis, GJ. & Kaur,P. (2011). MicroRNAs in chronic lymphocytic leukemia. *Exp Mol Pathol*, Vol. 9, No.2, pp. 173-178. ISSN 1096-0945.

Wierda, WG.; Johnson, MM.; Do, KA., et al. (2003). Plasma interleukin 8 level predicts for survival in chronic lymphocytic leukaemia. *Br J Haematol*, Vol.120, No.3, pp. 452-456. ISSN 0007-1048.

Wierda, WG.; O'Brien, S.; Wang, X., et al. (2007). Prognostic nomogram and index for overall survival in previously untreated patients with chronic lymphocytic leukemia. *Blood*, Vol.109, No.11, pp. 4679-4685. ISSN 0006-4971.

Yi, S.; Yu, Z.; Zhou, K., et al. (2011). TOSO is overexpressed and correlated with disease progression in Chinese patients with chronic lymphocytic leukemia. *Leuk Lymphoma*, Vol.52, No.1, pp. 72-78. ISSN 1029-2403.

Zenz, T.; Fröling, S.; Mertens, D., et al. (2010). Moving from prognostic to predictive factors in chronic lymphocytic leukaemia (CLL). *Best Pract Res Clin Haematol*, Vol.23, No.1, pp. 71-84.ISSN 1532-1924.

# Part 2

# CLL Therapy

# 3

# Immune Response and Immunotherapy in Chronic Lymphocytic Leukemia

Leticia Huergo-Zapico[1], Ana P. Gonzalez-Rodríguez[2], Juan Contesti[3],
Azahara Fernández-Guizán[1], Andrea Acebes Huerta[1],
Alejandro López-Soto[1] and Segundo Gonzalez[1]

[1]Functional Biology Department, Instituto Universitario Oncologico del Principado de
Asturias (IUOPA), University of Oviedo, Oviedo,
[2]Hematology Department, Hospital Universitario Central de Asturias, Oviedo
[3]Hematology Department, Hospital Cabueñe, Gijón,
Spain

## 1. Introduction

The contribution of the immune system to the pathogenesis of chronic lymphocytic leukemia (CLL) is receiving increasing attention in recent years. This interest has been supported by population studies, which have shown the increase of cancer risk in immunodeficient individuals (Grulich et al., 2007; Smyth et al., 2006; Swann et al., 2007), and experimental studies, which have shown that deficiencies in key immunological molecules and cells increase the susceptibility to develop several types of solid tumors and hematological malignancies (Smyth et al., 2006; Swann et al., 2007). Additionally, the interest in the study of tumor immunology has been boosted by the increasing use of immunotherapy in the treatment of cancer, particularly in CLL. In this chapter, we review the role of the immune system in the elimination of CLL, the mechanisms that leukemia cells use to evade the immune response, and finally, we analyze the basis of the use of immunotherapy in the treatment of CLL patients.

## 2. Immune surveillance of cancer

The immune system is able to prevent cancer development by eliminating cancer cells prior to tumors becoming clinically detectable or by attenuating tumor growth and progression (Smyth et al., 2006; Swann et al., 2009). Both T cells and Natural Killer (NK) cells play a critical role in cancer immune surveillance (**Figure 1**). T cells are able to recognize tumor antigens, which differentiate cancer cells from their nontransformed counterparts. Several tumor antigens have been described such as mutation of oncogenic proteins (e.g. p53), over-expressed cellular antigens (such as HER-2), viral antigens, differentiation antigens and aberrantly expressed antigens (Smyth et al., 2006; Swann et al., 2007). Cytotoxic CD8 T cells and helper CD4 T cells may recognize transformed cells bearing these tumor antigens presented as peptides by MHC class I and class II molecules, respectively.

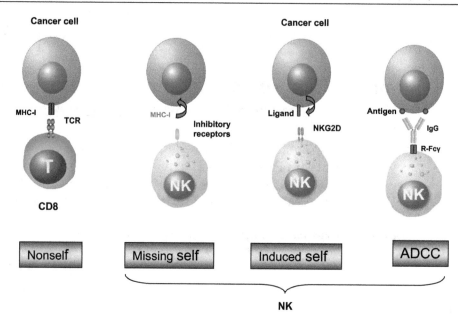

**NK**

Fig. 1. Mechanisms of cancer immune surveillance. T Cell Receptor (TCR) expressed by CD8 T cells is able to recognize tumor antigens presented as peptides by the Major Histocompatibility Complex class I proteins (MHC-I) (nonself recognition). NK cells use several mechanisms to recognize tumor cells. NK cells use inhibitory receptors to differentiate "*self*" from "*missing self*". The impairment of MHC class I expression observed in some tumor cells impairs the recognition by CD8 T cells. Nevertheless, MHC class I molecules have an inhibitory effect on the activation of NK cells. Consequently, the lack of expression of MHC class I molecules (*missing self*) promotes the activation of NK cells and the lysis of the target cell. NK cells also express activating receptors, such as NKG2D, which is able to recognize several ligands induced in transformed cells (*induced self*). NK cells also express the FcγRIII receptor (also named CD16), which is able to recognize tumor cells that have been bound by specific IgG antibodies. This mechanism of recognition is termed Antibody-Dependent Cell-Mediated Cytotoxicity (ADCC).

NK cells do not directly recognize tumor antigens, but instead, they recognize changes in cells caused by transformation. Several mechanisms of cancer recognition by NK cells have been described (Gonzalez et al., 2011). NK cells use a set of inhibitory receptors, such as killer cell immunoglobulin-like receptors (KIRs), to differentiate and eliminate cancer cells that lack MHC class I expression ("missing self" recognition) (Figure 1) (Gonzalez et al., 2011). NK cells also express activating receptors which recognize stress-induced molecules expressed on tumor cells ("induced self" recognition). The activating receptor NKG2D plays a pivotal role in the immune response against cancer. This receptor is expressed by NK cells, γδT cells and CD8 T cells, and recognizes several tumor-associated ligands named MICA, MICB and ULBP1-5 molecules. NKG2D ligands are restrictedly expressed in healthy cells, but they are induced in stressed and transformed cells, allowing the elimination of these cells by the immune system (Das *et al.*, 2001; Raulet et al., 2003; Bauer et al., 1999; Lopez-Larrea et al., 2008; Bahram et al., 1994 ; Cosman et al., 2001; González et al., 2008; Guerra et al., 2008). NK cells may also lyse target cells that have been bound by specific IgG antibodies. They are able to recognize the Fc region of the antibody through FcγRIII receptor (also named CD16). This mechanism of recognition is termed Antibody-Dependent Cell-Mediated Cytotoxicity (ADCC) and it is an important mechanism of action against tumors of therapeutic monoclonal antibodies, such as rituximab and alemtuzumab (Figure 1). These mechanisms of anti-tumor immune response may protect the host in the early stages of tumor initiation; however during cancer progression, tumors develop a plethora of mechanisms of immune evasion. Consequently, the anti-tumor response is ineffective in advanced tumors (Smyth *et al., 2006;* Swann *et al., 2007*).

## 3. Immune surveillance of chronic lymphocytic leukemia

There is little information related to the role of the immune response in the early stages of CLL progression. Nevertheless, it has widely been reported that the amounts of CD8 and CD4 T cells and NK cells are significantly elevated at diagnosis of the disease. The expansion of cytotoxic CD8 T cells is higher than CD4 T cells, and many CLL patients showed an inversion of CD4/CD8 ratio (Gonzalez-Rodriguez et al., 2010). Similar expansions of immune cells have been observed in other hematological malignancies and this increase of immune cells has been associated with a better prognosis of patients. Thus, higher absolute lymphocyte count predicts higher survival in lymphoma, acute myeloblastic leukemia and myeloma (Cox et al., 2008; Siddiqui et al., 2006; Porrata et al., 2007, 2009; Ray-Coquard et al., 2009; De Angulo et al., 2008; Behl et al. 2006, 2007; Ege et al., 2008). NK cell count has also been associated with clinical outcome in patients with diffuse large B-cell lymphoma (Plonquet et al., 2007). The expansion of immune cells observed in CLL and in other hematological malignancies may be compared to the expansion of tumor infiltrating lymphocytes in epithelial tumors. In several types of cancer, the presence of tumor infiltrating lymphocytes, mainly NK and CD8 T cells, has also been associated with the anti-tumor response and was found to be a better predictor of patient survival than traditional histopathological methods used to stage tumors (Dunn et al., 2004; Clemente et al., 1996; Scanlan et al., 2004; Rollins et al., 2006; Moore OS et al., 1949; Clark et al., 1969; Pagès et al., 2005)

In agreement with an anti-tumor role of the immune system, the expansion of NK and T cells has been associated with the time to treatment in CLL (Palmer et al., 2008). Furthermore, the relative numbers of CD8 and CD4 T cells at diagnosis are independent predictors for survival, and higher CD8 count is associated with significantly higher median time of survival of CLL patients (Gonzalez-Rodriguez et al., 2010). This suggests that the expansion of immune cells observed at diagnosis of CLL patients may be due, at least in part, to the expansion of anti-tumor immune cells. However, the analysis of the functionality of these cells is still lacking. Early studies showed that the expanded CD8 T cells have an activated phenotype and cytotoxic function and appear to have restricted clonality, which were originally interpreted as evidence of an autologous T cell response against leukemia cells. Furthermore, a subset of γδT cells with anti-tumor activity is one type of the immune cells expanded in CLL patients (Poggi et al., 2004). These T cells express the activating receptor NKG2D, which is able to mediate the lysis of CLL cells expressing NKG2D ligands (*"induced self" recognition*) (**Figure 1**). Leukemia cells from most patients lack NKG2D ligands expression and are highly resistant to NK cell-mediated lysis, but NKG2D ligands expression may be induced in leukemia cells by treatment with trans-retinoic acid or histone deacetilases (HDACs) inhibitors, rendering leukemia cells susceptible to lysis by immune cells (Kato et al., 2007; Del Giudice et al., 2009). The expansion of γδT cells has been associated with a better prognosis of CLL patients, supporting the hypothesis that the increase of T cells observed at diagnosis of CLL patients may be due, at least in part, to the expansion of anti-tumor T cells.

The activation of the immune system in CLL patients has not only been associated with improved prognosis, but also with tumor regression. The natural history of stage A disease is generally indolent or only slowly progressive. However, it is less known that CLL may undergo spontaneous regression (Del Giudice et al., 2009). There are no data about the functional role of the immune system in these remissions; however the activation of immune system has been associated with spontaneous remissions in other types of cancers (Smyth et al., 2006; Swann et al., 2007). This suggests that the activation of the anti-tumor immune response may have a significant impact on the progression of CLL, however further analyses about the functionality of immune cells in CLL are clearly warranted.

The role of immune system in CLL is further highlighted by the analysis of cancer risk in immunodeficient individuals. However, the deficiency of CD8 T cells is not compatible with life and most of the studies about the role of other immune deficiencies on cancer susceptibility are nonpopulation-based and of small sample size, making difficult to draw definite conclusions. Nevertheless, primary immune deficiency patients have been associated with a marked increased risk of cancer. Some types of cancers appear to be associated with specific forms of immunodeficiency including stomach cancer with common variable immune deficiency (CVID) (Kinlen et al., 1985; Mellemkjaer et al., 2002), leukemia with ataxia-telangiectasia (Morrell et al., 1986), and nonmelanocytic skin cancer with cartilage-hair hypoplasia (Taskinen et al., 2008). In a recent population-based study, the association of antibody deficiency with an increasing risk of leukemia, non-Hodgkin lymphoma and gastric cancer has been described (Vajdic et al., 2010). In agreement with clinical data, deficiencies in T cells and NK cells have also been associated with increased susceptibility of cancer in a diversity of experimental models of cancer (Smyth et al., 2006; Swann et al., 2007).

Nevertheless, the most compelling evidence about the potential role of the immune system in the pathogenesis of CLL is the increasing use of immunotherapy in the treatment of this disease. This highlights the capacity of the activation of the immune system to eliminate CLL cells and the potential role of immune system to cure this disease. Thus, the therapeutic effect of allogeneic hematopoietic stem cell transplantation in CLL relies on the ability of the immune cells of the graft to recognize and eliminate leukemia cells (Mehta et al., 1996; Ritgen et al., 2008). Similarly, the therapeutic use of immunomodulatory drugs, such as lenalidomide, is not directly based on a cytotoxic effect on CLL cells, but instead, lenalidomide exerts its therapeutic effect through the stimulation of the immune system.

## 4. Immune defects in chronic lymphocytic leukemia patients

In spite of the existence of compelling evidences about the ability of the immune system to eliminate nascent tumors, when the immune system is unable to eliminate all cancer cells, it sculpts or edits the phenotype of cancer cells, eliminating the most immunogenic ones and selecting the less immunogenic tumor cells, which are able to evade or suppress the immune response. The consequence of this process, named cancer immunoediting, is the development of numerous mechanisms of immune evasion and immune suppression in advanced tumors (Smyth et al., 2006; Swann et al., 2007). Accordingly, there is a progressive acquisition of a wide variety of immune defects in the course of the progression of CLL. As a result, patients progressively acquire a immunodeficiency status, which increases the incidence of opportunistic infections and the development of secondary neoplasias (Hamblin et al., 2008). The corollary of immune defects also includes the development of several autoimmune reactions. CLL patients have a 5-10% risk of development of an autoimmune complication, which primarily cause cytopaenia (Zent et al., 2010). The most common autoimmune disease affecting CLL patients is hemolytic anemia, with a lower frequency of immune thrombocytopenia and pure red blood cell aplasia and only rarely, autoimmune granulocytopaenia.

Practically all components of the immune system are impaired in CLL patients. The most obvious and well-known immune defect is hypogammaglobulinemia, which is present in up to 85% of patients (Hamblin *et al.*, 1987). Hypogammaglobulinemia is observed in other lymphoid malignancies, but the impairment of the humoral immune response is far greater in CLL. The clinical consequence of hypogammaglobulinemia is the increase of susceptibility of CLL patients to infection with extracellular bacterias, commonly affecting respiratory tract, skin and urinary tract, and the reactivation of some latent virus infections, mainly belonging to *Herpesviridae* family.

The defects in the humoral immunity are accompanied by several abnormalities in the cellular immune response, including quantitative and qualitative alterations of NK cells, CD4 and CD8 T cells, dendritic cells, neutrophils, monocytes and cytokines. The activity of NK cells against leukemia cells is frequently reduced and lymphoid neoplasms are quite resistant to NK cell-mediated cytotoxicity (Foa et al., 1984; Jewell et al., 1992; Kato et al., 2007). All effector mechanisms of NK cells analyzed are impaired in some degree in advanced CLL patients (Katrinakis et al., 1996; Caligaris-Cappio et al., 1999; Wierda et al., 1999). A partial down-regulation of MHC class I molecules, which allow leukemic cells to escape from cytotoxic T cell attack, has been reported (Demanet et al., 2004). However, the "missing self" recognition by NK cells (**Figure 1**) is limited in CLL by the aberrant expression of HLA-G in leukemia cells. HLA-G is a non classical MHC class I molecule that is physiologically expressed on fetal derived placental cells. Classical MHC class I molecules (HLA-A, -B and -C) are not expressed in fetal placental cells, but HLA-G inhibits NK cells activation against placental cells by interacting with several inhibitory receptors expressed by NK cells and cytotoxic T lymphocytes. Likewise, the aberrant expression of HLA-G on leukemia cells impairs the anti-leukemia immune response mediated by these cells. Accordingly, the expression of HLA-G on leukemia cells correlated with progression free survival and the level of immunosuppression of CLL patients (Nückel et al., 2005; Erikci et al., 2009).

There are also defects on the expression of NKG2D and its ligands in CLL (Gasser et al., 2005; Groh et al., 1996, 1999; Diefenbach et al., 2001; Cerwenka et al., 2001; González et al., 2006). The expression of NKG2D ligands in leukemia cells is low or absent in most of patients, which confers them with a high resistance to lysis by immune cells (Poggi et al., 2004). Furthermore, leukemia cells may also counter the anti-tumor activity of NKG2D by shedding some of its soluble ligands. Serum levels of soluble MICA, MICB and ULBP2 are significantly increased in

CLL patients and are associated with a poor treatment-free survival (Nückel et al., 2010). The shedding of soluble MICA has been described in many types of cancer and elevated levels of soluble MICA correlated with advanced stage tumors, metastasis and poor prognosis (Salih et al. 2002, 2003; Raffaghello et al., 2004; Rebmann et al., 2007), because soluble MICA impairs the recognition of cancer cells by immune cells and suppress the immune response (Groh et al., 2002, 2006). Of relevance, some of the immune defects observed in CLL patients may be reversible. For instance, leukemia cells which express low levels of NKG2D ligands may be rendered susceptible to immune cells when are treated with trans-retinoic acid or histone deacetylase inhibitors inhibitors, which restored the expression of NKG2D ligands on leukemia cells (**Salih et** al., 2002). This clearly suggests that therapeutic approaches that can bypass the immune evasion mechanisms of CLL patients may have therapeutic application in this disease.

T cell function is also impaired in CLL. There are defects on antigen presentation (Cantwell et al., 1997), T cell activation, in differentiation and function of CD4 T cells and defects in the cytotoxic activity of CD8 cells that are caused by direct contact with leukemia cells (Gorgun et al., 2005; Rossi et al., 1996; Junevik et al., 2007; Mackus et al., 2003). Regulatory T cells, a specialized subpopulation of T cells which suppresses the activation of the immune system and thereby maintains tolerance to self antigens, are increased in number in CLL and this increase is more significantly in most advanced patients (Beyer *et al.*, 2006). It is not yet clear whether inhibitory T cells may promote the tolerance of leukemia cells by the immune system and may contribute to the immune deficiency. Nevertheless, it is noticeable that this population is exquisitely sensitive to treatment with fludarabine. It has been proposed that the elimination of these inhibitory T cells might be one of the mechanisms that favors the development of autoimmune hemolytic anemia after treatment of CLL patients with fludarabine (Hamblin *et al.*, 2006).

The defects of cellular immunity observed in CLL increase the susceptibility of patients to virus infections, opportunistic infections and second malignancies, and may contribute to impair the anti-leukemia immune response. Additionally, the use of chemotherapy agents may complicate the clinical course of CLL since may exacerbate the pre-existing immunodeficiency. Nevertheless, the development of drugs and therapeutic strategies that can either bypass immune evasion mechanisms or rescue immune suppressor pathways may significantly benefit CLL patients. Thus, the increasing understanding of the molecular and cellular events underlying the immune dysfunction in CLL is of key importance in the development of novel immune-based therapies.

## 5. Immunotherapy

CLL is generally considered as an incurable disease, but it frequently progresses slowly. Early-stage CLL is, in general, not treated since there are no clear evidences that early therapeutic intervention improves survival time or quality of life. Instead, the disease is monitored over time to detect changes in disease progression. Determining when to start the treatment and by what means is often difficult. The National Cancer Institute Working Group has issued guidelines for treatment (Cheson et al., 1996; Hallek et al., 1996).

Until recently, chemotherapy has been the keystone of treatment of CLL. Alkylating agents have been considered the first line in the treatment of CLL patients for a long time. They can induce complete responses, but it is not considered curative. Chlorambucil slows disease progression, but does not prolong survival (Dighiero et al., 1998; Eichhorst et al., 2006; Hallek, 2010) (**Figure 2**). The purine analogue fludarabine was shown to give superior response rates to chlorambucil as primary therapy (Steurer et al., 2006; Rai et al., 2000), but there are no evidences that the early use of fludarabine improves overall survival. Treatment combinations of Fludarabine with the alkylating agent Cyclophosphamide (FC) result in higher response rates, in longer median progression-free survival and longer treatment-free survival than single agents (Maloney et al., 1999). Thus far, no difference in median overall survival has been observed.

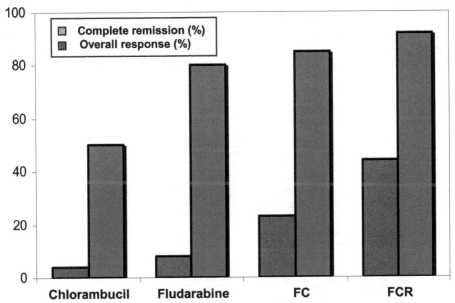

Fig. 2. Chronic lymphocytic leukemia therapy. The figure shows rates of complete remissions and overall response in CLL first line treatment. (F=Fludarabine, C=Cyclophosphamide, R= Rituximab).

In spite of the fact that chemotherapy provides benefits for CLL patients, it is palliative, and treated patients frequently develop recurrent disease. Likewise treatment induces myelosuppression and selection of chemotherapy resistant clones. Additionally, it can worsen immune function, increasing the immunodeficiency status of CLL patients. Prognosis for patients treated with chemotherapy regimens remains poor, prompting the development of new targeted agents. In line with this idea, the activation of the immune system to fight against CLL cells has opened new vistas in the treatment of CLL. Immunotherapy may potentially provide curative treatment and some immunotherapeutic approaches may mitigate disease complications caused by the defects of the immune system observed in CLL patients. In this sense, monoclonal antibodies, allogeneic hematopoietic stem cell transplantation and immunomodulatory drugs have successfully been used in the treatment of CLL. Immune-based therapy represents an exciting mode of treatment since it may be able to eliminate leukemia cells without myelosuppression.

## 5.1 Monoclonal antibodies

Monoclonal antibodies have the ability to target specific antigens expressed preferentially on the surface of malignant cells. Due to their specificity, the therapeutic efficacy of monoclonal antibodies is not generally associated with a high non-specific toxicity. Thus, they are increasingly being used in the treatment of hematological malignancies and solid tumors. In CLL, the use of **rituximab**, a chimeric murine/human monoclonal antibody directed against CD20, has improved the treatment of patients. Unlike other B cells antigens, CD20 is neither shedded nor internalized in resting normal B cells. Therefore it is an ideal target for antibody-based therapy in mature B cell malignancies. Rituximab treatment induces a significant reduction in B cell count within 3 days followed by a slow recovery over 9-12 months (Maloney et al., 1997; Onrust et al., 1999). The mechanism of B cell killing has not completely been elucidated, but rituximab acts through Antibody-Dependent Cell-Mediated Cytotoxicity, complement-mediated cytotoxicity, the activation of macrophages, and direct apoptosis of leukemia cells both caspase dependent and independent (Jaglowski et al., 2010) **(Figure 3)**.

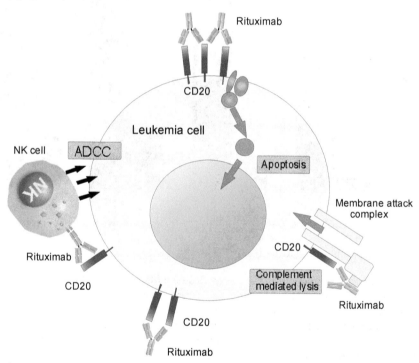

Fig. 3. Mechanism of action of rituximab. Rituximab is a monoclonal antibody directed against CD20 antigen, which is expressed on the surface of B cells. The recognition of the Fc portion of rituximab through the FcγRIII receptor mediates the lysis of leukemia cells by NK cells; a process named Antibody-Dependent Cell-Mediated Cytotoxicity (ADCC). The Fc portion of rituximab also induces the activation of the classical pathway of complement. The activation of complement cascade forms a transmembrane channel, which causes the osmotic lysis of the leukemia cell. Rituximab may also cause a direct apoptosis of CD20 cells.

The efficacy of rituximab monotherapy in CLL is lower than in other B cell malignancies. The resistance to rituximab is frequently associated with a low CD20 expression. Nevertheless, the addition of rituximab to chemotherapy has proven to be very efficacious therapy for CLL. Treatment combinations of Fludarabine, Cyclophosphamide and Rituximab (FCR) obtain the highest response, but they are not still considered curative (Byrd et al., 2005; Tam et al., 2008; Wierda et al., 2005) (**Figure 2**). FCR therapy shows superiority for response rates and progression-free survival when compared to FC chemotherapy (Hallek et al., 2009; Robak et al., 2008), and it is becoming the first-line choice for younger patients (Casak et al., 2011). Additionally, rituximab represents one of the most active therapies for the treatment of autoimmune complications of CLL not responding to initial steroid treatment. The use of monoclonal antibodies for purging of leukemia cells *ex vivo* also improves the results of autologous stem cell transplantation (Gribben et al., 2005; Montillo et al., 2006).

The therapeutic efficacy of rituximab is minimally hampered by non-specific toxicity; however it has been associated with adverse events such as immunosuppression, reactivation of latent virus and infusion-related. Combination with chemotherapy may be associated with more profound immunosuppression. Management of these adverse events is a critical component of the treatment strategy for CLL since they can greatly affect the quality of life of patients and the ability to tolerate this therapy.

**Alemtuzumab**, a CD52-target humanized monoclonal antibody, has demonstrated benefits in the treatment of CLL patients (Gribben et al., 2009). CD52 is a protein highly expressed on both normal and malignant lymphocytes (B and T cells) and it is also found in other immune cells such as monocytes, macrophages and eosinophils; but it is not expressed on hematopoietic progenitors. The administration of alemtuzumab results in a severe lymphopenia with a reduction in both B and T cells, but it also affects other healthy CD52-expressing immune cells, which likely exacerbate the pre-existing immunodeficiency. After treatment, there is a slow recovery of immune cells, except for B cells, which remain at low level at 18 months. Alemtuzumab acts through Antibody-Dependent Cell-Mediated Cytotoxicity (Crowe et al., 1992) (**Figure 1**), complement-mediated cytotoxicity (Golay et al., 2004; Zent et al., 2004), and induces direct cell death through a mechanism that is independent of p53 status and caspase activation (Mone et al., 2006), and is effective in patients with deletion (17p)(13.1).

A significant difference between the efficacy of alemtuzumab and rituximab is based on the fact that the level of CD52 expression in normal and malignant B cells is far greater than the level of CD20 expression in CLL cells. The high expression of CD52 may contribute to the improved clinical activity of alemtuzumab as a single-agent compared to rituximab in CLL (Ashraf et al., 2007). Alemtuzumab is currently approved for first-line treatment of CLL, and it is a good option for symptomatic patients, previously untreated patients and relapsed patients with poor prognostic features (Keating et al., 2002; Osterborg et al., 1996; Lundin et al., 2002 ; Hillmen et al., 2007).

New monoclonal antibodies directed against CD20, such as ofatumumab and GA101, have been developed. **Ofatumumab** and rituximab bind to different epitopes, and, in theory, ofatumumab has greater capacity of activation of complement-dependent cytotoxicity than rituximab (Teeling et al., 2004). *In vitro* studies have demonstrated that ofatumumab is significantly more effective than rituximab at lysing CLL cells and B cell lines, especially those with low CD20 copy numbers. It is currently approved for treating CLL patients who are refractory to fludarabine and alemtuzumab.

The novel third generation humanized monoclonal antibody **GA101** also binds with high affinity to CD20, and as a result it promotes greater induction of Antibody-Dependent Cell-Mediated Cytotoxicity (Jaglowski et al., 2010) and induces more efficient NK cell activation than rituximab (Bologna et al., 2011). The development of new monoclonal antibodies is probably the best demonstration of the therapeutic efficacy that these agents have obtained in CLL and other hematological malignancies.

### 5.2 Hematopoietic stem cell transplantation

About 20% of patients who need treatment develop an aggressive disease despite early institution of intensive chemotherapy. Efforts to develop curative treatment for these CLL patients have focused on autologous and allogeneic hematopoietic stem cell transplantation (Dreger et al., 2009). Both approaches show some methodological similarities, but the bases of both treatments are significantly different. Most patients may achieve a complete molecular response followed by **autologous stem cell transplantation,** a lower-risk form of treatment using the patient's own blood cells, which restores the hematopoietic system after an intensive chemotherapy regimen. The increase of the dose chemotherapy regimen is the base of the efficacy of autografting, and consequently, it is not an immune-based therapy. This therapy is not curative and subsequent clinical progression is inevitable (Provan et al., 1996; Milligan et al., 2005). The results of a phase 3 randomized European Group for Blood and Marrow Transplantation trial of autologous stem cell transplantation show the reduction of the risk of progression of CLL by more than 50%, but it does not have an effect on overall survival (Michallet et al., 2011), and it is particularly concerning the high incidence of myelodysplastic syndrome (9-12%) (Kharfan-Dabaja et al., 2007). Therefore, it is necessary to look for other solutions of treatment in this disease different from the chemotherapy and to move toward alternative non-chemotherapy-based treatment approaches.

**Allogeneic stem cell transplantation** offers a chance of definite cure of CLL, but is only feasible in a minority of patients. The basis of therapeutic response of allogeneic stem cell transplantation relies on the ability of immune cells of the graft to recognize and eliminate leukemia cells, a process known as graft-versus-leukemia effect (GvL) (Mehta et al., 1996; Ritgen et al., 2008) **(Figure 4)**. Thus, allogeneic stem cell transplantation is a cellular-based immunotherapy completely different from autografting. The immunology of allogeneic stem cell transplantation is different from other types of transplants, such as heart or kidney transplants, because the graft, in addition to stem cells, contains and generates mature immune cells including T cells, NK cells and dendritic cells. These cells repopulate the recipient's immune system, restoring the response to infections and eliminating leukemia cells. The donor immune cells exert its graft-versus-leukemia effect through T cell-mediated alloreaction against the histocompatibility antigens displayed on leukemia cells. However, as histocompatibility antigens are shared by all cells of individual, recipient tissues may also be attacked by donor's immune system causing graft-versus-host-disease (GvHD) (rejection), a life-threatening condition. For this reason, matching donor and recipient HLA molecules is crucial to minimize graft-versus-host-disease. Mismatches in HLA-A, -B, -C and HLA class II alleles are significant risk factors for graft-versus-host-disease. Due to the high number of HLA alleles is quite difficult to find a HLA-matched unrelated donor, but nearly 25% of siblings share both HLA haplotypes, because all HLA genes are closely linked in a small region of chromosome 6, known as Major Histocompatibility Complex (MHC). However, even in HLA-matched recipient and donor, graft-versus-host-disease may occur due to minor histocompatibility antigens, which are derived from differences between donor and recipient in other polymorphic genes different from HLA, differences in the level of expression of proteins or are derived from genome differences between male and female (such as H-Y antigens encoded by Y chromosome, which is absent in females).

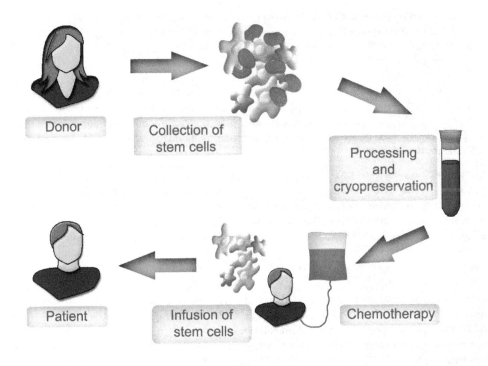

Fig. 4. Allogeneic stem cell transplantation. Hematopoietic stem cells are collected from the bone marrow or blood of the donor. Bone marrow or blood is taken to the processing laboratory where stem cells are concentrated and may be frozen (cryopreservation). High dose chemotherapy and/or radiation are given to the patient. To restore the patient's immune system, thawed or fresh stem cells are infused into the patient. The donor immune cells eliminate leukemia cells (graft-versus-leukemia) through a T cell-mediated alloreaction against patient's histocompatibility antigens displayed on leukemia cells.

If a HLA-matched sibling is not available, the use of unrelated umbilical blood units or an unrelated matched donor are viable options. Umbilical blood units offer the advantage that a higher number of mismatches in HLA antigens does not preclude transplant feasibility since naïve T cells in cord blood are less able to cause graft-versus-host-disease than mature donor T cells in bone marrow or peripheral blood, however graft-versus-leukemia is also less intense. Family donors, who matched a HLA haplotype, but fully mismatched the other ("haploidentical") is another option to obtain hemopoietic stem cells. The haploidentical transplant recipients have high risk of T-cell mediated graft-versus-host-disease (Velardi et al., 2010). This is controlled by an extensive immunosuppressive intensity in the conditioning regimen and extensive T cell depletion of the graft to prevent graft-versus-host-disease. The immune suppression and the depletion of T cells might be expected to result in weak or no graft-versus-leukemia effect, as it is conventionally achieved through T cell-mediated alloreactivity directed against recipient's histocompatibility antigens. Surprisingly, another immune cell influences the outcome of allogeneic stem cell transplantation in a favorable way. In these transplants, NK cell-mediated alloreactivity may control leukemia relapse without causing graft-versus-host-disease. This alloreaction is due to the fact that NK cells express specific inhibitory receptors, such as KIR or CD94/NKG2, for groups of HLA class I alleles. Inhibitory receptors and HLA class I genes structure individual NK cell repertoires during development. To establish a self-tolerance, each individual selects NK cells carrying inhibitory receptor combinations for their self HLA class I molecules. NK cells from those individuals that express inhibitory receptors for a HLA class I group, which is absent on allogeneic transplants, sense the missing expression of their self HLA class I molecules and mediate alloreactions against leukemia cells by "missing self" recognition (Figure 1).

Several nonrandomized prospective trials have demonstrated the potential efficacy of allogeneic stem cell transplantation in CLL; however even with reduced-intensity conditioning allogeneic stem cell transplantation is associated with significant morbidity and mortality. Nevertheless, it is a reasonable treatment option for poor-risk CLL patients. Allogeneic stem cell transplantation can overcome treatment resistance of poor-risk CLL defined as purine analogue refractoriness, early relapse after purine analogue combination therapy or autologous stem cell transplantation, and CLL with p53 deletion/mutation requiring treatment (Dreger et al., 2007). Nonmyeloablative allogeneic stem cell transplantation resulted in sustained remissions and prolonged survival in patients who had chemotherapy-refractory CLL (Sorror et al., 2008) and in high risk patients (Schetelig et al., 2008). Myeloablative allogeneic stem cell transplantation consistently results in a plateau in survival after 1 year, and the development of undetectable minimal residual disease (Pavletic et al., 2005). Evidence for graft-versus-leukemia in CLL can result in a complete and durable suppression of the leukemic clone (Ritgen et al., 2008; Rondón et al., 1996; Dreger et al., 2005; Farina et al., 2009; Sorror et al., 2005; Gribben et al., 2005). A prospective clinical trial is currently being performed in patients with high-risk CLL. This trial will finish in 2012 and will probably give us some guidance when and how to use allogeneic stem cell transplantation in poor-risk CLL.

In summary, there is convincing evidence that allogeneic stem cell transplantation can provide long-term disease control and possibly cure in selected patients with CLL, including those with a biologically highly unfavorable risk profile. Even patients who relapsed after allogeneic transplant may achieve durable remission following **donor lymphocyte infusion** without further chemotherapy or radiation chemotherapy (Hoogendoorn et al., 2007; Schetelig et al., 2003; Delgado et al., 2006; Marina et al., 2010). This further highlights the capacity of the donor-derived immunity in eradicating tumors (Marina et al., 2010).

## 5.3 Immune modulating drugs

Lenalidomide is a new immunomodulatory drug used in the treatment of CLL that is receiving considerable interest. It is a small molecular analog of thalidomide that was originally selected based on its ability to effectively inhibit tumor necrosis factor α (TNF-α) production. The mechanism of action of lenalidomide is complex and not yet fully understood. In CLL, lenalidomide has not a direct anti-tumor effect by inducing of apoptosis, but it has a significant anti-angiogenic and immune effects. It represents an exciting drug since it is able to eliminate CLL cells without immunosuppression.

Lenalidomide is clinically used in combination with dexamethasone in patients with multiple myeloma who have received prior therapy, in myelodysplasic syndrome, and in addition, there are current clinical trials analyzing the therapeutic effect of this drug in other types of cancers. In CLL, lenalidomide is clinically effective as a single agent in relapsed and refractory patients (Ferrajoli et al., 2008 ; Chanan-Khan et al., 2006), and ongoing trials are demonstrating that lenalidomide is clinically active as first-line CLL therapy (Chen et al., 2010). The responses achieved with lenalidomide are durable, even in patients with high-risk disease, with poor risk cytogenetics and with high-risk cytogenetics [del(11q)(q22.3) or del(17p)(p13.1)] (Sher et al., 2010).

The immunomodulatory mechanism of action of lenalidomide in CLL is poorly understood. Lenalidomide improves the humoral and cellular immune response of CLL patients (**Figure 5**). Lenalidomide treatment is associated with a significant increase in immunoglobulin

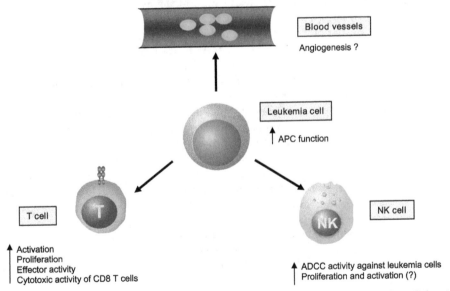

Fig. 5. Mechanism of action of lenalidomide in chronic lymphocytic leukemia. Lenalidomide does not have a direct cytotoxic effect on leukemia cells. Lenalidomide favors antigen presentation, activation, proliferation and functional activity of T cells. It also enhances Antibody-Dependent Cell-Mediated Cytotoxicity (ADCC) against rituximab-exposed leukemia cells. Other effects on angiogenic status remain to be elucidated.

levels. For instance, IgG levels were normalized in 7 out of 12 (58%) CLL patients with hypogammaglobulinemia (Badoux et al., 2009). Lenalidomide enhances antigen presentation to T cells (Aue et al., 2009; Chanan-Khan et al., 2006) and increases proliferation, activation and effector activity of T cells, which as mentioned before is impaired in CLL patients (Ramsay et al., 2008). Thalidomide and lenalidomide also have a significant immunomoudulatory effect on NK cells. In some experimental models, the antitumor effect of lenalidomide was mediated by NK cell stimulation (Awan et al., 2010). There is little information about the effect of lenalidomide on NK cells *in vivo*. Nevertheless, lenalidomide treatment increased the number of NK cells in CLL patients and increased Antibody-Dependent Cell-Mediated Cytotoxicity against leukemia cells (Wu et al., 2008). Lenalidomide induces a unique and previously uncharacterized immune response called tumor flare reaction associated with immune mediated antitumor response. Tumor flare reaction with lenalidomide appears to be disease-specific to CLL, may reflect clinical manifestation of tumor cell activation and correlates with clinical response (Chanan-Khan et al., 2010). Combination of lenalidomide with rituximab may act synergistically if the timing and sequencing strategies are optimized. An exciting new therapeutic strategy may be targeting tumor cell with chemotherapy or monoclonal antibodies and the microenvironment with lenalidomide (Ramsay et al., 2009).

## 6. Conclusion

In spite of the existence of little information about the role of the immune system in the pathogenesis of CLL, the current data clearly support the hypothesis that the activation of the anti-tumor immune response, particularly in the early stages of the disease, may have a significant impact on tumor progression. However, CLL patients progressively acquire a wide variety of immune evasion mechanisms. As a result, patients acquire a progressive immunodeficiency status, which increases the incidence of opportunistic infections and the development of secondary neoplasias. Chemotherapy has been the keystone of treatment of CLL, but it is palliative and may worsen the immunodeficiency status of patients. Nevertheless, the development of drugs and therapeutic strategies that can either bypass the immune evasion mechanisms or rescue immune suppressor pathways may significantly benefit CLL patients. Thus, immunotherapy may provide curative treatment and may mitigate disease complications caused by the defects of the immune system observed in CLL patients. In this sense, monoclonal antibodies, allogeneic hematopoietic stem cell transplantation and immunomodulatory drugs have successfully been used in the treatment of CLL. Immune-based therapy represents an exciting mode of treatment since it may be able to eliminate leukemia cells without inducing immune suppression. The elucidation of the molecular and cellular events underlying the immune dysfunction in CLL is of key importance to further develop novel immune-based therapies. It is presumably that a deeper knowledge of the immune response in CLL may open new frontiers in the treatment of these patients.

## 7. Acknowledgement

This work was supported by the Spanish grant of Fondo de Investigaciones Sanitarias (Institute Carlos III) PS09/00420.

# 8. References

Ashraf, U, Elefante AN, Cruz R, Wallace PK, Czuczman MS,Hernandez-llizaliturri FJ Emergence of rituximab-fludarabine resistance is associated with changes in CD20 antigen expression and improved response to alemtuzumab therapy in patients with chronic lymphocytic leukemia (chronic lymphocytic leukaemia). Blood 2007;110, 612a (abstract 2054).

Aue G, Njuguna N, Tian X, Soto S, Hughes T, Vire B, Keyvanfar K, Gibellini F, Valdez J, Boss C, Samsel L, McCoy JP Jr, Wilson WH, Pittaluga S, Wiestner A. Lenalidomide-induced upregulation of CD80 on tumor cells correlates with T-cell activation, the rapid onset of a cytokine release syndrome and leukemic cell clearance in chronic lymphocytic leukemia. Haematologica. 2009;94(9):1266-73.

Awan FT, Johnson AJ, Lapalombella R, Hu W, Lucas M, Fischer B, Byrd JC. Thalidomide and lenalidomide as new therapeutics for the treatment of chronic lymphocytic leukemia. Leuk Lymphoma. 2010;51(1):27-38.

Badoux, X., Reuben, J., Lee, B., Jorgensen, J., Estrov, Z., Yerrow, K. Ferrajoli, A. (2009). Lenalidomide therapy is associated with normalization of lymphocyte populations and increase in immunoglobulin levels in elderly patients with chronic lymphocytic leukemia [Abstract 10.31]. *Haematologica, 94*(3, Suppl.), S94.

Bahram S, Bresnahan M, Geraghty DE, Spies T. A second lineage of mammalian major histocompatibility complex class I genes, Proc Natl Acad Sci USA 1994; 91:6259-63.

Bauer S, Groh V, Wu J, Steinle A, Phillips JH, Lanier LL, Spies T. Activation of NK cells and T cells by NKG2D, a receptor for stress-inducible MICA. Science 1999; 285: 727-9.

Behl D, Porrata LF, Markovic SN, Letendre L, Pruthi RK, Hook CC, et al. Absolute lymphocyte count recovery after induction chemotherapy predicts superior survival in acute myelogenous leukemia. Leukemia. 2006;20:29-34.

Behl D, Ristow K, Markovic SN, Witzig TE, Habermann TM, Colgan JP,et al. Absolute lymphocyte count predicts therapeutic efficacy of rituximab therapy in follicular lymphomas. Br J Haematol. 2007;137:409-15.

Beyer M, Kochanek M, Darabi K, et al. Reduced frequencies and suppressive function of CD4+ CD25hi regulatory T cells in patients with chronic lymphocytic leukemia after therapy with fludarabine. Blood 2006;106:2018-2025.

Bologna L, Gotti E, Manganini M, Rambaldi A, Intermesoli T, Introna M, Golay J. Mechanism of Action of Type II, Glycoengineered, Anti-CD20 Monoclonal Antibody GA101 in B-Chronic Lymphocytic Leukemia Whole Blood Assays in Comparison with Rituximab and Alemtuzumab. J Immunol. 2011 Feb 4.

Byrd JC, Rai K, Peterson BL, Appelbaum FR, Morrison VA, Kolitz JE, Shepherd L, Hines JD, Schiffer CA, Larson RA. Addition of rituximab to fludarabine may prolong progression-free survival and overall survival in patients with previously untreated chronic lymphocytic leukemia: an updated retrospective comparative analysis of CALGB 9712 and CALGB 9011. Blood. 2005;105(1):49-53.

Caligaris-Cappio F, Hamblin TJ. B-cell chronic lymphocytic leukemia: a bird of a different feather. J Clin Oncol. 1999;17:399-408.

Cantwell M, Hua T, Pappas J, Kipps TJ. Acquired CD40-ligand deficiency in chronic lymphocytic leukemia. Nat Med. 1997;3:984-9.

Casak SJ, Lemery SJ, Shen YL, Rothmann MD, Khandelwal A, Zhao H, Davis G, Jarral V, Keegan P, Pazdur R. U.S. Food and drug administration approval: rituximab in combination with fludarabine and cyclophosphamide for the treatment of patients with chronic lymphocytic leukemia. Oncologist. 2011;16(1):97-104.

Cerwenka A, Baron JL, Lanier LL. Ectopic expression of retinoic acid early inducible-1 gene (RAE-1) permits natural killer cell-mediated rejection of a MHC class I-bearing tumor in vivo. Proc Natl Acad Sci USA 2001; 98:11521-11526.

Chanan-Khan A, Miller KC, Lawrence D, Padmanabhan S, Miller A, Hernandez-Illatazurri F, Czuczman MS, Wallace PK, Zeldis JB, Lee K. Tumor flare reaction associated with lenalidomide treatment in patients with chronic lymphocytic leukemia predicts clinical response. Cancer. 2010 Nov 29.

Chanan-Khan A, Miller KC, Musial L, Lawrence D, Padmanabhan S, Takeshita K, Porter CW, Goodrich DW, Bernstein ZP, Wallace P, Spaner D, Mohr A, Byrne C, Hernandez-Ilizaliturri F, Chrystal C, Starostik P, Czuczman MS. Clinical efficacy of lenalidomide in patients with relapsed or refractory chronic lymphocytic leukemia: results of a phase II study. J Clin Oncol. 2006;24(34):5343-9.

Chanan-Khan A, Porter CW. Immunomodulating drugs for chronic lymphocytic leukaemia. Lancet Oncol. 2006;7(6):480-8.

Chen CI, Bergsagel PL, Paul H, Xu W, Lau A, Dave N, Kukreti V, Wei E, Leung-Hagesteijn C, Li ZH, Brandwein J, Pantoja M, Johnston J, Gibson S, Hernandez T, Spaner D, Trudel S. Single-Agent Lenalidomide in the Treatment of Previously Untreated Chronic Lymphocytic Leukemia. J Clin Oncol. 2010 Dec 28.

Cheson BD, Bennett JM, Grever M, et al. (1996). "National Cancer Institute-sponsored Working Group guidelines for chronic lymphocytic leukemia: revised guidelines for diagnosis and treatment". Blood 87 (12): 4990-7.

Clark WH Jr, From L, Bernardino EA, Mihm MC. The histogenesis and biologic behavior of primary human malignant melanomas of the skin. Cancer Res 1969;29:705-27.

Clemente CG, Mihm MC Jr, Bufalino R, Zurrida S, Collini P, Cascinelli N. Prognostic value of tumor infiltrating lymphocytes in the vertical growth phase of primary cutaneous melanoma. Cancer 1996;77:1303-10

Cosman D, Mullberg J, Sutherland CL, Chin W, Armitage R, Fanslow W, Kubin M, Chalupny NJ. ULBPs, novel MHC class I-related molecules, bind to CMV glycoprotein UL16 and stimulate NK cytotoxicity through the NKG2D receptor. Immunity 2001; 14: 123-33.

Cox MC, Nofroni I, Ruco L, Amodeo R, Ferrari A, La Verde G, et al. Low absolute lymphocyte count is a poor prognostic factor in diffuse-large-B-cell-lymphoma. Leuk Lymphoma. 2008;49:1745-51.

Crowe JS, Hall VS, Smith MA, Cooper HJ, Tite JP. Humanized monoclonal antibody CAMPATH-1H: myeloma cell expression of genomic constructs, nucleotide sequence of cDNA constructs and comparison of effector mechanisms of myeloma and Chinese hamster ovary cell-derived material. Clin Exp Immunol. 19927(1):105-10.

Das H, Groh V, Kuijl C, Sugita M, Morita CT, Spies T, Bukowski JF. MICA engagement by human Vgamma2Vdelta2 T cells enhances their antigen-dependent effector function. Immunity 2001; 15:83-93.

De Angulo G, Yuen C, Palla SL, Anderson PM, Zweidler-McKay PA. Absolute lymphocyte count is a novel prognostic indicator in ALL and AML: implications for risk stratification and future studies. Cancer. 2008;112:407-15.

Del Giudice I, Chiaretti S, Tavolaro S, De Propris MS, Maggio R, Mancini F, Peragine N, Santangelo S, Marinelli M, Mauro FR, Guarini A, Foà R. Spontaneous regression of chronic lymphocytic leukemia: clinical and biologic features of 9 cases. Blood. 2009;114:638-46.

Delgado J, Thomson K, Russell N, et al. Results of alemtuzumab-based reduced-intensity allogeneic transplantation for chronic lymphocytic leukemia: a British Society of Blood and Marrow Transplantation Study. Blood 2006;107(4):1724-1730

Demanet C, Mulder A, Deneys V, Worsham MJ, Maes P, Claas FH, Ferrone S. Down-regulation of HLA-A and HLA-Bw6, but not HLA-Bw4, allospecificities in leukemic cells: an escape mechanism from CTL and NK attack? Blood. 2004;103(8):3122-30.

Diefenbach A, Jensen ER, Jamieson AM, Raulet DH. Rae1 and H60 ligands of the NKG2D receptor stimulate tumor immunity. Nature 2001; 413, 165-171.

Dighiero G, Maloum K, Desablens B, Cazin B, Navarro M, Leblay R, Leporrier M, Jaubert J, Lepeu G, Dreyfus B, Binet JL, Travade P. Chlorambucil in indolentchronic lymphocytic leukemia. French Cooperative Group on Chronic Lymphocytic Leukemia. N Engl J Med. 1998;338(21):1506-14.

Dreger P, Brand R, Milligan D, et al. Reduced-intensity conditioning lowers treatment-related mortality of allogeneic stem cell transplantation for chronic lymphocytic leukemia: a population-matched analysis. Leukemia 2005;19(6):1029-1033.

Dreger P, Corradini P, Kimby E, et al. Indications for allogeneic stem cell transplantation in chronic lymphocytic leukemia: the EBMT transplant consensus. Leukemia. 2007;21:12–17.

Dreger P. Allotransplantation for chronic lymphocytic leukemia Hematology 2009.

Dunn, GP, Old, LJ, Schreiber, RD. The three Es of cancer immunoediting. Annu Rev Immunol 2004; 22:329-60.

Ege H, Gertz MA, Markovic SN, Lacy MQ, Dispenzieri A, Hayman SR, Kumar SK, Porrata LF. Prediction of survival using absolute lymphocyte count for newly diagnosed patients with multiple myeloma: a retrospective study. Br J Haematol. 2008;141(6):792-8.

Eichhorst BF, Busch R, Hopfinger G, Pasold R, Hensel M, Steinbrecher C, Siehl S, Jäger U, Bergmann M, Stilgenbauer S, Schweighofer C, Wendtner CM, Döhner H, Brittinger G, Emmerich B, Hallek M; German chronic lymphocytic leukaemia Study Group. Fludarabine plus cyclophosphamide versus fludarabine alone in first-line therapy of younger patients with chronic lymphocytic leukemia. Blood. 2006;107(3):885-91.

Erikci AA, Karagoz B, Ozyurt M, Ozturk A, Kilic S, Bilgi O. HLA-G expression in B chronic lymphocytic leukemia: a new prognostic marker? Hematology. 2009;14:101-5.

Farina L, Carniti C, Dodero A, et al. Qualitative and quantitative polymerase chain reaction monitoring of minimal residual disease in relapsed chronic lymphocytic leukemia: early assessment can predict long-term outcome after reduced intensity allogeneic transplantation. Haematologica 2009;94(5):654-662.

Ferrajoli A, Lee BN, Schlette EJ, O'Brien SM, Gao H, Wen S, Wierda WG, Estrov Z, Faderl S, Cohen EN, Li C, Reuben JM, Keating MJ. Lenalidomide induces complete and partial remissions in patients with relapsed and refractory chronic lymphocytic leukemia. Blood. 2008;111(11):5291-7.

Foa R, Lauria F, Lusso P, Giubellino MC, Fierro MT, Ferrando ML, et al. Discrepancy between phenotypic and functional features of natural killer T-lymphocytes in B-cell chronic lymphocytic leukaemia. Br J Haematol. 1984;58:509-16.

Gasser S, Orsulic S, Brown EJ, Raulet DH. The DNA damage pathway regulates innate immune system ligands of the NKG2D receptor. Nature 2005; 436:1186-90.

Golay J, Manganini M, Rambaldi A, Introna M. Effect of alemtuzumab on neoplastic B cells. Haematologica. 2004;89(12):1476-83.

Gonzalez S, Gonzalez-Rodríguez AP, Lopez-Soto A, Huergo-Zapico L, Lopez-Larrea C, Suarez-Alvarez B. Conceptual aspects of self and nonself discrimination. 2011, 2(1):1-7.

González S, Groh V, Spies T. Immunobiology of human NKG2D and its ligands. Curr To Microbiol Immunol 2006; 298:121-38.

González S, López-Soto A, Suárez-Álvarez B, López-Vázquez A, López-Larrea C. NKG2D ligands: key targets of the immune response. Trends Immunol 2008; 14:179-89.

Gonzalez-Rodriguez AP, Contesti J, Huergo-Zapico L, Lopez-Soto A, Fernández-Guizán A, Acebes-Huerta A, Gonzalez-Huerta AJ, Gonzalez E, Fernandez-Alvarez C, Gonzalez S. Prognostic significance of CD8 and CD4 T cells in chronic lymphocytic leukemia. Leuk Lymphoma. 2010;51(10):1829-36

Gorgun G, Holderried TA, Zahrieh D, Neuberg D, Gribben JG. Chronic lymphocytic leukemia cells induce changes in gene expression of CD4 and CD8 T cells. J Clin Invest. 2005;115:1797-805.

Gribben JG, Hallek M. Rediscovering alemtuzumab: current and emerging therapeutic roles. Br J Haematol. 2009;144(6):818-31.

Gribben JG, Zahrieh D, Stephans K, Bartlett-Pandite L, Alyea EP, Fisher DC, Freedman AS, Mauch P, Schlossman R, Sequist LV, Soiffer RJ, Marshall B, Neuberg D, Ritz J, Nadler LM. Autologous and allogeneic stem cell transplantations for poor-risk chronic lymphocytic leukemia. Blood. 2005;106(13):4389-96.

Gribben JG, Zahrieh D, Stephans K, et al. Autologous and allogeneic stem cell transplantations for poor-risk chronic lymphocytic leukemia. Blood 2005;106(13):4389-4396

Groh V, Bahram S, Bauer S, Herman A, Beauchamp M, Spies T. Cell stress-regulated human major histocompatibility complex class I gene expressed in gastrointestinal epithelium. Proc Natl Acad Sci USA 1996; 93:12445-50.

Groh V, Rhinehart R, Secrist H, Bauer S, Grabstein KH, Spies T. Broad tumor-associated expression and recognition by tumor-derived gamma delta Tcells of MICA and MICB. Proc Natl Acad Sci USA 1999; 96:6879-6884.

Groh V, Smythe K, Dai Z, Spies T. Fas-ligand-mediated paracrine T cell regulation by the receptor NKG2D in tumor immunity. Nat Immunol 2006; 7:755-762.

Groh V, Wu J, Yee C, Spies T. Tumor-derived soluble MIC ligands impair expression of NKG2D and T-cell activation. Nature 2002; 419:734-738.

Grulich AE, van Leeuwen MT, Falster MO, Vajdic CM. Incidence of cancers in people with HIV/AIDS compared with immunosuppressed transplant recipients: a meta-analysis. Lancet 2007;370(9581):59-67.

Guerra N, Tan YX, Joncker NT, Choy A, Gallardo F, Xiong N, Knoblaugh S, Cado D, Greenberg NM, Raulet DH. NKG2D-deficient mice are defective in tumor surveillance in models of spontaneous malignancy. Immunity 2008; 28:571-80.

Hallek M, Cheson BD, Catovsky D, Caligaris-Cappio F, Dighiero G, Döhner H, Hillmen P, Keating MJ, Montserrat E, Rai KR, Kipps TJ; International Workshop on Chronic Lymphocytic Leukemia. Guidelines for the diagnosis and treatment of chronic lymphocytic leukemia: a report from the International Workshop on Chronic Lymphocytic Leukemia updating the National Cancer Institute-Working Group 1996 guidelines. Blood. 2008;111(12):5446-56.

Hallek M, Therapy of chronic lymphocytic lekemia. Best Pract Res Clin Haematol. 2010;23(1):85-96.

Hallek, M, Fingerle-Rowson G, Fink A-M, Busch R, Mayer J, Hensel M, Hopfinger G, Hess G, von Gruenhagen U et al. First-Line Treatment with Fludarabine (F), Cyclophosphamide (C), and Rituximab (R) (FCR) Improves Overall Survival (OS) in Previously Untreated Patients (pts) with Advanced Chronic Lymphocytic Leukemia (chronic lymphocytic leukaemia): Results of a Randomized Phase III Trial On Behalf of An International Group of Investigators and the German chronic lymphocytic leukaemia Study Group. Blood. ASH Annual Meeting Abstracts 2009; 114 (22): 535.

Hamblin AD, Hamblin TJ. The immunodeficiency of chronic lymphocytic leukaemia. Br Med Bull. 2008;87:49-62.

Hamblin TJ. Autoimmune complications of chronic lymphocytic leukemia. Semin Oncol 2006;33:230-239.

Hamblin TJ.. Chronic lymphocytic leukaemia. Balliere's Clin Haematol 1987;1:449-491.

Hillmen, P., Skotnicki, A.B., Robak, T., Jaksic, B., Dmoszynska, A., Wu, J., Sirard, C. & Mayer, J. (2007) Alemtuzumab compared with chlorambucil as first-line therapy for chronic lymphocytic leukemia. Journal of Clinical Oncology 2007;25:5616–5623.

Hoogendoorn M, Jedema I, Barge RM, et al. Characterization of graft-versus-leukemia responses in patients treated for advanced chronic lymphocytic leukemia with donor lymphocyte infusions after in vitro T-cell depleted allogeneic stem cell transplantation following reduced-intensity conditioning. Leukemia 2007;21(12):2569-2574

Jaglowski SM, Alinari L, Lapalombella R, Muthusamy N, Byrd JC. The clinicalapplication of monoclonal antibodies in chronic lymphocytic leukemia. Blood. 2010;116(19):3705-14.

Jaglowski SM, Byrd JC. Rituximab in chronic lymphocytic leukemia. Semen Hematol. 2010;47(2):156-69.

Jewell AP, Worman CP, Giles FJ, Goldstone AH, Lydyard PM. Resistance of chronic lymphocytic leukaemia cells to interferon-alpha generated lymphokine activated killer cells. Leuk Lymphoma. 1992;7:473-80.

Junevik K, Werlenius O, Hasselblom S, Jacobsson S, Nilsson-Ehle H, Andersson PO. The expression of NK cell inhibitory receptors on cytotoxic T cells in B-cell chronic lymphocytic leukaemia (B-chronic lymphocytic leukaemia). Ann Hematol. 2007;86:89-94.

Kato N, Tanaka J, Sugita J, Toubai T, Miura Y, Ibata M, et al. Regulation of the expression of MHC class I-related chain A, B (MICA, MICB) via chromatin remodeling and its impact on the susceptibility of leukemic cells to the cytotoxicity of NKG2D-expressing cells. Leukemia. 2007;21:2103-8.

Kato N, Tanaka J, Sugita J, Toubai T, Miura Y, Ibata M, Syono Y, Ota S, Kondo T, Asaka M, Imamura M. Regulation of the expression of MHC class I-related chain A, B (MICA, MICB) via chromatin remodeling and its impact on the susceptibility of leukemic cells to the cytotoxicity of NKG2D-expressing cells. Leukemia. 2007;21(10):2103-8.

Katrinakis G, Kyriakou D, Papadaki H, Kalokyri I, Markidou F, Eliopoulos GD. Defective natural killer cell activity in B-cell chronic lymphocytic leukaemia is associated with impaired release of natural killer cytotoxic factor(s) but not of tumour necrosis factor-alpha. Acta Haematol. 1996;96:16-23.

Keating MJ, Flinn I, Jain V, Binet JL, Hillmen P, Byrd J, Albitar M, Brettman L, Santabarbara P, Wacker B,Rai KR..Therapeutic role of alemtuzumab (Campath-1H) in patients who have failed fludarabine: results of a large international study. Blood 2002;9:3554-3561.

Kharfan-Dabaja MA, Kumar A, Behera M, Djulbegovic B. Systematic review of high dose chemotherapy and autologous haematopoietic stem cell transplantation for chronic lymphocytic leukaemia: what is the published evidence? Br J Haematol. 2007;139(2):234-42.

Kinlen LJ, Webster AD, Bird AG, Haile R, Peto J, Soothill JF, Thompson RA. Prospective study of cancer in patients with hypogammaglobulinaemia. Lancet 1985;1(8423):263-266.

leukemia include nonmutated B-cell antigens. Cancer Res. 2010 Feb 15;70(4):1344-55.

leukemia include nonmutated B-cell antigens. Cancer Res. 2010 Feb 15;70(4):1344-55.

Lopez-Larrea C, Suarez-Alvarez B, Lopez-Soto A, Lopez-Vazquez A, Gonzalez S. The NKG2D receptor: sensing stressed cells. Trends Mol Med 2008; 14:179-89.

Lundin J., Kimby E., Bjorkholm M, Broliden, PA, Celsing F, Hjalmar V, Mollgard L, Rebello P, Hale G, Waldmann H, Mellstedt H, Osterborg A. Phase II trial of subcutaneous anti-CD52 monoclonal antibody alemtuzumab (Campath-1H) as first-line treatment for patients with B-cell chronic lymphocytic leukemia (B-chronic lymphocytic leukaemia). Blood 2002;100:68–773.

Mackus WJ, Frakking FN, Grummels A, et al. Expansion of CMV-specific CD8 + CD45RA + CD27- T cells in B-cell chronic lymphocytic leukemia. Blood 2003;102:1057-1063.

Mackus WJ, Frakking FN, Grummels A, Gamadia LE, De Bree GJ, Hamann D, et al. Expansion of CMV-specific CD8+CD45RA+CD27- T cells in B-cell chronic lymphocytic leukemia. Blood. 2003;102:1057-63.

Maloney DG, Grillo-López AJ, Bodkin DJ, White CA, Liles TM, Royston I, Varns C, Rosenberg J, Levy R.IDEC-C2B8: results of a phase I multiple-dose trial in patients with relapsed non-Hodgkin's lymphoma. J Clin Oncol. 1997;15(10):3266-74.

Marina O, Hainz U, Biernacki MA, Zhang W, Cai A, Duke-Cohan JS, Liu F, Brusic V,

Mehta J, Powles R, Singhal S, Iveson T, Treleaven J, Catovsky D. Clinical and hematologic response of chronic lymphocytic and prolymphocytic leukemia persisting after allogeneic bone marrow transplantation with the onset of acute graft-versus-host disease: possible role of graft-versus-leukemia. Bone Marrow Transplant. 1996;17(3):371-5.

Mellemkjaer L, Hammarstrom L, Andersen V, Yuen J, Heilmann C, Barington T, Bjorkander J, Olsen JH. Cancer risk among patients with IgA deficiency or common variable immunodeficiency and their relatives: a combined Danish and Swedish study. Clin Exp Immunol 2002;130(3):495-500

Michallet M, Dreger P, Sutton L, Brand R, Richards S, van Os M, Sobh M, Choquet S, Corront B, Dearden C, Gratwohl A, Herr W, Catovsky D, Hallek M, de Witte T, Niederwieser D, Leporrier M, Milligan D; on behalf of the EBMT Chronic Leukemia Working Party. Autologous hematopoietic stem cell transplantation in chronic lymphocytic leukemia: results of European intergroup randomized trial comparing autografting versus observation. Blood. 2011; 117(5):1516-1521.

Milligan DW, Fernandes S, Dasgupta R, Davies FE, Matutes E, Fegan CD, McConkey C, Child JA, Cunningham D, Morgan GJ, Catovsky D; National Cancer Research Institute Haematological Studies Group. Results of the MRC pilot study show autografting for younger patients with chronic lymphocytic leukemia is safe and achieves a high percentage of molecular responses. Blood. 2005; 105(1):397-404.

Mone AP, Cheney C, Banks AL, Tridandapani S, Mehter N, Guster S, Lin T, Eisenbeis CF, Young DC, Byrd JC. Alemtuzumab induces caspase-independent cell death in human chronic lymphocytic leukemia cells through a lipid raft-dependent mechanism. Leukemia. 2006;20(2):272-9.

Montillo M, Tedeschi A, Miqueleiz S, Veronese S, Cairoli R, Intropido L, RicciF, Colosimo A, Scarpati B, Montagna M, Nichelatti M, Regazzi M, Morra E. Alemtuzumab as consolidation after a response to fludarabine is effective in purging residual disease in patients with chronic lymphocytic leukemia. J Clin Oncol. 2006;24(15):2337-42.

Moore OS Jr, Foote FW Jr. The relatively favourable prognosis of medullary carcinoma of the breast. Cancer 1949;2:635-42.

Morrell D, Cromartie E, Swift M. Mortality and cancer incidence in 263 patients with ataxia-telangiectasia. J Natl Cancer Inst 1986;77(1):89-92.

Neuberg D, Kutok JL, Alyea EP, Canning CM, Soiffer RJ, Ritz J, Wu CJ. Serologic markers of effective tumor immunity against chronic lymphocytic

Nückel H, Rebmann V, Dürig J, Dührsen U, Grosse-Wilde H. HLA-G expression is associated with an unfavorable outcome and immunodeficiency in chronic lymphocytic leukemia. Blood. 2005;105:1694-8.

Nückel H, Switala M, Sellmann L, Horn PA, Dürig J, Dührsen U, Küppers R, Grosse-Wilde H, Rebmann V. The prognostic significance of soluble NKG2D ligands in B-cell chronic lymphocytic leukemia Leukemia. 2010;24(6):1152-9.

Onrust SV, Lamb HM, Balfour JA. Rituximab. Drugs. 1999;58(1):79-88; discussion 89-90.

Osterborg A., Fassas AS, Anagnostopoulos A, Dyer MJ, Catovsky D, Mellstedt H. Humanized CD52 monoclonal antibody Campath-1H as first-line treatment in chronic lymphocytic leukaemia. British Journal of Haematology 1996;93:151–153.

Pagès F, Berger A, Camus M, Sanchez-Cabo F, Costes A, Molidor R, et al. Effector memory T cells, early metastasis, and survival in colorectal cancer. N Engl J Med 2005; 353:2654–66.

Palmer S, Hanson CA, Zent CS, et al. Prognostic importance of T and NK-cells in a consecutive series of newly diagnosed patients with chronic lymphocytic leukemia. Br J Haematol 2008; 141:607-614.

Pavletic SZ, Khouri IF, Haagenson M, King RJ, Bierman PJ, Bishop MR, Carston M, Giralt S, Molina A, Copelan EA, Ringdén O, Roy V, Ballen K, Adkins DR, McCarthy P, Weisdorf D, Montserrat E, Anasetti C. Unrelated donor marrow transplantation for B-cell chronic lymphocytic leukemia after using myeloablative conditioning: results from the Center for International Blood and Marrow Transplant research. J Clin Oncol. 2005;23(24):5788-94.

Plonquet A, Haioun C, Jais JP, Debard AL, Salles G, Bene MC, Feugier P, Rabian C, Casasnovas O, Labalette M, Kuhlein E, Farcet JP, Emile JF, Gisselbrecht C, Delfau-Larue MH; Groupe d'étude des lymphomes de l'adulte Peripheral blood natural killer cell count is associated with clinical outcome in patients with aaIPI 2-3 diffuse large B-cell lymphoma. Ann Oncol. 2007;18(7):1209-15.

Poggi A, Venturino C, Catellani S, Clavio M, Miglino M, Gobbi M, Steinle A, Ghia P, Stella S, Caligaris-Cappio F, Zocchi MR.Vdelta1 T lymphocytes from B-chronic lymphocytic leukaemia patients recognize ULBP3 expressed on leukemic B cells and up-regulated by trans-retinoic acid. Cancer Res. 2004;64(24):9172-9.

Porrata LF, Ristow K, Habermann TM, Witzig TE, Inwards DJ, Markovic SN. Absolute lymphocyte count at the time of first relapse predicts survival in patients with diffuse large B-cell lymphoma. Am J Hematol. 2009;84:93-7.

Porrata LF, Ristow K, Witzig TE, Tuinistra N, Habermann TM, Inwards DJ et al. Absolute lymphocyte count predicts therapeutic efficacy and survival at the time of radioimmunotherapy in patients with relapsed follicular lymphomas. Leukemia. 2007;21:2554-6.

Provan D, Bartlett-Pandite L, Zwicky C, Neuberg D, Maddocks A, Corradini P, Soiffer R, Ritz J, Nadler LM, Gribben JG. Eradication of polymerase chain reaction-detectable chronic lymphocytic leukemia cells is associated with improved outcome after bone marrow transplantation. Blood. 1996; 88(6):2228-35.

Raffaghello L, Prigione I, Airoldi I, Camoriano M, Levreri I, Gambini C, Pende D, Steinle A, Ferrone S, Pistoia V. Downregulation and/or release of NKG2D ligands as immune evasion strategy of human neuroblastoma. Neoplasia 2004; 6:558-68.

Rai KR, Peterson BL, Appelbaum FR, et al. (2000). "Fludarabine compared with chlorambucil as primary therapy for chronic lymphocytic leukemia". N. Engl. J. Med. 343 (24): 1750-7.

Ramsay AG, Gribben JG. Immune dysfunction in chronic lymphocytic leukemia T cells and lenalidomide as an immunomodulatory drug. Haematologica. 2009;94(9):1198-202.

Ramsay AG, Johnson AJ, Lee AM, Gorgün G, Le Dieu R, Blum W, Byrd JC, Gribben JG. Chronic lymphocytic leukemia T cells show impaired immunological synapse formation that can be reversed with an immunomodulating drug. J Clin Invest. 2008;118(7):2427-37.

Raulet DH. Roles of the NKG2D immunoreceptor and its ligands. Nat Rev Immunol 2003; 3:781-90.

Ray-Coquard I, Cropet C, Van Glabbeke M, Sebban C, Le Cesne A, Judson I,et al; European Organization for Research and Treatment of Cancer Soft Tissue and Bone Sarcoma Group. Lymphopenia as a prognostic factor for overall survival in advanced carcinomas, sarcomas, and lymphomas. Cancer Res. 2009 ;69:5383-91.

Rebmann V, Schütt P, Brandhorst D, Opalka B, Moritz T, Nowrousian MR, Grosse-Wilde H.Soluble MICA as an independent prognostic factor for the overall survival and progression-free survival of multiple myeloma patients. Clin Immunol 2007; 123:114-20.

Ritgen M, Böttcher S, Stilgenbauer S, Bunjes D, Schubert J, Cohen S, Humpe A, Hallek M, Kneba M, Schmitz N, Döhner H, Dreger P; German chronic lymphocytic leukaemia

Study Group. Quantitative MRD monitoring identifies distinct GVL response patterns after allogeneic stem cell transplantation for chronic lymphocytic leukemia: results from the Gchronic lymphocytic leukaemiaSG chronic lymphocytic leukaemia3X trial. Leukemia. 2008;22:1377–1386.

Robak T, Moiseev SI, Dmoszynska A, Solal-Céligny P, Warzocha K, Loscertales J et al. Rituximab, Fludarabine, and Cyclophosphamide (R-FC) Prolongs Progression Free Survival in Relapsed or Refractory Chronic Lymphocytic Leukemia (chronic lymphocytic leukaemia) Compared with FC Alone: Final Results from the International Randomized Phase III REACH Trial. Blood. ASH Annual Meeting Abstracts. 2008; 112 (11):1.

Rollins BJ. Inflammatory chemokines in cancer growth and progression. Eur J Cancer 2006;42:760-7.

Rondón G, Giralt S, Huh Y, Khouri I, Andersson B, Andreeff M, Champlin R. Graft-versus-leukemia effect after allogeneic bone marrow transplantation for chronic lymphocytic leukemia. Bone Marrow Transplant. 1996 Sep;18(3):669-72.

Rossi E, Matutes E, Morilla R, Owusu-Ankomah K, Heffernan AM, Catovsky D. Zeta chain and CD28 are poorly expressed on T lymphocytes from chronic lymphocytic leukemia. Leukemia. 1996;10:494-7.

Salih HR, Antropius H, Gieseke F, Lutz SZ, Kanz L, Rammensee HG, Steinle A. Functional expression and release of ligands for the activating immunoreceptor NKG2D in leukemia. Blood 2003; 102:1389-1396.

Salih HR, Rammensee HG, Steinle A. Cutting edge: down-regulation of MICA on human tumors by proteolytic shedding. J Immunol 2002; 169:4098-4102.

Scanlan MJ, Simpson AJ, Old LJ. The cancer/testis genes: review, standardization, and commentary. Cancer Immun 2004;4:1.

Schetelig J, Thiede C, Bornhauser M, et al. Evidence of a graft-versus-leukemia effect in chronic lymphocytic leukemia after reduced-intensity conditioning and allogeneic stem-cell transplantation: the Cooperative German Transplant Study Group. J Clin Oncol 2003;21(14):2747-2753.

Schetelig J, van Biezen A, Brand R, et al. Allogeneic hematopoietic cell transplantation for chronic lymphocytic leukemia with 17p deletion: a retrospective EBMT analysis. J Clin Oncol. 2008;5094–5100.

Sher T, Miller KC, Lawrence D, Whitworth A, Hernandez-Ilizaliturri F, CzuczmanMS, Miller A, Lawrence W, Bilgrami SA, Sood R, Wood MT, Block AW, Lee K, Chanan-Khan AA. Efficacy of lenalidomide in patients with chronic lymphocytic leukemia with high-risk cytogenetics. Leuk Lymphoma. 2010;51(1):85-8.

Siddiqui M, Ristow K, Markovic SN, Witzig TE, Habermann TM, Colgan JP, et al. Absolute lymphocyte count predicts overall survival in follicular lymphomas. Br J Haematol. 2006;134:596-601.

Smyth MJ, Dunn GP, Schreiber RD. Cancer immunosurveillance and immunoediting: the roles of immunity in suppressing tumor development and shaping tumor immunogenicity. Adv Immunol. 2006;90:1-50.

Sorror ML, Maris MB, Sandmaier BM, et al. Hematopoietic cell transplantation after nonmyelo-ablative conditioning for advanced chronic lymphocytic leukemia. J Clin Oncol 2005;23(16):3819-3829.

Sorror ML, Storer BE, Sandmaier BM, Maris M, Shizuru J, Maziarz R, Agura E, Chauncey TR, Pulsipher MA, McSweeney PA, Wade JC, Bruno B, Langston A, Radich J, Niederwieser D, Blume KG, Storb R, Maloney DG. Five-year follow-up of patients with advanced chronic lymphocytic leukemia treated with allogeneic hematopoietic cell transplantation after nonmyeloablative conditioning. J Clin Oncol. 2008;26(30):4912-20.

Steurer M, Pall G, Richards S, Schwarzer G, Bohlius J, Greil R. Purine antagonists for chronic lymphocytic leukaemia. Cochrane database of systematic reviews (Online) 2006; 3: CD004270.

Swann JB, Smyth MJ. Immune surveillance of tumors. J Clin Invest. 2007;117(5):1137-46.

Tam CS, O'Brien S, Wierda W, Kantarjian H, Wen S, Do KA, Thomas DA, Cortes J, Lerner S, Keating MJ. Long-term results of the fludarabine, cyclophosphamide, and rituximab regimen as initial therapy of chronic lymphocytic leukemia. Blood. 2008;112(4):975-80.

Taskinen M, Ranki A, Pukkala E, Jeskanen L, Kaitila I, Makitie O. Extended follow-up of the Finnish cartilage-hair hypoplasia cohort confirms high incidence of non-Hodgkin lymphoma and basal cell carcinoma. Am J Med Genet A 2008;146A(18):2370-2375.

Teeling JL, French RR, Cragg MS, van den Brakel J, Pluyter M, Huang H, Chan C, Parren PW, Hack CE, Dechant M, Valerius T, van de Winkel JG, Glennie MJ. Characterization of new human CD20 monoclonal antibodies with potent cytolytic activity against non-Hodgkin lymphomas. Blood. 2004;104(6):1793-800.

Totterman TH, Carlsson M, Simonsson B, Bengtsson M, Nilsson K. T-cell activation and subset patterns are altered in B-chronic lymphocytic leukaemia and correlate with the stage of the disease. Blood. 1989;74:786-92.

Vajdic CM, Mao L, van Leeuwen MT, Kirkpatrick P, Grulich AE, Riminton S. Are antibody deficiency disorders associated with a narrower range of cancers than other forms of immunodeficiency? Blood. 2010;116(8):1228-34.

Velardi A. Natural Killer cells and allogeneic haematopoietic cell transplantation. Natural Killer cells. Basic science and clinical application. London 2010, Pag543-53.

Wierda W, O'Brien S, Wen S, Faderl S, Garcia-Manero G, Thomas D, Do KA, Cortes J, Koller C, Beran M, Ferrajoli A, Giles F, Lerner S, Albitar M, Kantarjian H,Keating M. Chemoimmunotherapy with fludarabine, cyclophosphamide, and rituximabfor relapsed and refractory chronic lymphocytic leukemia. J Clin Oncol. 2005;23(18):4070-8.

Wierda WG, Kipps TJ. Chronic lymphocytic leukemia. Curr Opin Hematol. 1999;6:253-61.

Wu L, Adams M, Carter T, Chen R, Muller G, Stirling D, Schafer P, Bartlett JB. Lenalidomide enhances natural killer cell and monocyte-mediated antibody-dependent cellular cytotoxicity of rituximab-treated CD20+ tumor cells. Clin Cancer Res. 2008;14(14):4650-7.

Zent CS, Chen JB, Kurten RC, Kaushal GP, Lacy HM, Schichman SA. Alemtuzumab (CAMPATH 1H) does not kill chronic lymphocytic leukemia cells in serum free medium. Leuk Res. 2004;28(5):495-507.

Zent CS, Kay NE. Autoimmune complications in chronic lymphocytic leukaemia. Best Pract Res Clin Haematol. 2010;23(1):47-59.

# 4

# Interactions of the Platinum(II) Complexes with Nitrogen- and Sulfur-Bonding Bio-Molecules in Chronic Lymphocytic Leukemia

Jovana Bogojeski, Biljana Petrović and Živadin D. Bugarčić*
*University of Kragujevac, Faculty of Science, Department of Chemistry*
*Serbia*

## 1. Introduction

Transition metals and their reactions are in general important in the environment, in technical processes (catalysis, extraction and purification of metal complexes) and in biology and medicine (biological electron transfer, toxicology and use of metal complexes as drugs). Moreover, nonessential metal ions are very often used in biological systems either for therapeutic application or as diagnostic aids. For instance, metal complexes have been used for the treatment of many diseases (cancer, arthritis, diabetes, Alzheimer, *etc.*), but with little understanding of their mechanism of action in biological systems.(Ronconi & Sadler, 2007; Bruijnincx & Sadler, 2009) Biochemical studies have not clearly established the molecular basis for the activity and mechanism of action. The growing field of bioinorganic chemistry is presently dealing with the clarification of the mechanisms of action of metal complexes in biological systems.(Ronconi & Sadler,2007; Bruijnincx & Sadler, 2009; Jakupec et al., 2008)

Research in the area of application of metal complex compounds in medicine began with the discovery of antitumor properties of cisplatin. (Rosenberg, 1965, 1967, 1969, 1970) Today cisplatin is in routine use as therapeutics worldwide. Following the success of cisplatin a large number of analogous compounds were synthesized. All these compounds have a several common characteristics:

1.  bifunctional complex compounds with *cis*-geometry
2.  $PtX_2(amin)_2$ is general formula of this compounds, where $X_2$ are two labile monodentate or one labile bidentate ligand, and $(amine)_2$ are inert nitrogen-donor ligands
3.  nitrogen-donor ligands have to contain at least one NH bond.

Despite the large number of synthesized compounds only a few of them entered the medicinal use and most are still in preclinical investigation. (Jakupec et al., 2003; Reedijk, 2009) At the Fig. 1. are presented some of platinum complexes that are in the medicinal use worldwide.

Chronic lymphocytic leukemia is the most frequent type of leukemia and it accounts for approximately 25% of all leukemias. (Chiorazzi et al., 2005) Although at the present there is no curative treatment, combinations of cytotoxic agents and of immunotherapies that generate high complete remission rates hold promise for altering the natural history of this disease. (Wierda et al., 2005) Fludarabine (9-beta-D-arabinofuranosyl-2-fluoroadenine 5′-phosphate) is the most effective purine nucleoside analogue for the treatment of indolent lymphoproliferative disorders, including Chronic lymphocytic leukemia, low-grade lymphoma, and prolymphocytic leukemia. (Eichhorst et al., 2005)

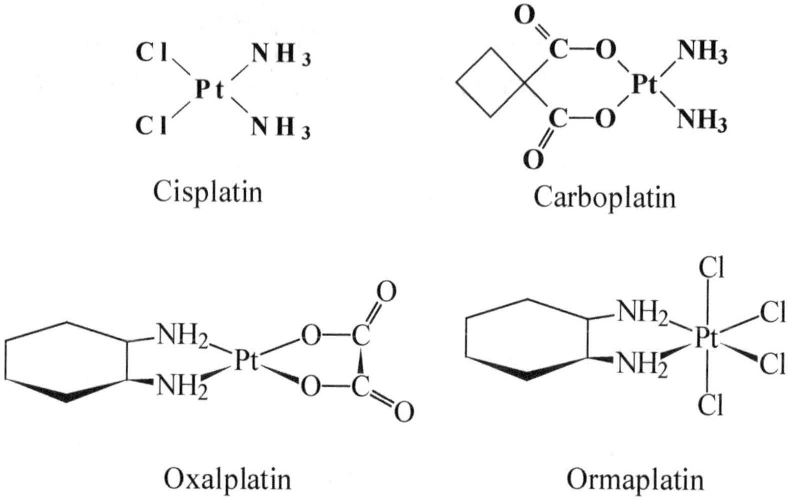

Cisplatin

Carboplatin

Oxalplatin

Ormaplatin

Fig. 1. The structures of some platinum complexes which are in clinical use worldwide.

The studies show that among the best drugs in the treatment of Chronic lymphocytic leukemia are the combination of Pt(II) complexes (cisplatin and oxaliplatin) and alkylating agents and nucleoside analogues such as fluradabine. (Zecevic et al., 2011) The nonoverlapping side effect profiles of oxaliplatin and fludarabine and their different but potentially complementary mechanisms of action provide a basis for investigation of the activity of the drugs in combination. The rationale for combining oxaliplatin with fludarabine is based on preclinical data showing synergistic cytotoxicity between cisplatin in combination with the nucleoside. (Wang et al., 1991; Yamauchi et al., 2001)

Consequently, knowledge of the interaction of the different Pt(II) complexes and nitrogen- and sulfur-bonding bio-molecules, and the results obtained from *in vitro* studies of this type of interactions will help in finding of good antitumor drug for the treatment of many tumors including the Chronic lymphocytic leukemia. The main topic of this chapter will be to show the results obtained in numerous studies of the interactions of the potential antitumor Pt(II) complexes and different biomolecules.

Platinum(II) has a high affinity for sulphur, so after administrating Pt(II) complex in the human body there is a strong possibility for binding with sulphur-donor bio-molecules. Sulphur-donor bio-molecules are present in large amounts in the form of peptides, proteins and enzymes. Binding of platinum complexes with sulphur-donor bio-molecules are responsible for the occurrence of toxic effects. (Lippert, 1999; Reedijk, 1999) However, a certain amount of platinum complexes being bound to nitrogen-donor bio-molecules (amino acids or DNA). Today it is generally accepted that the anti-tumor activity of platinum drugs can be ascribed to interactions between the metal complex and DNA, primarily with the

Interactions of the Platinum(II) Complexes with Nitrogen- and Sulfur-Bonding Bio-Molecules in Chronic Lymphocytic Leukemia

77

genetic DNA, which is located in the nucleus. The interactions with mitochondrial DNA are less responsible for the antitumor activity of the platinum complexes. (Fuertes et al., 2003) When the Pt(II) complexe reach the DNA, the possibilities for coordination are different. Binding of Pt(II) complexes to DNA primarily occurs through the N7 atoms of guanine, while a binding to N7 and N1 of adenine and N3 of cytosine occurs in small amount. (Lippert, 1999; Reedijk, 1999) Since the DNA molecule containing a different sequence of purine and pyrimidine bases, it was found that with 60% represented the coordination of the type 1,2-(GPG), i.e., the coordination realizes *via* two molecules of guanosine-5'-monophosphate (5'-GMP), which are located on opposite strands of DNA. About 25% is represented by coordination of the type 1,2-(APG), i.e. coordination with adenosine-5'-monophosphate (5'-AMP) and 5'-GMP placed on opposite DNA strands. Other ways of coordinations (monofunctional binding of the type 1,3-(GPG), coordination *via* guanosine located on the same chain of DNA, etc.) are less frequent. On the Fig. 2. is shown the different ways of coordination of cisplatin to DNA. (Jakupec et al., 2003; Kozelka et al., 1999)

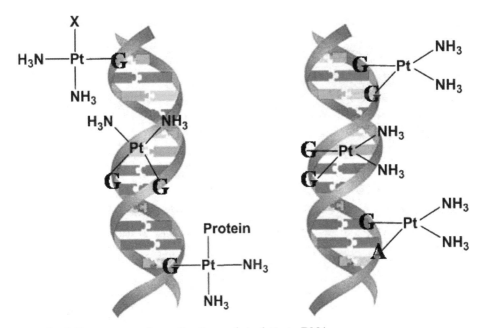

Fig. 2. The different ways of coordinations of cisplatin to DNA.

However, as noted above, the cells contain other bio-molecules which can also react with platinum complexes. High affinities for the platinum complexes show the bio-molecules that contain sulphur, as the thiols and the thioethars. Namely, Pt(II) as "soft" acid forms very stable compounds with sulphur donor ("soft" bases). The resulting compounds are responsible for the occurrence of toxicity (nephrotoxicity, neurotoxicity, resistance, etc.). Since the concentration of thiols, including glutathione (GSH) and L-cysteine, in intracellular liquid is about 10 mM, it is assumed that most of the platinum complex bound to sulphur before it comes to the molecules of DNA. (Jakupec et al., 2003; Reedijk, 2009; Lippert, 1999; Reedijk, 1999) Binding of platinum complexes to sulphur from thioethars are the kinetically favored process. The resulting Pt-S(thioethar) bond may be terminated in the presence of DNA, i.e. N7 atom of 5′-GMP can substitute the molecule of thioethar. (Reedijk, 1999; Soldatović & Bugarčić, 2005) For these reasons the compounds of the type Pt-S(thioethers) are believe to be the reservoirs of "platinum complexes" in the body, i.e. they are suitable intermediates in the reaction of Pt(II) complexes and DNA. Pt-S(thioethers) bond can be terminated in the presence of thiol molecules. The product of this substitution is thermodynamically stable. Also, Pt(II) complex can direct bind to sulphur from thiol molecules and the resulting Pt-S(thiol) bond is very stable and can not be easy broken. It is believed that compounds of the type Pt-S(thiol) are responsible for the occurrence of toxic effects during the use of Pt(II) complexes as anticancer reagents. The Pt-S(thiol) bond can be terminated in the presents of compounds known as "rescue agents", which are compounds with sulphur and they are very strong nucleophiles (diethyldithiocarbamate, thiourea, thiosulfate, GSH, cysteine, biotin, etc.). (Jakupec et al., 2003; Fuertes et al., 2003; Soldatović & Bugarčić, 2005)

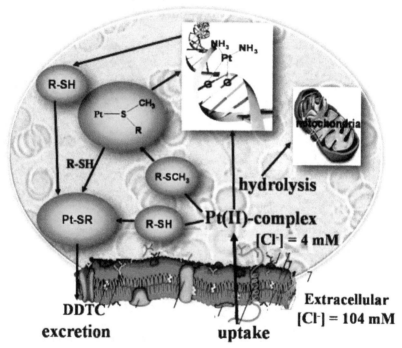

Scheme 1. Schematic presentation of the levels of action of cisplatin in the cell and possible biological consequences.

In recent years a much attention has given to studies of the antitumor activity of polynuclear Pt(II) complexes structurally similar to cisplatin.(Harris et al., 2005) The bridge ligand can be diamine ligands of the type $NH_2(CH_2)nNH_2$ (n = 6). (Mambanda et al., 2010) In the reaction with DNA primarily is obtained compound in which complex is bound simultaneously to both spirale. (Mambanda et al., 2010; Berners-Price et al., 2003) It was found that the presence of the hydrophobic part of the molecule enhances the absorption of these compounds on the cell membrane, where their activity decrease. Also, the polynuclear Pt(II)

Interactions of the Platinum(II) Complexes with Nitrogen- and Sulfur-Bonding Bio-Molecules in Chronic
Lymphocytic Leukemia

79

complexes with heterocyclic nitrogen compounds as bridge ligands were synthesized. (Lakomska et al., 2009)

Pt(IV) complexes are also very interesting. They react more slowly than the corresponding Pt(II) complexes.(Ali et al., 2005) It assumed that first Pt(IV) complexes by reduction translate to Pt(II) complexes and then the mechanism of action is the same as in the case of Pt(II) complexes. (Talman et al., 1997) For the reduction of Pt(IV) complexes can serve GSH, L-cysteine, L-methionine, DL-penicilamin (Lemma et al., 2000a) or ascorbic acid. (Lemma et al., 2000b)

Besides the already mentioned complexes of Pt(II), there are other platinum compounds such as $trans$-[PtCl$_2$(NH$_3$)$_2$] which does not show antitumor activity. (Jolley et al., 2001) These complexes were also intensively studied, (Natile & Coluccia, 2001) as well as some dinuclear complexes of $trans$-geometry. (Jansen et al., 2002) Special attention in recent years were given to the investigation of dinuclear complexes of platinum and paladium. (Mock et al., 2001)

## 2. Interaction of monofunctional Pt(II) complexes with sulphur- and nitrogen-donor bio-molecules

Monofunctional complexes of Pt(II) are a complexes which in structure contains a stable tridentate ligand, while the fourth coordination place is occupied with labile ligand, mostly chloride ligand. Because of this structure these complexes are not able to bind bifunctionaly to the DNA molecule. Accordingly to this monofunctional complexes of Pt(II) do not exhibit antitumor properties. However, one place for coordination greatly simplifies testing of substitution reactions of these complexes. For these reasons monofunctional complexes present model molecules for the study of interactions of Pt(II) complexes and bio-molecules which contain sulphur- and nitrogen-donor ligands.

Probably the greatest interest in examining substitution reactions of the monofunctional complexes are for complexes of general formula [Pt(NNN)X], where NNN represents a tridentate ligand coordinated $via$ three nitrogen donor atoms, while X is a labile ligand, usually chlorido ion. Most intensively studied compounds from this group are [Pt(dien)Cl]$^+$, where $dien$ is diethylentriamine or 1,5-diamino-3-azapentane, [Pt(bpma)Cl]$^+$, where $bpma$ is bis-(2-pyridylmethyl)amine, and [Pt(terpy)Cl]$^+$, where $terpy$ is (2,2':6',2''-terpyridine).

### 2.1 Interaction of [Pt(dien)Cl]$^+$ complex with sulphur- and nitrogen-donor bio- molecules

There are a large number of studies of substitution reactions of the [Pt(dien)Cl]$^+$ complex and his aqua analog, with different ligands and in different experimental conditions. This studies including investigations of the substitution reactions of the [Pt(dien)Cl]$^+$ complex with sulphur-donor ligands, especially with thiols and thioethers and nitrogen-donor ligands.

In the substitution reactions of [Pt(dien)Cl]$^+$ with GSH it was observed that substitution process depends on the pH value at which the reaction is studied. (Đuran et al. 1991; Bose et al., 1995; Tauben et al. , 2000; Petrović B. & Bugarčić, 2001) At pH > 7 as the only reaction product are obtained mononuclear complexes [Pt(dien)GS]$^+$, while at pH < 7 a binuclear complex [{Pt(dien)$_2$GS}]$^{3+}$ with GSH as the bridging ligand forms. Also, the process of substitution is followed by deprotonation of GSH, which is observed in the reactions of other Pt(II) complexes with thiols. (Bugarčić & Đorđević, 1998) When the ligand is thioetar, S-methyl-glutathione, reactions are much faster, but the product with thiol is thermodynamically more stable. (Tauben et al., 2002) Comparing the values of rate constants of substitution reactions of [Pt(dien)Cl]$^+$ complexes with different thiols and thioethers, (Tauben et al. , 2000; Petrović B. & Bugarčić, 2001; Bugarčić & Đorđević, 1998; Lampers & Reedijk, 1990) it was noted a discrepancy of GSH compared to other thiols. GSH is a tripeptide that contains an unusual peptide linkage between the amine group of L-cysteine (which is attached by normal peptide linkage to a L-glycine) and the carboxyl group of the glutamate side-chain, with a L-cysteine molecule at the center. It was assumed that the substitution process was much slower compared to L-cysteine. However, the experimentally obtained values showed a much higher reactivity of GSH. This is explained by a suitable geometrical structure of molecules, which cause the formation of intramolecular hydrogen bond involving the proton from the thiol groups, resulting in significantly increased nucleophelicity of the sulphur atoms and therefore higher reactivity. (Bugarčić et al., 2004a; Petrović B. & Bugarčić, 2001; Bugarčić & Đorđević, 1998)

During the substitution reaction of the [Pt(dien)Cl]$^+$ complexes with L-methionine (Petrović B. & Bugarčić, 2001; Lampers & Reedijk, 1990; Barnham et al. , 1994) as a reaction product primarily has been formed complex [Pt(dien)(L-methionine)]$^{2+}$. It was noted that only in very acidic solutions (pH < 1) there is a possibility for protonation of the terminal amino groups of *dien* ligand, which leads to the opening of one chelate ring and the creation of *S,N*-chelat. (Chen et al., 1998) Reaction between [Pt(dien)Cl]$^+$ complexes and L-methionine was studied in the presence of 5'-GMP, assuming the existence of competition of this two ligands.(Lampers & Reedijk, 1990; Soldatović & Bugarčić, 2005) The [Pt(dien)Cl]$^+$ first reacts with L-methionine and form [Pt(dien)(L-methionine)]$^{2+}$ product. Then 5'-GMP molecule coordinated to Pt(II) by substitution of coordinated L-methionine forming thermodynamically more stable [Pt(dien)(N7-GMP)]$^{2+}$ complex.

INO, 5'-IMP and 5'-GMP can coordinate to metal ions *via* N1 and N7. (Arpalahti & Lehikoinen, 1990; Arpalahti & Lippert, 1990; Caradonna & Lippard, 1988; Bose et al., 1986; Martin, 1999) Under pH = 2.5 only the N7 position of INO, 5'-IMP and 5'-GMP will be free for coordination to the central metal atom, since at this pH the N1 position is protonated. (Sigel et al., 1994) Binding through the N7 position in a neutral or weakly acidic medium has been verified. (Bugarčić et al., 2004a) 5'-GMP is more reactive toward Pt(II) complexes than either INO or 5'-IMP. Furthermore, the pH at which anti-tumor complexes bind to DNA is significantly higher than this one. It is expected that at neutral pH the phosphate residue on the nucleotide will also bind to the central metal atom as a result of its deprotonation. (Jacobs et al., 1992)

From a comparison of the reactivity of GSH or L-methionine with INO, 5'-IMP and 5'-GMP in the reaction with [Pt(dien)(H$_2$O)]$^{2+}$, [Pt(dien)Cl]$^+$ and [Pt(dien)Br]$^+$ (Soldatović & Bugarčić, 2005) can be concluded that these N-bonding ligands are good nucleophiles. This small difference in the reactivity of N-bondining (INO, 5'-IMP and 5'-GMP) and S-bonding nucleophiles (GSH and L-methionine) is not usually. The complex formation reactions have been studied at pH 2.5 were GSH and L-methionine are protonated. On the other hand, at pH 2.5, N7 sites of N-bonding ligands are not protonated. However, at

Interactions of the Platinum(II) Complexes with Nitrogen- and Sulfur-Bonding Bio-Molecules in Chronic
Lymphocytic Leukemia

81

neutral pH, although less than 10% of thiols are deprotonated, the N-bonding ligand cannot compete with the thiols. The second-order rate constant for GSH is $10^2$ times higher than for the 5′-GMP. (Bugarčić et al., 2004b) Also, from obtained results, (Soldatović & Bugarčić, 2005) could be concluded that L-methionine is the best nucleophile for the Pt(II) complexes. This could be explaining by positive inductive effect of the methyl group on the sulphur. However, this is in agreement with the previous results. (Petrović B. & Bugarčić, 2001)

Competitive reactions of [Pt(dien)Cl]+ with L-methionine and 5′-GMP demonstrated initially rapid formation of [Pt(dien)(L-methionine)]$^{2+}$ followed by displacement of L-methionine by 5′-GMP. In the later stages the concentration of [Pt(dien)(N7-GMP)]$^{2+}$ is predominant. (Soldatović & Bugarčić, 2005)

The reactions of [Pt(dien)Cl]+ (10 mM) with L-methionine and 5′-GMP in a molar ratio: [Pt(dien)Cl]+: L-methionine : 5′-GMP = 1:1:3 were also studied. (Soldatović & Bugarčić, 2005)

In the initial stage of the reactions (< 40 h) $^1$H NMR peak for the free L-methionine (d 2.142 ppm) decrease in the intensity and new peak of the [Pt(dien)(L-methionine)]$^{2+}$ appeared in the spectrum (d 2.544 ppm), whereas a little of the 5′-GMP reacted. In the later stages (72 h), the peaks for the bounded L-methionine and free 5′-GMP (d 8.208 ppm) decreased in intensity, whereas those for free L-methionine increased in intensity, as did those assignable to bound 5′-GMP in [Pt(dien)(N7-GMP)]$^{2+}$ (d 8.624 ppm) as shown in Fig. 3

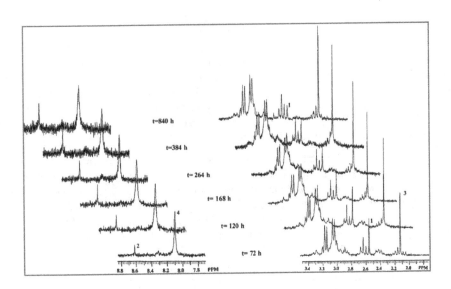

Fig. 3. $^1$H NMR spectra of the reactions of [Pt(dien)Cl]+ (10 mM) with mixture of L-methionine and 5′-GMP in the ratio 1:1:3 (where 1 is the signal for the [Pt(dien) (L-methionineh)]$^{2+}$, 2 is the signal for the [Pt(dien)(N7-GMP)]$^{2+}$, 3 is the signal for the free L-methionine and 4 is the signal for the free 5′-GMP. (Soldatović & Bugarčić, 2005)

Moreover, Pt–thioether adducts are more easily converted into Pt–thiolate adduct than Pt–N7–GMP adduct. (Teuben et al., 2000) On the other hand, it has been known that 5'-GMP cannot substitute thiols from Pt–thiolate adduct. (Bugarčić et al., 2004a) These findings could have implications for the mechanism of action of platinum anticancer drugs. Sulphur-bonding ligands have a much higher affinity for Pt(II) complexes than nitrogen-bonding ligands. (Bugarčić et al., 2004a; Bugarčić et al., 2002a) Moreover, nephrotoxicity has been explained by the formation of Pt-S(GSH) aduct.

Product in reactions of the [Pt(dien)Cl]+ complexes with thioethers or nucleotides in the presence of glutathione is a very stable complexes of the type [Pt(dien)SG]+, which confirms the fact that the Pt-S(thiol) bond is the most stable. (Bose et al., 1995) The Pt-S(thiol) bond can be terminated only in the presence of certain nucleophiles with sulphur, such as diethyldithiocarbamate, thiosulphate, thiourea. (Bugarčić et al., 2004a) Interesting is attempt to hydrolysed Pt-S(GSH) bond in the presence of transition metal ions Cu(II) and Zn(II). (Cheng & Pai, 1998)

## 2.2 Interaction of [Pt(terpy)Cl]+ complex with sulphur- and nitrogen-donor bio-molecules

In addition, [Pt(terpy)Cl]+ complex was also extensively studied. [Pt(terpy)Cl]+ complex has some biological activity. (Becker et al., 2001) In square-planar planes it contains tridentate-coordinated terpyridine system (terpy = 2,2':6',2''-terpyridine), while the fourth coordination site occupies chloro ligand.

Tridentate-coordinated terpyridine system, because of the presence of the aromatic pyridine unit and because of their bulkiness, strongly affects on the characteristics of this complex. In fact, [Pt(terpy)Cl]+ complex is much more reactive than complex with *dien* ligand. (Hofmann et al., 2003) The obtained values for lengths of chemical bonds between the platinum(II) and three nitrogen donor atoms of terpyridine system show that the shortest connection is to the secondary nitrogen atom. This feature is certainly reflected on its reactivity in the processes of substitution. In addition, the presence of electrostatic interactions between the pyridine units and metal ions has been observed in crystal structures of various Pt-terpy complexes. (Bailey et al., 1995)

Although the high reactivity of the complex depend on the electronic interactions between the terpyridine system and Pt(II), (Hofmann et al., 2003) bulkiness of the *terpy* ligand has great influence on the characteristics of this complex. The substitution reactions of the [Pt(terpy)Cl]+ complexes with different thioethers has been confirmed that there is no reaction, (Petrović B. et al., 1999; Bugarčić et al., 1997) which can be attributed to the strong steric effect. Although, the reactions of [Pt(terpy)Cl]+ complexes with some S-methyl-thioethers and thiones may occur, but in this case as the product of reactions appear dinuclear platinum complexes in which the bridge ligand is S-methyl-group. (Annibale et al., 1999) High reactivity of the [Pt(terpy)Cl]+ complex in substitution reactions with thiols is explained by formation of intramolecular hydrogen bonds between protons from the thiol-group and outgoing chloro ligand, which further stabilizes the transition state. (Annibale et al., 1998; Petrović B. et al., 1999; Bugarčić et al., 1997)

In the reaction between biologically relevant ligands and Pt(II) complexes, DNA fragments usually coordinated through the N7 atom to Pt(II). (Bugarčić et al., 2004b) Several products

Interactions of the Platinum(II) Complexes with Nitrogen- and Sulfur-Bonding Bio-Molecules in Chronic
Lymphocytic Leukemia

83

of the reaction between [Pt(terpy)Cl]$^+$ complex and DNA fragments were synthesized and characterized by X-ray analysis, in which the presence of strong intramolecular hydrogen bonds are observed. The role of these bonds are to further stabilizes the products of the reaction. (Wong & Lippard, 1977)

The kinetics of the complex-formation reactions between [Pt(terpy)H$_2$O]$^{2+}$, with thiols: L-cysteine, DL-penicillamine, GSH, and with thiourea were studied. (Bugarčić et al., 2002a) Rate constants and activation parameters derived from these experiments are summarized in Table 1.

| L | $k_1^{298}$/M$^{-1}$ s$^{-1}$ | $\Delta H^{\neq}$/kJ mol$^{-1}$ | $\Delta S^{\neq}$/J K$^{-1}$ mol$^{-1}$ | $\Delta V^{\neq}$/cm$^3$ mol$^{-1}$ |
|---|---|---|---|---|
| L-Cysteine | 37.8 ± 0.1 | 25 ± 0.5 | –132 ± 2 | –9.3 ± 0.4 |
| L-Glutathione | (5.8 ± 0.1)×10$^2$ | 23 ± 1 | –116 ± 3 | –12.4 ± 0.6 |
| DL-Penicillamine | 12.8 ± 0.1 | 38 ± 1 | –98 ± 3 | –20.6 ± 1.0 |
| Thiourea | (1.72 ± 0.02)×10$^5$ | 22 ± 1$^b$ | –73 ± 1$^b$ | –6.0 ± 0.3$^b$ |

$^a$All values refer to 0.10 M HClO$_4$(Bugarčić et al., 2002a) $^b$ Data from Jaganyi et al., 2001

Table 1. Rate constants and activation parameters for the reaction of [Pt(terpy)H$_2$O]$^{2+}$ with thiols and thiourea.

From Table 1. can be seen that although the thiol ligands are good entering groups for the Pt(II) complex, thiourea is the best nucleophile. From a comparison of the thiols used, it can be concluded that the variation in size, bulkiness and salvation of the entering ligands reflect in their properties as nucleophiles. The difference in nucleophilicity of the selected ligands is obvious and their reactivity follows the order; DL-penicillamine < L-cysteine < GSH < thiourea. The sensitivity of the reaction rate towards the σ-donor properties of the entering ligands is in line with that expected for an associative mode of activation. In addition, steric effects are very important as well. For example, DL-penicillamine has the lowest reactivity of the thiols used. This can be attributed to the steric effects involving the two methyl groups on carbon near the sulphur atom. At the same time, GSH is considerably more reactive than expected. This anomaly seems to suggest an appreciable anchimeric effect capable of reducing the activation energy of the substitution reaction, arising from hydrogen bonding interactions between the acidic group located in a suitable position of the nucleophile. The anchimeric effect has been reported for other reactions at Pt(II) complexes and is well known for organic reactions. (Wilkins, 1991) This clearly demonstrates that the versatile kinetic behaviour is controlled by steric hindrance on the tridentate ligand and the nucleophilicity of the entering nucleophiles. Increasing steric hindrance is expected to slow down the ligand substitution reactions, whereas increasing nucleophilicity is expected to speed up this process in terms of an associative mechanism.

A trigonal bipyramidal transition state for reaction of [Pt(terpy)H$_2$O]$^{2+}$ with thiols, is probably stabilized by hydrogen bonding between the entering thiol and the leaving water ligand as already proposed for the reaction of [Pd(H$_2$O)$_4$]$^{2+}$ with monodentate acetate, propionate, glycolate, and carboxylic acids (Shi & Elding, 1996, 1997) and for [Pt(H$_2$O)$_4$]$^{2+}$ with thioglycolic acid. (Bugarčić & Đorđević, 1998) These findings indicate that bond-making with the entering thiol is important in the activation process and that water is still tightly bound to the metal centre in the transition state.

Also, the reactions between [Pt(terpy)Cl]$^+$ and thiols, such as GSH, L-cysteine, DL-penicillamine and thioglycolic acid have been studied. (Petrović B. et al., 1999) These thiols are very good entering groups for Pt(II) complex. The reaction of the Pt(II) complex and DL-pencillamine is also the slowest one (Table 2.).

The complex [Pt(terpy)Cl]$^+$ appears to be more reactive than [Pt(dien)Cl]$^+$ (Table 2.) in accordance with the greater possibility of π-interaction and π-*trans* effect probably operating as well. The Pt-N distance to the middle nitrogen atom of the terpyridine ligand, 1.930(4) A is slightly shorter than the distances of Pt to the other two nitrogen atoms, N1, 2.018(5) and N3 2.030(5). (Hofmann et al., 2003)

| | $k_2/M^{-1}s^{-1}$ [Pt(dien)Cl]$^+$ | $k_2/M^{-1}s^{-1}$ [Pt(terpy)Cl]+ |
|---|---|---|
| Thiglycolic acid | $7.86 \times 10^{-3}$ | $5.62 \times 10^{-2}$ |
| L-Cysteine | $1.43 \times 10^{-3}$ | $1.06 \times 10^{-2}$ |
| D-penicillamine | $8.04 \times 10^{-4}$ | $6.02 \times 10^{-3}$ |
| Glutathione | $3.85 \times 10^{-3}$ | $7.77 \times 10^{-2}$ |

Table 2. The second-order rate constants for the reactions between thiols and Pt(II) complexes at T = 295 K. (Petrović B. et al., 1999)

As in the case of [Pt(dien)H$_2$O]$^{2+}$, the kinetic data clearly show that 5′-GMP is more reactive to [Pt(terpy)H$_2$O]$^{2+}$ than either INO and 5′-IMP in 0.1 M NaClO$_4$ and at pH = 2.5. (Bugarčić et al., 2004a) On the contrary, in the reactions of [Pd(SMC)(H$_2$O)$_2$]$^{2+}$ with the same nucleophiles, (Bugarčić et al., 2002b) the most reactive one was INO, which can be attributed to a primary process that involves partial preassociation of the metal complex with the phosphate group in 5′-GMP and 5′-IMP. Furthermore, the pH at which antitumour complexes bind to DNA is significantly higher than used in this study. It is expected that at neutral pH the phosphate residue on the nucleotide will also bind to the central metal atom as a result of its deprotonation. (Jacobs et al., 1992) From a comparison of the reactivity of thiols (L-cysteine, DL-penicillamine and GSH) (Bugarčić et al., 2002a), with INO, 5′-IMP and 5′-GMP in the reaction with [Pt(terpy)H$_2$O]$^{2+}$, it can be concluded that these N-bonding ligands are even better nucleophiles than the mentioned thiols. The preference of these N-bonding nucleophiles over thiols in acidic solutions needs to be addressed. It must be kept in mind that the reactions with thiols have been investigated at pH 1, where all thiols were protonated. On the other hand, at pH 2.5 the N7 sites of INO, 5′-IMP and 5′-GMP are not protonated. However, at or near neutral pH, although less than 10% of thiols are deprotonated, the N-bonding bases cannot compete with the thiol containing amino acids and peptides. (Bose et al., 1995; Volckova et al., 2002) Therefore, binding primarily takes place through the sulphur donor sites. However, for the GSMe system, rapid coordination to the sulphur atom followed by migration to the N7 site of the purine was observed. (Teuben et al., 1977) Similar competition experiments of the bifunctional platinum complex, *cis*-dichloro-(ethylendiamine)platinum(II) and its hydrolysed forms with a mixture of 5′-GMP or dGpG and thioether containing di- and tri-peptides, also afforded sulphur bound intermediates, followed by the formation of N7 coordinated guanine products. (Barnhham et al., 1996)

Interactions of the Platinum(II) Complexes with Nitrogen- and Sulfur-Bonding Bio-Molecules in Chronic
Lymphocytic Leukemia

85

Several sulphur donor ligands are usually co-administered with platinum drugs to reduce the toxicity. (Chen et al., 1998; Berners-Price et al., 1996) Some of them, such as GSH, DEDTC, thiosulfate and thiourea, were used in the study with [Pt(terpy)(cyst-$S$)]$^{2+}$ and [Pt(terpy)(gua-$N7$)]$^{2+}$ complexes. (Bugarčić et al., 2004a) The X-ray structure of the [Pt(terpy)(cyst-$S$)]$^{2+}$ and [Pt(terpy)(gua-$N7$)]$^{2+}$ complexes were determinated. (Bugarčić et al., 2004a)

The [Pt(terpy)(cyst-$S$)]$^{2+}$ complex is unreactive toward nitrogen binding ligands and cysteine cannot be replaced by N7 from INO, 5'-IMP and 5'-GMP. However, very strong sulphur-donor nucleophiles, such as DEDTC, thiosulfate and thiourea, could reverse the Pt–cysteine bond under pH *ca.* 6. (Bugarčić et al., 2004a) This results clearly show that therapeutic nucleophilic agents for platinum drugs, such as DEDTC, thiosulfate and thiourea, may help to displace Pt from Pt–cysteine adducts and in that way could reduce nephrotoxicity.

It is widely accepted that, once formed, the Pt–nucleobase complexes are inert under mild conditions and in the absence of strong *trans*-labilising ligands. (Lippert, 1999) In contrast, the presence of strong nucleophiles, for instance sulphur-containing bio-molecules, could facilitate the dissociation of N-coordinated nucleobases from the Pt(II) complex. In particular, various sulphur-containing molecules have aroused considerable interest owing to their important roles in the biological processing of anticancer platinum drugs. (Reedijk,1999) The substitution reactions of monofunctional [Pt(dien)(L-$N7$)]$^{2+}$ (L = adenosine or guanosine) with thiourea have been studied in acidic aqueous solution. (Mikola et al., 1999) The substitution of guanosine from [Pt(terpy)(guo-$N7$)]$^{2+}$ by some sulphur-donor nucleophiles which have been used as protecting agents were studied. (Bugarčić et al., 2004a) This result strongly indicate that all studied sulphur-donor nucleophiles could substitute guanosine from the Pt(II) complex. Also it is noticed that DEDTC and thiosulfate are the strongest nucleophiles and that these nucleophiles can very easily substitute guanosine from [Pt(terpy)(guo-$N7$)]$^{2+}$. However, the tripeptide GSH is a very efficient nucleophile as well. This observation could be very important since it is already known that GSH has numerous cellular functions, including the detoxification of chemotherapeutic agents. However, GSH has been used as protecting agent and administered before or after cisplatin. (Reedijk, 1999) Cisplatin readily reacts with GSH and as much as 67% of the administered platinum has been found to coordinate to GSH. However, the role of GSH appears to be dual: GSH deactivates and activates cisplatin. (Volckova et al., 2002) The higher effectiveness of cisplatin has also been demonstrated by co-administering cisplatin and GSH in patients. However, it is not clear whether this increase in effectiveness is due to the reduced toxicity or due to the modification of the platinum drug by binding to the metal. Currently there is much interest in the mechanisms responsible for the development of resistance. Such resistance is often associated with increased cellular GSH, consistent with the view that GSH protects cells against foreign compounds and the effects of radiation. (Jaganyi & Tiba, 2003) From our results we can conclude that the employed rescue or protecting agents such as thiourea, thiosulfate and DEDTC can much easier substitute guanosine than L-cysteine form the [Pt(terpy)X]$^{2+}$ complex (X is guo-$N7$ or cyst-$S$). This is in excellent agreement with previous investigations, where has been shown that the Pt-S (cysteine) bond is very stable. (van Boom et al., 1999; Teuben et al., 2000; Pitteri et al., 2001) The thiolate ion is capable of providing a stronger binding affinity owing to its better σ-donating ability. Such a Pt-S bond is considered relatively inert may cause the inhibition of the anticancer activity of platinum drugs.

The kinetics for the complex formation of the [Pt(terpy)Cl]$^+$ with 5'-GMP in the presence and absence of GSH at pH *ca.* 6, with a concentration ratio [Pt(terpy)Cl]$^+$ : GSH : 5'-GMP = 1 : 2 : 10 were studied. (Bugarčić et al., 2004b) The second order rate constants, obtained from linear least-squares analysis of the kinetic data (Bugarčić et al., 2004b) clearly point to a kinetic preference of [Pt(terpy)Cl]$^+$ toward the GSH at pH *ca.* 6. 5'-GMP is also a very good nucleophile for Pt(II) complexes, but at neutral pH cannot compete with GSH. The second-order rate constant for GSH is $10^2$ times higher than for 5'-GMP. This is also reflected in the competition reactions utilizing mixtures of GSH and GMP. Also, proton and $^{195}$Pt NMR data did not show any N7 coordination of GMP, in spite of its excess, in the presence of thiols. (Teuben et al., 2000) However, at or near neutral pH, although less than 10% of thiols are deprotonated, the N-bonding bases cannot compete with the thiol containing amino acids and peptides. (Bugarčić et al., 2004a; Teuben et al., 2000) Therefore, binding primarily takes place through the sulphur donor sites. However, for the GSMe system, rapid coordination to the sulphur atom followed by migration to the N7 site of the purine was observed. (van Boom et al., 1999; Barnham et al., 1994)

The progress of the reaction of [Pt(terpy)Cl]$^+$ with other compounds over extended periods of time can be monitored with techniques such as HPLC which allows aliquots separated from the reaction mixture at programmed times to be analyzed. The studied reactions were carried out in water, without any buffer, since buffer ions (*e.g.* phosphate) are potential ligands for Pt(II). The pH of each solution was regularly checked over the reaction time, and was shown to be kept between 4.5 and 5.5. The products formed were isolated by reversed-phase HPLC and characterized by MALDI-TOF mass spectrometry. As expected, the products obtained corresponded to the adducts [Pt(terpy)(GS)]$^+$ and [Pt(terpy)(5'-GMP)]$^+$ (*m/z* 734,2 and 789,8, respectively). The reaction between [Pt(terpy)Cl]$^+$, GSH and 5'-GMP was then followed by HPLC. The ratio of the three compounds in the repeated assays was 1:1:12, respectively. It was observed that [Pt(terpy)Cl]$^+$ reacted much faster with GSH than with 5'-GMP, but this did not prevent a small amount (< 16%) of [Pt(terpy)(5'-GMP)]$^+$ from being formed at the very beginning of the process. The relative proportion of this adduct remained virtually constant throughout the reaction process, which indicates that once formed it remains unaltered. The possibility that [Pt(terpy)(GS)]$^+$ reactes with the excess of 5'-GMP present in the reaction mixture to give [Pt(terpy)(5'-GMP)]$^+$ can be ruled out, unless GSH can replace 5'-GMP from [Pt(terpy)(5'-GMP)]$^+$ at the same reaction rate. The identity of the formed adducts was confirmed by mass spectrometric analysis of the products isolated from the reaction mixture by HPLC (Fig. 4.). (Bugarčić et al., 2004b)

## 2.3 Interaction of [Pt(bpma)Cl]$^+$ complex with sulphur- and nitrogen-donor bio-molecules

In recent years, an intensive investigation of the substitution reactions of Pt(II) complexes which containing an inert tridentate nitrogen donor ligand with two or three pyridine units was performed. The role of these studies is to explain the effect of present pyridine on the reactivity of these compounds. For example, the complex [Pt(bpma)Cl]$^+$, contains tridentate nitrogen donor ligand consisting of two pyridines connected *via* amide.

This complex in substitution reactions react faster than the [Pt(dien)Cl]$^+$ complex, but slower compared to [Pt(terpy)Cl]$^+$ complex. The substitution reactions of this complex with thiols. (Jaganyi & Tiba, 2003) pyridine, derivatives of pyridine (Pitteri et al., 2001), 5'-GMP, azoles

Interactions of the Platinum(II) Complexes with Nitrogen- and Sulfur-Bonding Bio-Molecules in Chronic
Lymphocytic Leukemia

87

and diazines (Bogojeski and Bugarčić, 2011) were studied. It is interesting that the aqua complex, $[Pt(bpma)(H_2O)]^{2+}$, which crystallizes with perchlorate as external ions, acts as a double base acid, because in the process of deprotonation the second stage involved coordinated amido group. (Pitteri et al., 2002)

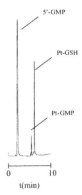

Fig. 4. HPLC profile of an aliquot of the reaction mixture [Pt(terpy)Cl]+/glutathione/5'-GMP = 1:1:12 after 1 week reaction time.

The substitution reactions of $[Pt(bpma)Cl]^+$ and $[Pt(bpma)(H_2O)]^{2+}$ with L-methionine, GSH and 5'-GMP were studied. (Bugarčić et al., 2007) The reactions of the chloro complexes were followed in the presence of 10 mM NaCl and at pH ≈ 5, whereas the reactions of the aqua complexes were studied at pH 2.5.The nucleophilic attack of these ligands occurs *via* the sulphur donor of the thioether group in the case of L-methionine and of the thiol group in the case of GSH. L-methionine appears to be a better nucleophile than GSH under these experimental conditions. This could be explained by the positive inductive effect of the methyl group on the sulphur donor. (Bugarčić et al., 2007)

Transformation from Pt–S(thioether) to Pt–N7(GMP) coordination seems to be common. (Reedijk, 1999; Soldatović & Bugarčić, 2005) To obtain more quantitative data for the stability differences between Pt–DNA and Pt–S(thioether) adducts, it was performed DFT calculations applying the model reaction (Eq. 1.) (L3 is terpy, bpma, dien, gly-met-S,N,N), where guanine approximates the guanosine-based interactions and $SR_2$ represents a generic thioether:

$$[L_3Pt\text{-}(N7\text{-guanine})]^{2+} + S(CH_3)_2 \longrightarrow [L_3Pt\text{-}S(CH_3)_2]^{2+} + guanine \qquad (1)$$

In all cases guanine coordination to the L3Pt fragment is much more favored than thioether coordination. As shown in Table 3.

The $[Pt(bpma)Cl]^+$ and $[Pt(bpma)(H_2O)]^{2+}$ complexes are more reactive than [PtCl(gly-met-S,N,N)] and [Pt(glymet-S,N,N)(H₂O)]+. This can be explained by the steric effect of the coordinated S–CH₃ group in the *cis* position in [Pt(gly-met-S,N,N)(H₂O)]+ and [PtCl(gly-met-S,N,N)]. Moreover, another reason for the higher reactivity of the [Pt(bpma)(H₂O)]²+ and [Pt(bpma)Cl]+ complexes is the presence of two pyridine rings in the coordination sphere. This has been studied in detail for a set of monofunctional Pt(II) complexes with tridentate ligands in which the number and position of the amine and pyridine groups were systematically varied. (Hofmann et al., 2003) The presence of π-acceptor ligands promotes the electrophilicity of the metal center and thereby the nucleophilic attack. (Hofmann et al., 2003; Jaganyi et al., 2001) This behavior distinguishes these complexes from classic platinum drugs where such effects are not present.

| $L_3$ | B3LYP/LANL2DZp | B3LYP(CPCM)/LANL2DZp// B3LYP/LANL2DZp |
|---|---|---|
| terpy | running (ca. 27 kcal/mol) | Still running kcal/mol |
| bpma | +28.7 kcal/mol | +12.8 kcal/mol |
| dien | +34.1 kcal/mol | +11.0 kcal/mol |
| Gly-Met-N,N,S | +21.5 kcal/mol | +9.5 kcal/mol |
| Gly-Met-N,N,S (without H-bond) | +17.5 kcal/mol | +8.5 kcal/mol |

Table 3. DFT results for model eq. (1)

[1]H NMR spectroscopy was used to investigate the substitution reactions of the chloro complexes [Pt(bpma)Cl][+] and [PtCl(gly-met-S,N,N)] with 5'-GMP. The substitution reactions were studied in $D_2O$ at 298 K. (Bugarčić et al., 2007)

The reaction of [PtCl(gly-met-S,N,N)] with 5'-GMP is approximately 50 times slower than the reactions of this complex with L-methionine or GSH. This could be accounted for in terms of steric effects of the incoming 5'-GMP and the complex as well. On the other hand, for the reactions with [Pt(bpma)Cl][+] the rate constants are of the same order of magnitude, but L-methionine is the best nucleophile and 5'-GMP is the poorest one. However, the [Pt(bpma)Cl][+] complex is much more reactive towards 5'-GMP than [PtCl(gly-met-S,N,N)]. (Bugarčić et al., 2007) This is in agreement with earlier published findings. (Volckova et al., 2002; Tauben et al., 2000)

Substitution reactions of the complex [Pt(bpma)($H_2O$)][2+] with TU, DMTU and TMTU $Cl^-$, $Br^-$, $I^-$ and $SCN^-$, were studied in aqueous 0.10 M $NaClO_4$ at pH 2.5. (Jaganyi et al., 2006) Based on the second order rate constants, $k_2$, it can be concluded that the reactivity of the nucleophiles towards the complex follows the order: TMTU < TU < DMTU. The observed trend for the platinum complex was also reported earlier in the literature for the substitution reactions of the coordinated water molecule from [Pt(dien)($H_2O$)][2+], [Pt(terpy)($H_2O$)][2+] and [Pt(bpma)($H_2O$)][2+] complexes. (Shoukry et al., 1998; Bugarčić et al., 2004c)

The observed trends can be attributed to the different structures (in terms of steric and inductive effects) of these three nucleophiles. The order of increasing steric hindrance for these nucleophiles is: TMTU < DMTU < TU. Theoretically, it would be expected that TU would react much faster than the other two nucleophiles. Instead, it turns out that DMTU is a much better nucleophile than TMTU and TU. This enhanced reactivity is due to the inductive effect introduced by the two methyl groups in the case of the DMTU, which over compensate the steric effect. (Jaganyi et al., 2006)

Interactions of the Platinum(II) Complexes with Nitrogen- and Sulfur-Bonding Bio-Molecules in Chronic
Lymphocytic Leukemia

89

## 3. Interaction of bifunctional Pt(II) complexes with sulphur- and nitrogen-donor bio-molecules

In order to achieve the best possible strategy in the designing of antitumor platinum complexes, it is necessary to know how mentioned compounds react with various sulfur- and nitrogen-donor bio-molecules. Significant information about these interactions were obtained from a number of studies implemented in *vitro*, among which are investigation of the substitution reactions of bifunctional platinum complexes with various bio-molecules at different conditions.

Cisplatin is most investigated bifunctional Pt(II) complex. (Redijk, 1999, 2009; Lippert, 1999) In details has been described how cisplatin coordinate to a molecule of DNA. (Redijk, 1999, Lippert, 1999) In addition to investigate the interaction with the classical nucleoside (Barry et al., 2005; Anzellotti et al., 2005) The interactions with AMP, ADP and ATP were investigated, and the best reactivity toward Pt(II) complexes showed to be ATP. (Arpalahti & Lehikoinen, 1990; Arpalahti & Lippert, 1990; Caradonna & Lippard, 1988; Bose et al., 1986; Martin, 1999) Also, the interactions of cisplatin with sulfur-donor bio-molecules, L-cysteine, GSH, L-methionine were studied. GSH is more reactive than L-cysteine. (Bugarčić et al., 2004a) In reactions with L-methionine, amino acid coordinates bidentate to platinum building $S,N$-chelate. If the amino acids is presented in excess the reaction may lead to the bidentate coordination of two molecules of amino acid for Pt(II)-ion. (Norman et al., 1992) The competitive reaction between cisplatin, L-methionine and 5'-GMP in the mixture were also examined. A predominant product is complex [Pt(NH$_3$)$_2$(N7-GMP)$_2$], while compounds [Pt(N,L-methionine)(N7-GMP)(NH$_3$)] and [Pt(N,L-methionine)$_2$] are formed in a very small concentrations. (Kung et al., 2001) The competitive reactions between 5'-GMP and thiols were also studied, but only found product where is platinum coordinated to sulphur from thiols. (Volckova et al., 2002) The reactions of cisplatin with 5'-GMP and GSH were studied spectrophotometricaly at 37 °C. NMR technique was also applied to study the reactions of cisplatin with guanosine-5'-monophosphate. (Petrović D. et al., 2007) The rate constants for the reactions of cisplatin with 5'-GMP, obtained by [1]H NMR experiments and obtained by Uv–Vis experiments, are in a good agreement. However, these results are in a good agreement with the published results. (Barnham et al., 1994)

Fig. 5. show [1]H NMR spectra of the reaction between cisplatin and 5'-GMP. The peak for the free 5'-GMP is at d 8.22 ppm, and for the product the peaks are at d 8.69 and at 8.71 ppm. The peak at 8.69 ppm is smaller than the peak at 8.71 ppm at the later stage of the reaction. (Petrović D. et al., 2007)

During the reaction the peak at 8.71 ppm, which corresponds to the product, [Pt(NH$_3$)$_2$Cl(N7-GMP)]$^+$, increased in intensity, while the peak for the free 5'-GMP (d 8.22 ppm) decreased in intensity. At the end of the reaction all 5'-GMP is coordinated to Pt(II), and the peak for the free 5'-GMP disappears as shown in Fig. 5.

The reactions of cisplatin with GSH were studied spectrophotometricaly, and it has been found that GSH is better nucleophile for cisplatin than 5'-GMP, (Petrović D. et al., 2007) what is also in agreement with previously published results. (Soldatović & Bugarčić, 2005; Hagrman et al., 2004)

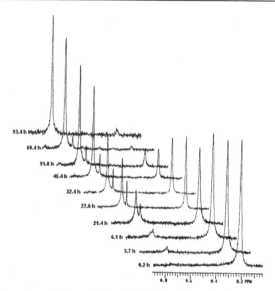

Fig. 5. ¹H HMR spectra of a solution of cisplatin (7.5 mM) and 5'-GMP (7.5 mM) in $D_2O$ at pH 7.4 and 298 K recorded as a function of time.

Substitution reactions of the complexes $cis$-[Pt(NH₃)₂Cl₂], [Pt(SMC)Cl₂]⁻, [Pt(en)Cl₂], and [Pt(dach)Cl₂], with selected biologically important ligands, $viz.$ 5'-GMP, L-histidine and 1,2,4-triazole, were studied. (Bogojeski et al., 2010) All reactions were studied in aqueous 25 mM Hepes buffer in the presence of 5 mM NaCl at pH = 7.2 under $pseudo$-first-order conditions as a function of concentration at 310 K by using Uv/Vis spectrophotometry. The substitution reactions were studied in the presence of 5 mM chloride to be close to the conditions in the cell where the concentration is ca. 4 mM. Two consecutive reaction steps, which both depend on the nucleophile concentration, were observed in all cases.

The most reactive N-donor nucleophile is 1,2,4 triazole. L-Histidine has the same order of reactivity as 5'-GMP and it is only slightly faster than 5'-GMP. The difference in the reactivity of these nucleophiles can be accounted in terms of electronic and steric effects. 5'-GMP is sterically more crowded than L-histidine and that can be the reason why the reactions with 5'-GMP are a bit slower. From a comparison of the values of the second-order rate constants for the first reaction step, $k_2$, it can be concluded that the order of reactivity of the complexes is: [Pt(SMC)Cl₂]⁻ > $cis$-[Pt(NH₃)₂Cl₂] > [Pt(en)Cl₂] > [Pt(dach)Cl₂]. The high reactivity of [Pt(SMC)Cl₂]⁻ can be attributed to the strong $trans$-labilization effect of the coordinated sulfur atom from the S-methyl-L-cysteine chelate. Such labilization has clearly been illustrated by an earlier study. (Bugarčić et al., 2004b) The reactivity of the complexes $cis$-[Pt(NH₃)₂Cl₂], [Pt(en)Cl₂] and [Pt(dach)Cl₂] depends on steric effects. The [Pt(dach)Cl₂] complex is the sterically most crowded one and the reactions are found to be slower than those with [Pt(en)Cl₂] and $cis$-[Pt(NH₃)₂Cl₂]. The reactions with [Pt(dach)Cl₂] were expected to be slower than those with [Pt(en)Cl₂], because the Pt(II) center should be less electrophilic due to the positive inductive effect of the cyclohexane ring. (Summa et al., 2006) The second step of the reaction are significantly slower than the reactions of the first step in all cases.

Interactions of the Platinum(II) Complexes with Nitrogen- and Sulfur-Bonding Bio-Molecules in Chronic
Lymphocytic Leukemia

91

Transformation from Pt–S(thioether) to Pt–N7(GMP) coordination seems to be common in biological processes. (Reedijk, 1999; Soldatović & Bugarčić, 2005; Jansen et al., 2002; van Boom et al., 1999; Tauben et al., 2000; Barnham et al., 1996) We performed quantum chemical calculations to gain more insight into this process. To obtain more quantitative data for the difference in stability between Pt–DNA and Pt–S(thioether) adducts, DFT calculations were performed.

In all cases guanine coordination to the fragments Pt(NH$_3$)$_2$, Pt(en) and Pt(dach) is much more favored than thioether coordination. For the first step in the gas phase Pt–N7(Gua) is more stable than Pt–S(thioether) by *ca.* 31–33 kcal/mol, and for the second step by 32–34 kcal/mol.

Finally, this result could be the first to clearly show how much the Pt–N7(Gua) adduct is more stable than the Pt–S(thioether) adduct. This is important since Pt–S(thioether) adducts have been postulated to be a drug reservoir for the binding of platinum to DNA, which may act as intermediates and then be transformed into Pt–N7(Gua) adduct. (Lippert, 1999; Reedijk, 1999; Jansen et al., 2002; van Boom et al., 1999; Jung & Lippard, 2007)

The kinetics and mechanism of ligand substitution reactions of [Pt(SMC)Cl$_2$] with biologically relevant ligands were studied as a function of chloride and nucleophile concentrations at pH 2.5 and 7.2. (Soldatović et al., 2009) It was observed that the slope and intercept obtained from the linear dependence of the observed rate constant on the nucleophile concentration strongly depend on the [Cl$^-$] for all the studied substitution reactions. At high [Cl$^-$], the rate constant for the forward reaction is almost zero and that for the back reaction follows the order: L-methionine > GSH ~ INO > 5'-GMP. Ion-pair formation between the positively charged Pt(II) complex and the chloride ion is suggested to account for the saturation kinetics observed for the back reaction.

At the highest [Cl$^-$] of 0.1 M the binding of the nucleophiles is drastically slowed down and almost completely suppressed. This will be the case during the transport of such anti-tumour complexes in blood. At low chloride concentrations as found in cells, effective binding of the studied nucleophiles will occur. The order of reactivity L-met > GSH ~ INO > 5'-GMP clearly shows the high affinity of the Pt(II) complex for thioether. These interactions are more favourable because the transformation from Pt–S(thioether) to Pt–N7 coordination was observed. (Soldatović & Bugarčić, 2005) In our earlier work we did not observe any measurable transformation from Pt–S(thiol) to Pt–N7 coordination. (Bugarčić et al., 2004b) The lower reactivity of 5'-GMP compared to INO can be explained by the fact that at pH 2.5 the N7 position of inosine is almost fully deprotonated whereas in 5'-GMP it is still partially protonated (N7 p$K$a = 2.33). (Bugarčić et al., 2004b) At pH = 7.2, it is possible that the 5'-monophosphate residue of the nucleotide (p$K$a a 6) binds to the metal center, which can lead to additional complications in the complex-formation at higher pH and slower second-order rate constants are obtained.

A set of three oxaliplatin derivatives containing 1,2-*trans*-R,R-diaminocyclohexane (dach) as a spectator ligand and different chelating leaving groups X–Y, *viz.*, [Pt(dach)(O,O-cyclobutane-1,1-dicarboxylate)], or Pt(dach)(CBDCA), [Pt(dach)(N,O-glycine)]$^+$, or Pt(dach)(gly), and [Pt(dach)(N,L-methioninehionine)]$^+$, or Pt(dach)(L-Met), where L-Met is L-methionine, were synthesized and the crystal structure of Pt(dach)(gly) was determined by X-ray diffraction. (Summa et al., 2007) The effect of the leaving group on the reactivity of the resulting Pt(II) complexes was studied for the nucleophiles thiourea, GSH and L-Met under *pseudo*-first-order conditions as a function of nucleophile concentration and temperature, using Uv–Vis spectrophotometric techniques. [1]H NMR spectroscopy was used to follow the substitution of the leaving group by guanosine 5′-monophosphate (5′-GMP[2-]). The rate constants for all reactions of direct substitution of the X–Y chelate by the selected nucleophiles, showing that the nature of the chelate, viz., O–O (CBDCA[2-]), N–O (glycine) or S–N(L-Met), respectively, plays an important role in the kinetic and mechanistic behavior of the Pt(II) complex.

The nature of the chelate, being O–O(CBDCA[2-]), N–O(glycine) or S–N(L-Met) was shown to play an important role in the kinetic and mechanistic behavior of the Pt(II) complexes. Pt(dach)(CBDCA) exhibits a higher reactivity towards the sulfur donor L-Met than Pt(dach)(gly), whereas the order is the opposite for the nitrogen donor 5′-GMP[2-] and the sulfur donors thiourea and GSH in the first reaction step. The Pt–N bond was always found to be very strong, especially for the reaction with 5′-GMP[2-], in which the 1:1 reaction product [Pt(N-gly)(N7-GMP)] is very stable and hardly (7%) reacts with another molecule of 5′-GMP[2-] to form the 1:2 product. By contrast, the liberation of H[2]CBDCA in Pt(dach)(CBDCA) in the second reaction step was faster than the rate-determining first reaction step and could not be analyzed under the selected experimental conditions. The mechanism of the substitution reactions is associative as supported by the large and negative values of $\Delta S^{\#}$.

Multinuclear complexes of platinum(II) represent a third generation of antitumor drugs as and platinum(IV) complexes. (Esposito & Najjar, 2002) The reason for the increasing interest in multinuclear complexes is their ability to form DNA adducts that differ significantly from those formed cisplatin and related complexes, (McGregor et al., 1999) which results in a completely different anti tumor behaviour. The biological activity of polynuclear platinum complexes maybe modulated by the geometry and number of leaving groups in the coordination sphere of platinum atoms as well as by the nature of linkers connecting the platinum centers. In contrast with the mononuclear complexes, such as antitumor cisplatin and clinically ineffective transplatin, in the dinuclear case both geometries are antitumor active. (Farrell, 2004)

We compared the cytotoxic capacity of platinum complexes (Fig. 6.) towards TOV21G, HCT 116 tumour human cell lines and human MSC, normal rapidly dividing cells (Fig. 7.). (Jovanović et al., 2011)

All complexes displayed a dose-dependent and time-dependent cytotoxicity towards the tested cell lines but the most cytotoxic effect showed towards TOV21G cells (Fig. 7). The complex [PtCl[4](dach)] at the lower concentrations induced significantly higher cytotoxic effect towards TOV21G cells then other four complexes.

HCT116 cells were more resistant to the cytotoxic effects of selected complexes (Fig. 7). Again, [PtCl[4](dach)] was the most efficient and exerted very similar activity towards HCT116 cells as cisplatin.

The complexes **Pt2** and **Pt3** displayed cytotoxicity towards MSC similar as cisplatin, but the other three complexes **Pt1**, [PtCl[4](dach)] and [PtCl[4](bipy)] were more toxic. (Jovanović et al., 2011)

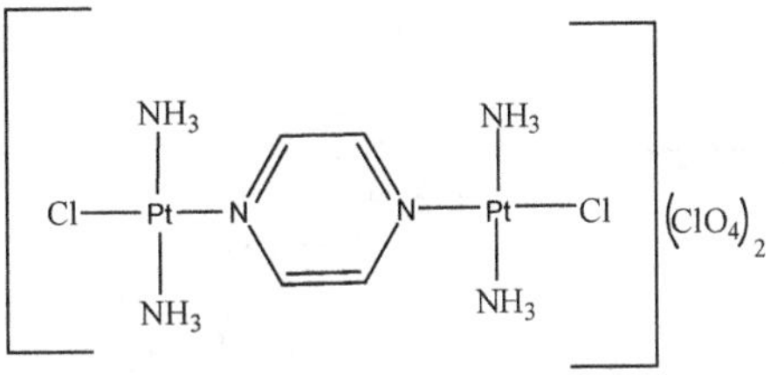

Interactions of the Platinum(II) Complexes with Nitrogen- and Sulfur-Bonding Bio-Molecules in Chronic
Lymphocytic Leukemia

93

[{*trans*-Pt(NH$_3$)$_2$Cl}$_2$($\mu$-pyrazine)](ClO$_4$)$_2$, **Pt1**

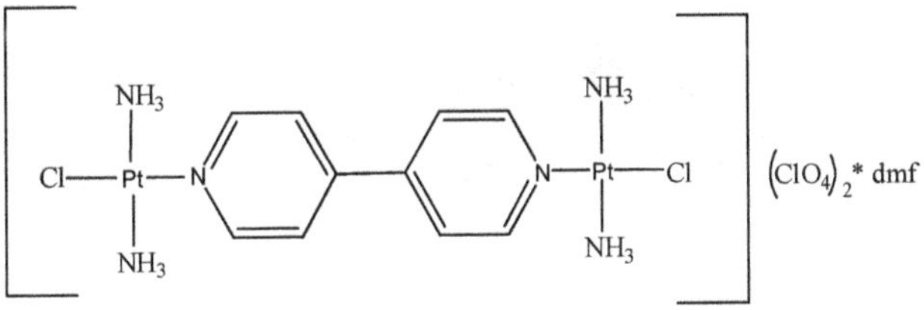

[{*trans*-Pt(NH$_3$)$_2$Cl}$_2$($\mu$-4,4'-bipyridyl)](ClO$_4$)$_2$·DMF, **Pt2**

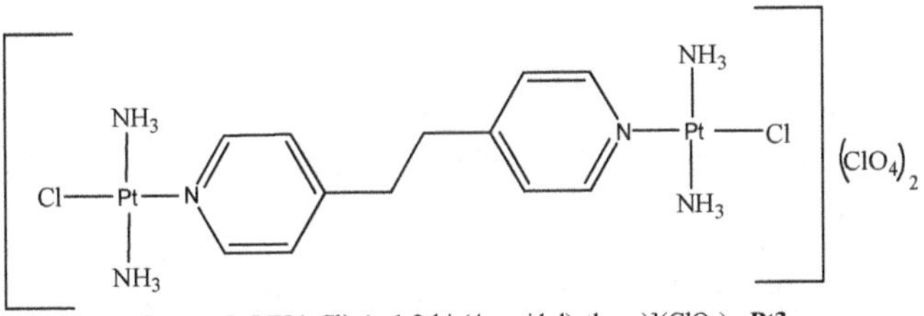

[{*trans*-Pt(NH$_3$)$_2$Cl}$_2$($\mu$-1,2-bis(4-pyridyl)ethane)](ClO$_4$)$_2$, **Pt3**

Fig. 6. Structures of investigated dinuclear platinum(II) complexes.

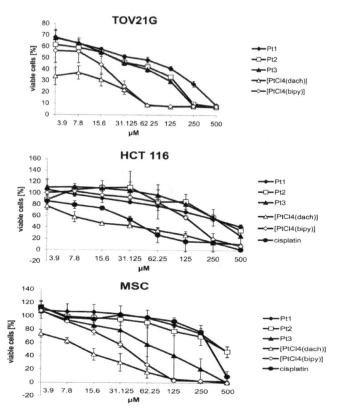

Fig. 7. Cytotoxic activity of tested complexes measured by MTT test (Mean+/-SE).

## 4. Conclusion

Results presented here, could contribute to a better understanding of the precise biochemical mechanism of some Pt(II) complexes. Moreover, the results of the substitution reactions with biologically relevant ligands could help to get more information on the possible interaction modes of Pt(II) complexes with *in vivo* targets and their representative application in the study of their anti-tumour properties. Detailed knowledge of the interactions between transition metal ions complexes with biomolecules and stability of final products under varying experimental conditions is fundamental for future investigations of new pharmacological agents and discovery of the alternative tumor treatment. Connecting theoretical calculations, chemistry, biochemistry and cellular biology and establishement of the structure-activity relationship Pt(II) complexes will help to solve some of the questions and will finally result in more tailored drug design. Numerous data imply that interactions of Pt(II) complexes and investigation of the mechanism of their reaction with DNA fragments (purine and pyrimidine bases, as well as oligonucleotides) are important for antitumor activity of Pt(II) complexes and the results of studies presented above contribute to that. Investigations of the interaction of Pt(II) complexes with other S-donor biomolecules can help us to get better insights in the destiny of anti-tumor drugs in

Interactions of the Platinum(II) Complexes with Nitrogen- and Sulfur-Bonding Bio-Molecules in Chronic
Lymphocytic Leukemia

95

the cells after their uptake, as well as to obtain more information about the inner cellular processes, which are affected by therapy.

Further research in this area will be based on the synthesis and investigation of the substitution reactions of the transition metals complexes especially Pt(II), Pt(IV), Au(III) and Ru(II/III) complexes. This complexes are investigated in order to find compounds that would demonstrate greater anti-tumour activity and less toxicity and resistance compared to cisplatin. It turned out that some complexes of Pt(IV) are toxic to cancers where cisplatin developed resistance. A good feature of the complexes of Pt(IV) is that some of them can be taken orally. When the complex of Pt(IV) enters the cell, it leads to the reduction of Pt(IV) to Pt(II) and binding to DNA. Au(III) is isoelectronic with Pt(II) and forms square planar complexes, and is therefore a good candidate for the synthesis of new complexes that could show better properties than the complexes of Pt(II). Also, complexes of Ru(II/III) are potential anti-cancer agents and consequently the study of these complexes is of great importance.

## 5. Acknowledgements

The authors gratefully acknowledge financial support from the Ministry of Education and Science of the Republic of Serbia, project No. 172011.

## 6. References

Ali M. S.; Khan S. R. A.; Ojima H.; Guzman I. Y.; Whitmire K. H.; Siddik Z. H. & Khokhar A. R. (2005). Model platinum nucleobase and nucleoside complexes and antitumor activity: X-ray crystal structure of [PtIV(trans-1R,2R-diaminocyclohexane)trans(acetate)2(9-ethylguanine)Cl]NO$_3$H$_2$O. *Journal of Inorganic Biochemistry*, Vol. 99, pp. 795-804, ISSN:0162-0134.

Annibale G.; Bergamini P.; Bertolasi V.; Cattabriga M.; Lazzaro A.; Marchi A. & Vertuani G. (1999). Platinum assisted cyclization of S-methyl 3-acyl-2-methyldithiocarbazates under mild conditions. Crystal structure of [Pt$_2$(μ-SMe)(terpy)$_2$][ClO$_4$]$_3$. *Journal of the Chemical Society, Dalton Transactions: Inorganic Chemistry*, No. 21, pp. 3877-3882, ISSN:0300-9246.

Annibale G.; Brandolisio M.; Bugarčić Ž. D. & Cattalini L. (1998). Nucleophilicity of thiols towards planar tetracoordinated platinum(II) complexes. *Transition Metal Chemistry*, Vol. 23, pp. 715-719, ISSN:0340-4285.

Anzellotti A. I.; Ma E. S. & Farell N. (2005). Platination of Nucleobases To Enhance Noncovalent Recognition in Protein-DNA/RNA Complexes. *Inorganic Chemistry*, Vol. 44, pp. 483-485, ISSN:0020-1669.

Arpalahti J. & Lehikoinen P. (1990). Kinetics of complexation of aquated (diethylenetriamine)platinum(II) with inosine and 1-methylinosine as a function of pH. *Inorganic Chemistry*, Vol. 29, pp. 2564-2567, ISSN:0020- 1669.

Arpalahti J. & Lippert B. (1990) Coordination of aquated cis-platinum(II) diamines to purine nucleosides. Kinetics of complex formation. *Inorganic Chemistry*, Vol. 29, pp. 104-110, ISSN:0020-1669.

Bailey J. A.; Hill M. G.; Marsh R. E.; Miskowski V. M.; Schaeefer W. P. & Gray H. B. (1995). Electronic Spectroscopy of Chloro(terpyridine)platinum(II). *Inorganic Chemistry,* Vol. 34, pp. 4591-4599, ISSN:0020-1669.

Barnham K. J.; Djuran M.I.; del Socorro P. & Sadler P.J. (1994). Intermolecular displacement of S-bound L-methionine on platinum(II) by guanosine 5'-monophosphate: implications for the mechanism of action of anticancer drugs. *Journal of the Chemical Society, Chemical Communications,* No. 6, pp. 721-722, ISSN:0022-4936.

Barnham K. J.; Guo Z. J. & Sadler P. J. (1996). Stabilization of monofunctional platinum-nucleotide adducts: reactions of N-acetyl-L-methionine complexes with guanosine 5'-monophosphate and guanylyl(3'-5')guanosine. *Journal of the Chemical Society, Dalton Transactions,* No. 13, pp. 2867-2876, ISSN:0300-9246.

Barnham K. J.; Djuran M. I.; Murdoch P. d. S.; Ranford J. D. & Sadler P. J. (1996). Ring-Opened Adducts of the Anticancer Drug Carboplatin with Sulfur Amino Acids. *Inorganic Chemistry,* Vol. 35, pp. 1065-1072, ISSN:0020-1669.

Barry C. G.; Day C. S. & Bierbach U. (2005). Duplex-Promoted Platination of Adenine-N3 in the Minor Groove of DNA: Challenging a Longstanding Bioinorganic Paradigm. *Journal of the American Chemical Society,* Vol. 127, pp. 1160-1169, ISSN:0002-7863.

Becker K.; Herold-Mende C.; Park J. J.; Lowe G. & Shirmer R. H. (2001). Human thioredoxin reductase is efficiently inhibited by (2,2':6',2"-terpyridine)platinum(II) complexes. Possible implications for a novel antitumor strategy. *Journal of medicinal chemistry,* Vol. 44, pp. 2784-2792, ISSN:0022-2623.

Berners-Price S. J.; Barnham K. J.; Frey U. & Sadler P. J. (1996). Kinetic analysis of the stepwise platination of single- and double-stranded GG oligonucleotides with cisplatin and cis-[PtCl(H$_2$O)(NH$_3$)$_2$]$^+$. *Chemistry--A European Journal,* Vol. 2, pp. 1283-1291, ISSN:0947-6539.

Berners-Price S. J.; Davies M. S.; Cox J. W.; Thomas D. S. & Farrell N. (2003) Competitive reactions of interstrand and intrastrand DNA-Pt adducts: A dinuclear-platinum complex preferentially forms a 1,4-interstrand cross-link rather than a 1,2 intrastrand cross-link on binding to a GG 14-mer duplex. *Chemistry--A European Journal,* Vol. 9, pp. 713-725, ISSN:0947-6539.

Bogojeski J.; Bugarčić Ž. D.; Puchta R. & van Eldik R. (2010). Kinetic studies on the reactions of different bifunctional platinum(II) complexes with selected nucleophiles. *European Journal of Inorganic Chemistry,* No. 34, 5439-5445, ISSN:1434-1948.

Bogojeski J. & Bugarčić Ž. D. (2011). Kinetic and thermodznamic studies on reactions of [Pt(bpma)Cl]$^+$ and [Pt(bpma)H$_2$O]$^{2+}$ (bpma = bis-(2-pyridylmethyl)amine) with some azoles and diazines. *Transaction Metal Chemistry,* Vol. 36, pp. 73-78, ISSN:0340-4285.

Bose N.; Cornelius R. D. & Viola R. E. (1986). Multinuclear NMR studies and the kinetics of formation of platinum(II)-adenine nucleotide complexes. *Journal of the American Chemical Society,* Vol. 108, pp. 4403-4408, ISSN:0002- 7863.

Bose N.; Moghaddas S.; Weaver E. L. & Cox E. H. (1995). Reactivity of Glutathione and Cysteine toward Platinum(II) in the Presence and Absence of Guanosine 5'-Monophosphate. *Inorganic Chemistry,* Vol. 34, pp. 5878-5883, ISSN:0020-1669.

Bruijnincx P. C. A. & Sadler P. J. (2009). Controlling platinum, ruthenium, and osmium reactivity for anticancer drug design. *Advances in Inorganic Chemistry,* Vol. 61, pp. 1-62, ISSN:0898-8838.

Interactions of the Platinum(II) Complexes with Nitrogen- and Sulfur-Bonding Bio-Molecules in Chronic
Lymphocytic Leukemia

97

Bugarčić Ž. D.; Đorđević B. V. & Đuran M. I. (1997). Mechanism of the reactions between chloro(2,2':6',2''-terpyridine)platinum(II) and ligands containing a thiol group. *Journal of the Serbian Chemical Society*, Vol. 62, pp. 1031-1036, ISSN:0352-5139.

Bugarčić Ž. D. & Đorđević B. V. (1998). Kinetics and mechanism of the reaction of platinum(II) complexes with thioglycolic acid. *Monatshefte fuer Chemie*, Vol. 129, pp. 1267-1274, ISSN:0026-9247.

Bugarčić Ž. D.; Liehr G. & van Eldik R. (2002). Kinetics and mechanism of the reactions of $[Pt(terpy)H_2O]^{2+}$ with thiols in acidic aqueous solution. Synthesis and crystal structure of $[Pt(terpy)(tu)](ClO_4)^2$ (tu = thiourea). *Journal of the Chemical Society, Dalton Transactions*, No. 14, pp. 2825-2830, SSN:1472-7773.

Bugarčić Ž. D.; Shoukry M. M. & van Eldik R. (2002). Equilibrium and kinetic data for the interaction of diaqua-(S- methyl-l-cysteine)palladium(II) with biologically relevant ligands. *Journal of the Chemical Society, Dalton Transactions*, No. 21, pp. 3945-3951, SSN:1472-7773.

Bugarčić Ž. D.; Heinemann F. W. & van Eldik R. (2004). Substitution reactions of $[Pt(terpy)X]^{2+}$ with some biologically relevant ligands. Synthesis and crystal structure of $[Pt(terpy)(cyst-S)](ClO_4)_2 \square 0.5H_2O$ and $[Pt(terpy)(guo-N7)](ClO_4)_2 \square 0.5guo \square 1.5H_2O$. *Dalton Transactions*, No. 2, pp. 279-286, ISSN:1477-9226.

Bugarčić Ž. D.; Soldatović T.; Jelić R.; Alguero B. & Grandas A. (2004). Equilibrium, kinetic and HPLC study of the reactions between platinum(II) complexes and DNA constituents in the presence and absence of glutathione. *Dalton Transactions*, No. 22, pp. 3869-3877, ISSN:1477-9226.

Bugarčić Ž. D.; Petrović B. & Zangrando E.(2004). Kinetics and mechanism of the complex formation of $[Pd(NNN)Cl]^+$ with pyridines in methanol: synthesis and crystal structure of $[Pd(terpy)(py)](ClO_4)_2$. *Inorganica Chimica Acta*, Vol. 357, pp. 2650-2656, ISSN:0020-1693.

Bugarčić Ž. D.; Rosić J.; Petrović B. V.; Summa N.; Puchta R. & van Eldik R. (2007). Kinetics and mechanism of the substitution reactions of $[Pt(bpma)Cl]^+$, $[PtCl(gly-met-S,N,N)]$ and their aqua analogs with L-methionine, glutathione and 5'-GMP. *Journal of Biological Inorganic Chemistry*, Vol. 12., pp. 1141-1150, ISSN:0949-8257.

Caradonna J. P. & Lippard S. J. (1988). Synthesis and characterization of [d(ApGpGpCpCpT)]2 and its adduct with the anticancer drug cis-diamminedichloroplatinum(II). *Inorganic Chemistry*, Vol. 27, pp. 1454-1466.

Chen Y.; Guo Z.; Murdoch P. S.; Zang E. & Sadler P. J. (1998). Interconversion between S- and N-bound L-methionine adducts of $Pt(dien)^{2+}$ (dien = diethylenetriamine) via dien ring-opened intermediates. *Journal of the Chemical Society, Dalton Transactions: Inorganic Chemistry*, No. 9, pp. 1503-1508.

Cheng C. C. & Pai C. H. (1998). Specific displacement of glutathione from the Pt(II)-glutathione adduct by Cu(II) in neutral phosphate buffer. *Journal of Inorganic Biochemistry*, Vol. 71, pp. 109-113.

Chiorazzi N.; Rai K. R. & Ferrarini M. (2005). Chronic lymphocytic leukemia. *New England Journal of Medicine*, Vol. 352, pp. 804-815, ISSN:0028-4793.

Eichhorst B. F.; Busch R. Hopfinger G. et al. (2005) Fludarabine plus cyclophosphamide versus fludarabine alone in first line therapy of younger patients with chronic lymphocytic leukemia. *Blood*, Vol. 107, pp. 885-891.

Esposito B.P. &  Najjar R. (2002). Interactions of antitumoral platinum- group metallodrugs with albumin, *Coordination Chemistry Reviews*, Vol. 232, pp. 137-149, ISSN 0010-8545.

Farrell N. (2004). Polynuclear platinum drugs in: A. Sigel, H. Sigel (Eds.), Metal ions in biological systems, New York and Basel Marcel Dekker Inc., New York, pp. 251-296.

Frey U.; Ranford J.D. & Sadler P.J. (1993). Ring-opening reactions of the anticancer drug carboplatin: NMR characterization of cis-[Pt(NH$_3$)$_2$(CBDCA-O)(5'-GMP-N7)] in solution. *Inorganic Chemistry*, Vol. 32, pp. 1333-1340, ISSN:0020-1669.

Fuertes M. A.; Alonso C. & Perez J. M. (2003). Biochemical modulation of cisplatin mechanisms of action: enhancement of antitumor activity and circumvention of drug resistance. *Chemical Reviews*, Vol. 103, pp. 645-662, ISSN:0009-2665.

Hagrman D.; Goodisman J. & Soud A-K. (2004). Kinetic study on the reactions of platinum drugs with glutathione. *Journal of Pharmacology and Experimental Therapeutics*, Vol. 308, pp. 658-666, ISSN:0022-3565.

Harris A.; Qu Y. & Farell N. (2005). Unique Cooperative Binding Interaction Observed between a Minor Groove Binding Pt Antitumor Agent and Hoeschst Dye 33258. *Inorganic Chemistry*, Vol. 44, pp. 1196-1198, ISSN:0020-1669.

Hofmann A.; Jaganyi D.; Munro O. Q.; Liehr G. & van Eldik R. (2003). Electronic Tuning of the Lability of Pt(II) Complexes through □ -Acceptor Effects. Correlations between Thermodynamic, Kinetic, and Theoretical Parameters. *Inorganic Chemistry*, Vol. 42, pp. 1688-1700, ISSN:0020-1669.

Jacobs R.; Prinsloo F. & Breet E. (1992). Kinetics of binding of DNA nucleotides to antitumor type complexes. *Journal of the Chemical Society, Chemical Communications*, No. 3, pp. 212-213, ISSN:0022-4936.

Jaganyi D.; Hofmann A. & van Eldik R. (2001). Controlling the lability of square-planar PtII complexes through electronic communication between □ -acceptor ligands. *Angewandte Chemie, International Edition*, Vol. 40, pp. 1680-1683, ISSN:1433-7851.

Jaganyi D. & Tiba F. (2003). Substitution of [Pt(terpy)H$_2$O]$^{2+}$ and [Pt(bpma)H$_2$O]$^{2+}$ with thiols in acidic aqueous solution. terpy = 2,2':6'2''-terpyridine; bpma = bis(2-pyridylmethyl)amine. *Transition Metal Chemistry*, Vol. 28, pp. 803-807, SSN:0340-4285.

Jaganyi D.; Tiba F.; Munro O. Q.; Petrović B. & Bugarčić Ž. D. (2006). Kinetic and mechanistic study on the reactions of [Pt(bpma)(H$_2$O)]$^{2+}$ and [Pd(bpma)(H$_2$O)]$^{2+}$ with some nucleophiles. Crystal structure of [Pd(bpma)(py)](ClO$_4$)$_2$. *Dalton Transactions*, No. 24, pp. 2943-2949, ISSN:1477-9226.

Jakupec M. A.; Galanski M. & Keppler B. K. (2003). Tumour-inhibiting platinum complexes-state of the art and future perspectives. *Reviews of Physiology, Biochemistry and Pharmacology*, Vol. 146, pp. 1-53, ISSN:0303-4240.

Jakupec M. A.; Galanski M.; Arion V. B.; Hartinger C. G. & Keppler B. K. (2008). Antitumor metal compounds: more  than theme and variations. *Dalton Transactions*, No. 2, pp. 183-194, ISSN:1477-9226.

Jansen B. A. J.; Brouwer J. & Reedijk J. (2002). Glutathione induces cellular resistance against cationic dinuclear platinum anticancer drugs. *Journal of Inorganic Biochemistry*, Vol. 89, pp. 197-202, ISSN:0162-0134.

Interactions of the Platinum(II) Complexes with Nitrogen- and Sulfur-Bonding Bio-Molecules in Chronic
Lymphocytic Leukemia

99

Jolley J. N.; Yanovsky A. I.; Kelland L. R. & Nolan K. B. (2001). Synthesis and antitumour activity of platinum(II) and platinum(IV) complexes containing ethylenediamine-derived ligands having alcohol, carboxylic acid and acetate substituents. Crystal and molecular structure of [PtL$_4$Cl$_2$] H$_2$O where L$_4$ is ethylenediamine-N,N'-diacetate. *Journal of Inorganic Biochemistry*, Vol. 83, pp. 91-100, ISSN:0162-0134.

Jovanović S.; Soldatović T.; Milovanović M.; Volarević V.; Čanović D.; Arsenijević N. & Bugarčić Ž. D. (2011). Ligand substitution reactions of Pt(IV) and dinuclear Pt(II) complexes with 5'-GMP and their cytotoxic properties. Submitted in European Journal of Medicinal Chemistry

Jung Y. & S. J. Lippard (2007). Direct Cellular Responses to Platinum-Induced DNA Damage. *Chemical Reviews*, Vol. 107, pp. 1387-1407, ISSN:0009-2665.

Kozelka J.; Legendre F.; Reeder F. & Chottard J. C. (1999). Kinetic aspects of interactions between DNA and platinum complexes. *Coordination Chemistry Reviews*, Vol. 190-192.

Kung A.; Strickman D. B.; Galanski M. & Keppler B. K. (2001). Comparison of the binding behavior of oxaliplatin, cisplatin and analogues to 5'-GMP in the presence of sulfur-containing molecules by means of capillary electrophoresis and electrospray mass spectrometry. *Journal of Inorganic Biochemistry*, Vol. 86, pp. 691-698, ISSN:0162-0134.

Lakomska I.; Kooijman H.; Spek A. L.; Shen W. & Reedijk J. (2009). Mono- and dinuclear platinum(II) compounds with 5,7-dimethyl-1,2,4-triazolo[1,5-a]pyrimidine. Structure, cytotoxic activity and reaction with 5'-GMP. *Dalton Transactions*, Vol. 48, pp. 10736-10741, ISSN:1477-9226.

Lampers L. M. & Reedijk J. (1990). Reversibility of binding of cisplatin-methionine in proteins by diethyldithiocarbamate or thiourea: a study with model adducts. *Inorganic Chemistry*, Vol. 29, pp. 217-222, ISSN:0020-1669.

Lemma K.; Shi T. & Elding L. I. (2000). Kinetics and mechanism for reduction of the anticancer prodrug trans,trans,trans-[PtCl$_2$(OH)$_2$(c-C$_6$H$_{11}$NH$_2$)(NH$_3$)] (JM335) by thiols. *Inorganic chemistry*, Vol. 39, pp. 1728-1734, ISSN:0020-1669.

Lemma K.; Sargeson A. M. & Elding L. I. (2000). Kinetics and mechanism for reduction of oral anticancer platinum(IV) dicarboxylate compounds by L-ascorbate ions. *Dalton Transaction*, No. 7, pp. 1167-1172, ISSN:1470-479X.

Lippert B. (1999). Cisplatin, Chemistry and Biochemistry of Leading Antitumor Drugs ,Wiley-VCH, Zuruch.

Lippert B. (1999). Impact of Cisplatin on the recent development of Pt coordination chemistry: a case study. *Coordination Chemistry Reviews*, Vol. 182, pp. 263-295, ISSN:0010-8545.

Mambanda A.; Jaganyi D.; Hochreuther S. & van Eldik R. (2010). Tuning the reactivity of chelated dinuclear Pt(II) complexes through a flexible diamine linker. A detailed kinetic and mechanistic study. *Dalton Transactions*, Vol. 39, 3595-3608, ISSN:1477-9226.

Martin R. B. , *Cisplatin, Chemistry and Biochemistry of Leading Antitumor Drugs*, ed. B. Lippert, Wiley-VCH, Zurich, 1999, p. 193-200.

McGregor T.D.; Balcarova Z.; Qu Y.; Tran M.-C.; Zaludova R.; Brabec V. & Farrell N. (1999). Sequence-dependent conformational changes in DNA induces by polinuclear platinum complexes. *Journal of Inorganic Biochemistry*, Vol. 77, pp. 43-46, ISSN:0162-0134.

Mikola M.; Klika K. D.; Hakala A. & Arpalahti J. (1999). Substitution Reactions of Platinum(II)-Nucleobase Complexes by Associative Mechanism Involving Pseudorotation of the Five-Coordinate Intermediate. *Inorganic Chemistry*, Vol. 38, pp. 571-578, ISSN:0020-1669.

Mock C.; Puscasu I.; Rauterkus M. J.; Tallen G.; Wolff J. E. A. & Krebs B. (2001). Novel Pt(II) anticancer agents and their Pd(II) analogues: syntheses, crystal structures, reactions with nucleobases and cytotoxicities. *Inorganica Chimica Acta*, Vol. 319, pp. 109-116, ISSN:0020-1693.

Natile G. & Coluccia M. (2001). Current status of trans-platinum compounds in cancer therapy. *Coordination Chemistry Reviews*, Vol. 216-217, pp. 383-410, ISSN:0010-8545.

Norman R. E.; Ranford J. D. & Sadler P. J. (1992). Studies of platinum(II) methionine complexes: metabolites of cisplatin. *Inorganic Chemistry*, Vol. 31, pp. 877-888,ISSN:0020-1669.

Petrović B. & Bugarčić Ž. D. (2001). Kinetics and mechanism of complex formation between [Pt(dien)Cl]+ and thiols and thioethers. *Journal of Coordination Chemistry*, Vol. 53, pp. 35-45, ISSN:0095-8972.

Petrović B. V.; Đuran M. I. & Bugarčić Ž. D. (1999). Binding of platinum(II) to some biologically important thiols. *Metal-Based Drugs*, Vol. 6, pp. 355-360, ISSN:0793-0291.

Petrović D.; Stojimirović B.; Petrović B.; Bugarčić Z. M. & Bugarčić Ž. D. (2007). Studies of interactions between platinum(II) complexes and some biologically relevant molecules. *Bioorganic & Medicinal Chemistry*, Vol. 15, pp. 4203-4211, ISSN:0968-0896.

Pitteri B.; Marangoni G.; Cattalini L.; Visentin F.; Bertolasi V. & Gilli P. (2001). The role of the non-participating groups in substitution reactions at cationic Pt(II) complexes containing tridentate chelating nitrogen donors. Crystal structure of {Pt[bis(2-pyridylmethyl)amine](py)}(CF$_3$SO$_3$)$_2$. *Polyhedron*, Vol. 20, pp. 869-880, ISSN:0277-5387.

Pitteri B.; Annibale G.; Marangoni G.; Bertolasi V. & Ferretti V. (2002). Base hydrolysis kinetics and equilibria of [bis(2-pyridylmethyl)amine]chloroplatinum(II) and crystal and molecular structures of [Pt(bpma)Cl]Cl H$_2$O and [Pt(bpma)(OH$_2$)](ClO$_4$)$_2$ 2H$_2$O. *Polyhedron*, 2002, Vol. 21, pp. 2283-2291, ISSN:0277-5387.

Reedijk J. (1999). Why does cisplatin reach guanine-N7 with competing S-donor ligands available in the cell? *Chemical Reviews*, Vol. 99, pp. 2499-2510, ISSN:0009-2665.

Reedijk J. (2009). Platinum anticancer coordination compounds: study of DNA binding inspires new drug design. *European Journal of Inorganic Chemistry*, No. 10, pp. 1303-1312, ISSN:1434-1948.

Ronconi L. & Sadler P. J. (2007). Using coordination chemistry to design new medicines. *Coordination Chemistry Reviews*, Vol. 251, pp. 1633-1648, ISSN:0010-8545.

Rosenberg B. & Camp L. V. (1965). INHIBITION OF CELL DIVISION IN ESCHERICHIA COLI BY ELECTROLYSIS PRODUCTS FROM A PLATINUM ELECTRODE, *Nature, Vol. 205, pp. 698-699*, ISSN:0028-0836.

Rosenberg B.; Camp L. V.; Trosko J. E. & Mansour V. H. (1969). Platinum compounds: a new class of potent antitumor agents. *Nature*, Vol. 222, pp. 385-386, ISSN:0028-0836.

Interactions of the Platinum(II) Complexes with Nitrogen- and Sulfur-Bonding Bio-Molecules in Chronic
Lymphocytic Leukemia

101

Rosenberg B. & Camp L. V. (1970). Successful regression of large solid sarcoma 180 tumors by platinum compounds. *Cancer Research*, Vol. 30, pp. 1799-1802, ISSN:0008-5472.

Rosenberg B.; Camp L. V.; Grimley E. B. & Thomson A. J. (1967). Inhibition of growth or cell division in Escherichia coli by different ionic species of platinum(IV) complexes. *Journal of Biological Chemistry*, Vol. 242, pp. 1347-1352, ISSN:0021-9258.

Shi T. & Elding L. I. (1996). Equilibrium and High-Pressure Kinetic Study of Formation and Proton-Assisted Aquation of Monodentate Acetate, Propionate, and Glycolate Complexes of Palladium(II) in Aqueous Solution. *Inorganic Chemistry*, Vol. 35, pp. 735-740, ISSN:0020-1669.

Shi T. & Elding L. I. (1997). Linear Free Energy Relationships for Complex Formation Reactions between Carboxylic Acids and Palladium(II). Equilibrium and High-Pressure Kinetics Study. *Inorganic Chemistry*, Vol. 34, pp. 528-536, ISSN:0020-1669.

Shoukry A.; Rau T.; Shoukry M. & van Eldik R. (1998). Kinetics and mechanisms of the ligand substitution reactions of bis(amine)(cyclobutane-1,1-dicarboxylato)palladium(II). *Journal of the Chemical Society, Dalton Transactions*, No. 18, pp. 3105-3112.

Sigel H.; Massoud S. S.; Corfu N. A. (1994). Comparison of the Extent of Macrochelate Formation in Complexes of Divalent Metal Ions with Guanosine (GMP$^{2-}$), Inosine (IMP$^{2-}$), and Adenosine 5'-Monophosphate (AMP$^{2-}$). The Crucial Role of N-7 Basicity in Metal Ion-Nucleic Base Recognition. *Journal of the American Chemical Society*, Vol. 116, pp. 2958-2971, ISSN:0002-7863.

Soldatović T. & Bugarčić Ž. D. (2005). Study of the reactions between platinum(II) complexes and -methionine in the presence and absence of 5'-GMP. *Journal of Inorganic Biochemistry*, Vol. 99, pp. 1472-1479, ISSN:0162-0134.

Soldatović T.; Bugarčić Ž. D. & van Eldik R. (2009). Influence of the chloride concentration on ligand substitution reactions of [Pt(SMC)Cl$_2$] with biologically relevant nucleophiles. *Dalton Transactions*, No. 23, pp. 4526-4531, ISSN:1477-9226.

Summa N.; Schiessl W.; Puchta R.; van Eikema Hommes N. & van Eldik R. (2006). Thermodynamic and Kinetic Studies on Reactions of Pt(II) Complexes with Biologically Relevant Nucleophiles. *Inorganic Chemistry*, Vol. 45, pp. 2948-2959, ISSN:0020-1669.

Summa N.; Soldatović T.; Dahlenburg L.; Bugarčić Ž. D. & van Eldik R. (2007). Kinetics and mechanism of the substitution reactions of [Pt(bpma)Cl]$^+$, [PtCl(gly-met-S,N,N)] and their aqua analogs with L-methionine, glutathione and 5'-GMP. *Journal of Biological Inorganic Chemistry*, Vol. 12, pp. 1141-1150, ISSN:0949-8257.

Talman E. G.; Bruning W.; Reedijk J.; Spek A. L. & Veldman N. (1997). Crystal and Molecular Structures of Asymmetric cis- and trans-Platinum(II/IV) Compounds and Their Reactions with DNA Fragments. *Inorganic Chemistry*, Vol. 36, pp. 854-861, ISSN:0020-1669.

Tauben J. M.; Rodrugez M.; Zubiri & Reedijk J. (2000). Glutathione readily replaces the thioether on platinum in the reaction with [Pt(dien)(GSMe)]$^{2+}$ (GSMe = S-methylated glutathione); a model study for cisplatin-protein interactions. *Dalton*, No. 3, pp. 369-372, ISSN:1470-479X.

Teuben J. M.; van Boom S. S. G. E. & Reedijk J. (1997). Intramolecular migration of coordinated platinum from a sulfur to N7 in the nucleopeptide Met-d(TpG) (5'-Omethioninate-N-ylcarbonylthymidine 2'-deoxyguanosine monophosphate). *Journal of the Chemical Society, Dalton Transactions,* No. 21, pp. 3979-3980, ISSN:0300-9246.

van Boom S.S.G.E.; Chen B.W; Tauben J.M. & Reedijk J. (1999). Platinum-Thioether Bonds Can Be Reverted by Guanine-N7 Bonds in Pt(dien)2+ Model Adducts. *Inorganic Chemistry,* Vol. 38, pp. 1450-1455.

Volckova E.; Dudones L. P. & Bose R. N. (2002). HPLC determination of binding of cisplatin to DNA in the presence of biological thiols: implications of dominant platinum-thiol binding to its anticancer action. *Pharmaceutical research,* Vol. 19, pp. 124-131, ISSN:0724-8741.

Wierda W.; O'Brien S.; Wen S.; Faderl S.; Garcia-Manero G.; Thomas D.; Do K-A.; Cortes J.; Koller C.; Beran M.; Ferrajoli A.; Giles F.; Lerner S.; Albitar M.; Kantarijan H. & Keating M. (2005) Chemoimmunotherapy with fludarabine, cyclophosphamide, and rituximab for relapsed and refractory chronic lymphocytic leukemia. *Journal of Clinical Oncology,* Vol. 23, pp. 4070-4078 ISSN:0732-183X.

Wang Y. F.; Curtis J. E.; Lipton J.; Minkin S. & McCulloch E. A. (1991) Cytosine arabinoside (ara-C) and cisdichlorodiammineplatinumII (cisplatin) alone and in combination: effects on acute myeloblastic leukemia blast cells in culture and in vivo. *Leukemia,* Vol. 5, pp. 522-527.

Wilkins R. G. (1991) *Kinetics and Mechanism of Reactions of Transition metal Complexes,* 2nd edn., Verlag, Berlin, p. 300.

Wong Y. S. & Lippard S. J. (1977). X-ray crystal structure of a 2:2 chloroterpyridineplatinum(II)-adenosine-5'-monophosphate intercalation complex. *Journal of the Chemical Society, Chemical Communications,* No. 22, pp. 824-825, ISSN:0022-4936.

Yamauchi T.; Nowak B. J.; Keating M. J. & Plunkett W. (2001). DNA repair initiated in chronic lymphocytic leukemia lymphocytes by 4-hydroperoxycyclophosphamide is inhibited by fludarabine and clofarabine. *Clinical Cancer Research,* Vol. 7, pp. 3580-3589.

Zecevic A.; Sampath D.; Ewald B.; Chen R.; Wierda W. & Plunkett W.. (2011) Killing of Chronic Lymphocytic Leukemia by the Combination of Fludarabine and Oxaliplatin Is Dependent on the Activity of XPF Endonuclease. *Clinical Cancer Research,* Vol. 17, pp. 4731-4741, ISSN:1078-0432.

# 5

# Infectious Diseases and Clinical Complications During Treatment in CLL

Farhad Abbasi
*Bushehr University of Medical Sciences*
*Iran*

## 1. Introduction

Infectious complications continue to be one of the major causes of morbidity and mortality in patients with chronic lymphocytic leukemia (CLL). The pathogenesis of infections in these patients is multifactorial (Wadhwa & Morrison, 2006). Predisposition to infection in CLL is mediated through various abnormalities including both the immune defects inherent in the primary disease (impairment in humoral and cellular immunity) and in the further immunosuppression related to management of CLL (Morra et al., 1999). Increased infectious events may arise from the multiple courses of immunosuppressive therapy and progressive deterioration of a patient's immune system over the course of disease (Elter et al., 2009). Hypogammaglobulinemia is an important predisposing factor for infection in patients with early-stage disease and for those treated with conventional alkylating agents (Wadhwa & Morrison, 2006). It is probably the most important immune defect increases the risk of severe bacterial infections and its frequency and severity has direct relationship with the duration of the disease (Morra, et al., 1999). The majority of disease-specific complications in CLL, notably infection and autoimmunity, relate to the underlying alterations in immune function. Both cellular and humoral immunity are impaired with qualitative and quantitative defects in B cells, T cells, NK cells, neutrophils and the monocyte/macrophage lineage. Virtually all patients have reduced immunoglobulin levels, even in early stages, and this is associated with an increased frequency and severity of infection (Dearden, 2008). The immunodeficiency chiefly manifests as hypogammaglobulinaemia but involves all elements of the immune system. It is caused by the interpolation of tumor cells among immunological cells and mediated by bi-directional cell contact and secretion of cytokines, which both sustain and invigorate the tumor and suppress immunity. CLL treatment generally makes the immunodeficiency worse (Hamblin & Hamblin, 2008). The proportion of patients treated with purine analogs and monoclonal antibodies such as rituximab and alemtuzumab is increasing. As a result of this therapy, these patients often experience profound and sustained T-cell immunodeficiency. Consequently, the spectrum of organisms causing infections in these patients is changing from common bacterial organisms to less common opportunistic pathogens such as Pneumocystis, Listeria, mycobacteria, herpesviruses and Candida (Wadhwa & Morrison, 2006). The early recognition of infections as well as prophylactic administration of appropriate antibiotics has been the mainstay of managing infections in patients with CLL. Hopefully, increasing understanding of the molecular events underlying the neoplastic change in CLL will lead to more targeted and less immunosuppressive therapeutic modalities (Ravandi & O'Brien S, 2006).

## 2. Infectious diseases in chronic lymphocytic leukemia

Patients with lymphoid malignancies such as chronic lymphocytic leukemia are at increased risk for infectious morbidity and mortality. Defects in cell-mediated immunity appear to be a major predisposing factor in these patients. An expanding spectrum of pathogens associated with lymphocytopenia and depletion of CD4 has been described in the setting of therapy with purine analogs. Infectious diseases in chronic lymphocytic leukemia are categorized as bacterial, viral, fungal and parasitic infection. CLL is characterized by progressive defects in humoral- and cell-mediated immunity. These defects are manifested as a propensity to develop infections with encapsulated, and less frequently, with gram-negative enteric bacteria. In addition, reactivation of viruses such as herpesvirus is not uncommon. Treatment of the disease exacerbates immunosuppression by depleting immune effectors and broadening the spectrum of potentially offending pathogens (Wierda, 2003). Neutrophil count, serum immunoglobulin G level and granulocyte chemotaxis are predicting factors of susceptibility to infections. Phagocytosis and intracellular killing of granulocytes are intact in patients with CLL (Itälä et al, 1996, 1998). Over the past decade, the introduction of nucleoside analogs and monoclonal antibodies into the treatment of patients with CLL has resulted in higher rates and longer duration of response. This is a significant step towards achieving the ultimate goal of disease-eradication and improved survival. A continuing problem, however, is the susceptibility of these patients to infections. Profound dysregulation of the host immune system in patients with CLL and its impact on the clinical course of the disease are well established. A number of investigators have sought to identify the mechanisms underlying this innate immune dysfunction, which is further exacerbated by the actions of the potent therapeutic agents (Ravandi & O'Brien S, 2006). A characteristic spectrum of infectious complications has been described for specific treatment agents. With chlorambucil, most infections are bacterial in origin, caused by common Gram-positive and -negative organisms. Recurrent infections are a hallmark, with the respiratory tract being the most common site of infection. The pathogenesis of infection with the purine analogues is related to the quantitative and qualitative T-cell abnormalities induced by these agents. Risk factors for infection identified in patients treated with fludarabine include advanced-stage disease, prior CLL therapy, response to therapy, elevated serum creatinine, hemoglobin < 12 g/dl, and decreased serum IgG. As compared with patients receiving chlorambucil, patients receiving fludarabine have more major infections and herpes virus infections. However, Pneumocystis, Aspergillus, and cytomegalovirus (CMV) infections are uncommon. The use of alemtuzumab is complicated by frequent opportunistic infections. CMV reactivation is especially problematic, occurring in 10%-25% of patients (Morrison, 2009). The humanized, anti-CD52 monoclonal antibody alemtuzumab has shown notable activity for both untreated and fludarabine-refractory CLL. The antibody not only targets malignant cells but also affects normal, healthy immune cells. The cumulative effects of the malignancy and successive courses of treatments adversely impinge on a patient's defense response to certain bacterial, fungal, and viral infections (Elter et al., 2009). Severe lymphopenia is one of the most profound hematologic effects of alemtuzumab, often predisposing patients to infectious complications such as herpes simplex virus, cytomegalovirus, and Pneumocystis jirovecii pneumonia. Opportunistic infections secondary to mycobacterial sources have been documented less frequently (Saadeh & Srkalovic, 2008).

## 2.1 Bacterial infection

Patients with chronic lymphocytic leukemia are at an increased risk for infections with bacteria which require complement for osponization (Heath & Cheson, 1985). Patients with chronic leukemias typically are affected by infections due to the underlying hematologic condition, particularly hypogammaglobulinemia in CLL patients. With active treatment, particularly those agents that cause defects in cell-mediated immunity, the incidence of opportunistic infections increases although endogenous bacterial, mycobacterial, and fungal infections also occur (Young, 2011). These defects are manifested as a propensity to develop infections with encapsulated bacteria, and less frequently, with gram-negative enteric bacteria. Bacterial pneumonia, urinary tract infection, sepsis, meningitis, typhlitis or neutropenic enterocolitis and soft tissue infections are common infections occur in CLL patients with bacterial source (Perkins et al., 2002). Staphylococcus spp., Streptococcus spp. (especially Streptocccoccus pneumonia) Enterococcus spp., Enterobacteriaceae, Hemophillus influenza, Pseudomonas spp. (especially Pseudomonas aeruginosa), Listeria monocytogenes, Nocardia, Vibrio vulnificus etc. are bacteria that cause infection in CLL patients (Travade et al, 1986; Barton & Ratard, 2006). Infections are one of the most important causes of mortality in CLL patients, and Streptococcus pneumoniae has been considered the most important single pathogen in this group (Sinisalo et al., 2007). In a survey on CLL patients with pneumonia, Pneumococcus was the most frequent agent followed by Pseudomonas aeruginosa, Pneumocystis carinii and Aspergillus fumigates. (Batlle et al., 2001).

## 2.2 Epstein-Bar virus infection

Epstein-Barr virus (EBV) is a gammaherpesvirus which infects greater than 90% of the world population. Infection is nonsymptomatic in healthy individuals, but has been associated with a number of lymphoproliferative disorders when accompanied by immunosuppression. Like all herpesviruses, EBV has both latent and lytic replication programs, which allows it to evade immune clearance and persist for the lifetime of the host (Bajaj et al., 2001). The most common primary symptoms of EBV infection are fever, skin eruption, lymphadenopathy, hepatosplenomegaly, eyelid edema, pharyngitis, cardiac arrhythmia and arthralgia (Li et al. 2004; C. Berger 2003). EBV can cause meningoencephalitis or central nervous system tumor-like lesion in immunocompromised patient (Khalil et al., 2008; Turkulov et al., 1999). This virus plays an important role in the etiology of nasopharyngeal carcinoma, adenocarcinoma of the parotid glands, gastric carcinoma, Burkitt's lymphoma and lymphoproliferative syndromes (Zahorodnia, 2011). EBV is pathogenically associated with a well defined group of lymphoid and epithelial tumors in which the virus directly drives transformation of infected cells. Recent evidence however indicates that this virus may infect a subpopulation of tumor cells in patients with chronic lymphocytic leukemia (Dordević, 2006). As one the most important clinical presentation of EBV and other herpesviruses is central nervous system (CNS) involvement; Rapid, sensitive and economical detection and identification of human herpesviruses as causative agents of CNS infections is clinically important. The traditional methods for the detection of herpesviruses in CNS infections all suffer from limitations. Polymerase chain reaction (PCR) is the best laboratory test. Multiplex nested consensus PCR provide a rapid, sensitive and economical method for detection of viral infections and is applicable to small volumes of CSF samples (Tafreshi, 2005). The spectrum of drugs active against EBV remains very limited. Gancyclovir and acyclovir are used in medical practice. The search of new compounds active against EBV remains necessary (Zahorodnia, 2011).

### 2.3 Cytomegalovirus infection

Human cytomegalovirus (CMV) is one of herpesviruses that commonly infect humans. Advances in molecular virology coupled with improvements in diagnostic methods and treatment options have vastly improved ability to manage CMV infection, but many uncertainties remain, including the mechanisms of persistence and pathogenesis and its hypothesized roles in a variety of human illnesses (Boeckh & Geballe, 2011). It is a recognized cause of morbidity and mortality in immunocompromised individuals (Emery, 2001). Primary infection with CMV is followed by persistence of the virus in a latent form. During life, the virus can reactivate, resulting in renewed shedding of the virus or development of disease. Significant progress has been made in detecting CMV, but in the immunocompromised patients, establishing the diagnosis of CMV infection can still be problematic (Vancíková & Dvorák, 2001).

Cellular immune responses are important against virus infections (Sester et al, 2002). CMV infection causes significant morbidity and mortality in the setting of immunodeficiency (Ozdemir et al, 2002). It can cause serious clinical complications in eye (retinitis), lung, central nervous system and other organs in immunocompromised individuals (Bronke et al, 2005; Reeves et al, 2005). For diagnosis the most sensitive molecular amplification methods such as PCR should be used. Treatment of infection depends mainly on the immune status of the host (Vancíková & Dvorák, 2001). The availability of sensitive diagnostic tests such as pp65 antigenemia has made the early diagnosis of CMV possible (Kusne et al, 1999). CMV should be suspected as a cause of pneumonia in immunocompromised patients and diagnosis may require invasive procedures bronchoalveolar lavage (BAL) and transbronchial lung biopsy (TBLB) may be required for diagnosis of CMV pneumonitis. (Yadegarynia et al, 2009). In immunocompetent patients only symptomatic treatment is recommended, while in immunocompromised patients antiviral therapy should be used. The most commonly used antiviral agents are: ganciclovir, foscarnet, cidofovir, valganciclovir and valaciclovir (Vancíková & Dvorák, 2001). Although it remains rare, ganciclovir-resistant CMV disease is increasingly seen in clinical practice, potentially fostered by the prolonged use of antiviral agents in high-risk patients. Treatment of drug-resistant CMV is currently non-standardized and may include foscarnet, cidofovir, CMV hyperimmune globulins or leflunomide (Eid & Razonable, 2010).

### 2.4 Herpes simplex virus infection

Herpes simplex viruses type 1 and 2 (HSV-1 and HSV-2) are alpha herpes viruses. Humans are the only natural host and they can be transmitted through oral or genital secretions. These viruses are ubiquitous all over the world, with different percentage rates (Dordević,

2006). They can infect both skin and nerves and develop latent infection within the dorsal root and trigeminal ganglia. Infection with these viruses is common and causes a wide range of clinical syndromes (Midak-Siewirska et al, 2010). HSV infections range in severity from common cutaneous outbreaks to life-threatening central nervous system and deep organ involvement (Higgins et al 1999). Atypical clinical manifestations of HSV may occur in immunocompromised patients. HSV-2 infection is responsible for significant neurological morbidity, perhaps more than any other virus (JR. Berger et al, 2008). Herpes esophagitis is common in immunosuppressed patients, but has rarely been reported in immunocompetent individuals, in whom it appears to be a self-limited illness (Canalejo Castrillero et al, 2010). Pneumonia, hepatitis, gasterointestinal involvement and disseminated infection may occur in immunocompromised patients (Longerich et al, 2005; Medlicott et al, 2005; Massler et al, 2011). Multiple herpes virus co-infection (HSV and EBV) may occur in patients with chronic lymphocytic leukemia (Mercadal et al, 2006). HSV infections have a severe and rapidly progressive course especially in immunocompromised patients, leading to significant morbidity and mortality. Therefore, rapid and reliable laboratory diagnosis of HSV infections is important for initiation of early antiviral therapy. PCR, direct fluorescein antibody (DFA) methods and cell culture are used for diagnosis (Cordes et al, 2011). There is evidence that acyclovir is effective for preventing and treating HSV infections. There is no evidence that valaciclovir is more effective than acyclovir, or that a high dose of valaciclovir is better than a low dose (Nolan, 2009). Antiviral-resistant herpes virus infection has become a great concern for immunocompromised patients (Shiota et al, 2011).

## 2.5 Hepatitis B virus infection

Recent studies emphasize the risk of hepatitis B virus (HBV) reactivation among patients with hematologic malignancies of B lineage, in which HBV has been recently hypothesized to play a pathogenetic role. Occult HBV infection is significantly more prevalent among patients with CLL and may contribute to the susceptibility of patients with CLL to HBV reactivation, whether exposed or not to biological agents (Rossi et al, 2009). Chemotherapy-induced HBV reactivation is a serious problem in chronic HBV carriers with hematologic malignancies. In Yağci's study all patients with chronic lymphocytic leukemia experienced chemotherapy-induced HBV reactivation regardless of the chemotherapy regimen. CLL patients who are HBV carriers are at significant risk of chemotherapy-induced HBV reactivation (Yağci et al, 2006). Reactivation of HBV in HBsAg-positive patients is a well-documented complication of cytotoxic or immunosuppressive therapy and has also been observed after treatment with rituximab (Heider et al, 2004). Patients may be treated with lamivudine or lamivudine plus adefovir dipivoxil combination therapy to control viral replication and allow for long-term anti-cancer chemotherapy (Cortelezzi et al, 2006). lamivudine is highly effective in inhibiting HBV proliferation and can be used to prevent HBV flare-up during chemotherapy in patients with positive HBs antigen (Heider et al, 2004).

## 2.6 Fungal infection

Opportunistic fungal infection may occur in patient with CLL. Candida and Aspergillus are common fungi. Invasive Candida infections are important causes of morbidity and mortality in immunocompromised patients. The cornerstone of diagnosis remains the detection of the organism by culture with identification of the isolate at the species level; in vitro susceptibility testing is mandatory for invasive isolates. Options for initial therapy of candidaemia and other invasive Candida infections in non-granulocytopenic patients include fluconazole or one of the three approved echinocandin compounds; liposomal amphotericin B. Voriconazole are secondary alternatives. In granulocytopenic patients, an echinocandin or liposomal amphotericin B is recommended as initial therapy. Indwelling central venous catheters serve as a main source of infection independent of the pathogenesis of candidaemia and should be removed whenever feasible. Dose reduction or discontinuation of pre-existing immunosuppressive treatment (particularly glucocorticosteroids) should be performed. Ophthalmoscopy is recommended prior to the discontinuation of antifungal chemotherapy to rule out endophthalmitis or chorioretinitis (Ruhnke et al, 2011).

Morbidity and mortality caused by invasive Aspergillus infections are increasing. This is because of the higher number of patients with malignancies treated with intensive immunosuppressive therapy regimens as well as their improved survival from formerly fatal bacterial infections. Clinical diagnosis is based on radiologic findings and non-culture based diagnostic techniques such as galactomannan or DNA detection in blood or bronchoalveolar lavage samples. Most promising outcomes can be expected in patients at high risk for aspergillosis in whom antifungal treatment has been started pre-emptively, backed up by laboratory and imaging findings. The gold standard of systemic antifungal treatment is voriconazole, which has been proved to be significantly superior to conventional amphotericin B and has led to a profound improvement of survival rates in patients with cerebral aspergillosis. Liposomal amphotericin B at standard dosages appears to be a suitable alternative for primary treatment, while caspofungin, amphotericin B lipid complex or posaconazole have shown partial or complete response in patients who had been refractory to or intolerant of primary antifungal therapy. Combination therapy with two antifungal compounds may be a promising future strategy for first-line treatment (Maschmeyer et al, 2007).

Cryptococcus neoformans is an important fungal pathogen of immunocompromised individuals. Lung and CNS are two important organs involved by Cryptococcus neoformans (Price et al, 2011). Diagnosis is based on direct microscopic examination of India ink preparations and PCR (Ndiaye et al, 2011; Sidrim et al, 2010; Mseddi et al, 2011). Amphotericin B and flucytosine is used for treatment (Thalla et al, 2009). Histoplasmosis (Van Koeveringe & Brouwer, 2010), fusariosis (Campo et al, 2010) and other uncommon fungal infection may be seen in immunocomromised patients.

### 2.7 Pnemocystis jirovecii infection

Pneumocystis jiroveci pneumonia (formerly Pneumocystis carinii pneumonia) occurs frequently in patients with immunodeficiency (Otahbachi et al, 2007). Pneumocystis carinii pneumonia (PCP) in patients with chronic lymphocytic leukaemia (CLL) who have not been treated with fludarabin are rare, although clinically relevant CD4 T-cell depletion can occur in longstanding CLL without prior treatment with purine analogues (Vavricka et al, 2004). It is associated with a wide spectrum of clinical presentations (Gal et al, 2002). The most frequent symptoms are: fever, dyspnea, non-productive cough, thoracic pain, chills and severe hypoxaemia (Pagano et al, 2002). For diagnosis of PCP bronchoalveolar lavage (BAL) cytology and transbronchial lung biopsy (TBLB) may be required (Bijur et al, 1996). Because Pneumocystis cannot be cultured, diagnosis relies on detection of the organism by colorimetric or immunofluorescent stains or by polymerase chain reaction. Trimethoprim-sulfamethoxazole is the preferred drug regimen for both treatment and prevention of PCP, although a number of alternatives are also available. Corticosteroids are an important adjunct for hypoxemic patients (Kovacs et al, 1994).

## 2.8 Mycobacterium avium complex infection

Mycobacterium avium complex (MAC) primarily causes respiratory infection in patients with underlying lung disease or disseminated disease in immunocompromised patients (Azzam et al, 2009). MAC is clinically important since it can cause severe infections in immunocompromised individuals (Rodrigues et al, 2009). Severe lymphopenia is one of the most profound hematologic effects of alemtuzumab, often predisposing patients to infectious complications such as herpes simplex virus, cytomegalovirus, and Pneumocystis jirovecii pneumonia. Opportunistic infections secondary to mycobacterial sources like mycobacterium avium complex have been documented less frequently (Saadeh & Srkalovic, 2008). A diagnosis requires a high index of suspicion in patients with immunocompromised status who present with prolonged fever, with or without organ-specific symptoms and signs. Therefore, clinical specimens must be sent for mycobacterial cultures for a definite diagnosis (Saritsiri et al, 2006). Microscopic evaluation, culture and PCR may be necessary for diagnosis (Haas et al, 1998). Combination of clarithromycin, rifabutin and ethambutol has proven to be the most efficacious therapy and therefore it is considered as standard therapy for disseminated MAC infection. Clarithromycin, rifabutin and azithromycin given as primary prophylaxis can diminish the risk of disseminated MAC infection (Fätkenheuer et al, 1998).

## 2.9 Adenovirus infection

Adenovirus infections are widespread in society and are occasionally associated with severe, but rarely with life-threatening, disease in otherwise healthy individuals. In contrast, adenovirus infections present a real threat to immunocompromised individuals and can result in disseminated and fatal disease (Andersson et al, 2010). It is an important cause of morbidity and mortality in the immunocompromised host (Gavin & Katz, 2002). Adenovirus infection has been reported following alemtuzumab treatment in CLL patients (Martin et al, 2006). There is no formally approved treatment of adenovirus infections today, and existing antiviral agents evaluated for their antiadenoviral effect give inconsistent results (Andersson et al, 2010). ribavirin and cidofovir are used for treatment of adenovirus infection (Gavin & Katz, 2002).

## 2.10 Other microorganism infection

Other opportunistic and non-opportunistic organisms like toxoplamosis, tuberculosis, non tuberculosis mycobacteria, herpes zoster infection, etc may infect CLL patients (Herrero et al, 1995; Mehta et al, 1997; Juliusson & Liliemark, 1996; Krebs et al, 2000)

# 3. Management

## 3.1 Diagnosis

Appropriate diagnosis is important for treatment. Different diagnostic methods may be needed to achieve diagnosis. Culture (blood, urine, sputum, etc.), search for antigens

(Legionella pneumophila serogroup 1, galactomannan, and Streptococcus pneumonia), CSF analysis, radiologic modality (x-ray, CT scan, MRI, etc.), broncoscopy, endoscopy, tissue biopsy and other diagnostic test may be used to find the etiologic agents (Batlle et al., 2001; Krebs et al, 2000).

## 3.2 Treatment

Appropriate antibacterial, antiviral and anti fungal treatment can be life saving (for specific treatment of each microorganism see above). Immunoglobulins are an important component of host defense against infections. They also play a central role in immune regulation. A wide spectrum of human diseases is associated with decreased or abnormal regulation of immunoglobulin levels. Recently intravenous (IV) preparations of immunoglobulin have become available for clinical studies. There are already substantial data indicating a useful role for IV immunoglobulin in patients with primary hypogammaglobulinemia, neonates predisposed to group B streptococcal infections, individuals with ITP, children with Kawasaki disease, bone marrow transplant patients predisposed to CMV infections and in individuals with CLL (Berkman et al, 1988). Intravenous immunoglobulin (IVIG) replacement therapy reduces the number of bacterial infections in CLL patients. However, due to the complexity of immunodeficiency in CLL and the cost-effectiveness of replacement therapy, it is important to identify patients who are likely to benefit from the treatment and to investigate which dose should be used. Low dose of gammaglobulin intravenously can restore normal serum IgG levels in hypogammaglobulinaemic B-CLL patients, and leads to a decreased number of febrile episodes and admissions to hospital due infections (Jurlander et al, 1994, 1995). IVIG has been shown to be a useful prophylactic therapy against infections (Gamm et al, 1994). Granulocyte colony stimulating factor (G-CSF) supplementation may improve the rate of infectious complications by reducing the duration of drug-induced neutropenia (Südhoff et al, 1997). It can be used safely and effectively in CLL-patients with severe bacterial infections to restore neutropenia (Hollander et al, 1991). Granulocyte macrophage colony stimulating factor (GM-CSF) is also effective in improving CLL associated chronic neutropenia and also enhances impaired granulocyte chemiluminescence. Thus, GM-CSF could be helpful for giving chemotherapy without neutropenic delays and for prophylaxis of infectious complications in CLL patients (Itälä et al, 1996, 1998).

## 3.3 Prophylaxis

Patients with advanced disease who receive cytotoxic therapy may benefit from antibacterial prophylaxis. Risk of infection can potentially be reduced by administration of intravenous immunoglobulin and use of prophylactic antibiotics for individuals who are at high risk (5). Treatments of CLL enhance the risk of myelosuppression and infection, so these patients may need antibiotic, antiviral, and antimycotic prophylaxis during and after their administration (Todisco, 2009). Antimicrobial prophylaxis, particularly anti-Pneumocystis prophylaxis, may be indicated in selected patients (Young, 2011). Consideration of primary prophylaxis against M. avium complex infections in aggressively treated patients with advanced B-CLL or other clinical indications may be warranted (Saadeh & Srkalovic, 2008). Some investigators recommend routine antibacterial and antiviral prophylaxis during and after purine nucleoside analogues treatment (Perkins et al.,

2002). An understanding of the patients at highest risk and duration of risk are important in developing recommendations for empirical management, antimicrobial prophylaxis and targeted surveillance (Thursky et al, 2006).

## 3.4 Vaccination

Routine vaccination should be maintained in CLL patients and vaccination early in the course of treatment may result in improve protection (Young, 2011). Antibody response rates to vaccine antigens are lower in patients with CLL compared to normal host. However, if the vaccine has been administered at an early stage of the disease and before starting chemotherapy and the development of hypogammaglobulinaemia, a significant vaccination response to antigens will be obtained in almost 40% of the CLL patients. Early administration of vaccine may be beneficial in CLL patients (Sinisalo et al., 2007). Bacterial polysaccharide vaccines would seem to be ineffective in antibody formation in patients with CLL. However, protein and conjugate vaccines appear to be more immunogenic and their responses may be further enhanced with ranitidine adjuvant treatment (Sinisalo et al, 2003). Response rate to Haemophilus influenzae type b (Hib) conjugate vaccine among adult and elderly patients with chronic lymphocytic leukaemia was 43% in Sinsalo's study (Sinisalo et al, 2002). It is recommended to vaccinate CLL patients with S. pneumoniae and Haemophilus influenzae type b (Hib) vaccines as soon as the diagnosis of CLL is made, early in the course of the disease with determination of post-vaccination antibody levels (Hartkamp et al, 2001). Antibody production after vaccination against common pathogen in CLL patients may improve by treatment histamine type-2 receptor blockade such as ranitidine (Jurlander et al, 1994, 1995). Influenza vaccination is recommended for patients with B-cell CLL however immune response to influenza vaccination appears to be poor (Van der Velden et al, 1995). New well-designed investigations are needed to develop appropriate vaccination strategies and evaluate vaccination efficacy in infection morbidity and mortality in CLL (Sinisalo et al, 2003).

## 4. Conclusion

Infectious complications are leading causes of morbidity and mortality in CLL patients. High index of suspicious and using appropriate diagnostic methods, treatment and prophylaxis can enhance survival of patients.

## 5. Acknowledgment

With special thanks to Dr Soolmaz Korooni.

## 6. References

Andersson EK, Strand M, Edlund K, Lindman K, Enquist PA, Spjut S, Allard A, Elofsson M, Mei YF, Wadell G. (2010). Small-molecule screening using a whole-cell viral replication reporter gene assay identifies 2-{[2-(benzoylamino)benzoyl]amino}-benzoic acid as a novel antiadenoviral compound. *Antimicrob Agents Chemother.* Vol.54, No.9, (September 2010), pp.3871-7, ISSN 0066-4804

Azzam HC, Gahunia MK, Sae-Tia S, Santoro J. (2009). Mycobacterium avium-avium-associated typhlitis mimicking appendicitis in an immunocompetent host. *Am J Med Sci.* Vol.337, No.3, (March 2009), pp. 218-20, ISSN 0002-9629

Bajaj BG, Murakami M, Robertson ES. (2001). Molecular biology of EBV in relationship to AIDS-associated oncogenesis. *Cancer Treat Res.* Vol.133, (2001), pp. 141-62, ISSN 0927-3042

Barton JC, Ratard RC. (2006).Vibrio vulnificus bacteremia associated with chronic lymphocytic leukemia, hypogammaglobulinemia, and hepatic cirrhosis: relation to host and exposure factors in 252 V. vulnificus infections reported in Louisiana. *Am J Med Sci.* Vol.332, No.4, (October 2006), pp. 216-20, ISSN 0002-9629

Batlle M, Ribera JM, Oriol A, Rodríguez L, Cirauqui B, Xicoy B, Grau J, Feliu J, Flores A, Millá F. (2001). Pneumonia in patients with chronic lymphocytic leukemia. Study of 30 episodes. *Med Clin (Barc).* Vol.116, No.19, (May 2001), pp. 738-40, ISSN 0025-7753

Berger C. Infectious mononucleosis. *Ther Umsch.* Vol.60, No.10, (October 2003), pp. 625-30, ISSN 0040-5930

Berger JR, Houff S. (2008). Neurological complications of herpes simplex virus type 2 infection. *Arch Neurol.* Vol.65, No.5, (May 2008), pp. 596-600. ISSN 0003-9942

Berkman SA, Lee ML, Gale RP. (1988). Clinical uses of intravenous immunoglobulins. *Semin Hematol.* Vol.25, No. 2, (April 1988), pp. 140-58, 0037-1963

Bijur S, Menon L, Iyer E, Deshpande J, Sivaraman A, Vaideeswar P, Mahashur AA. (1996). Pneumocystis carinii pneumonia in human immunodeficiency virus infected patients in Bombay: diagnosed by bronchoalveolar lavage cytology and transbronchial lung biopsy. *Indian J Chest Dis Allied Sci.* Vol.38, No.4, (October-December 1996), pp. 227-33, ISSN 0377-9343

Boeckh M, Geballe AP. (2011). Cytomegalovirus: pathogen, paradigm, and puzzle. *J Clin Invest.* Vol.121, No.5, (May 2011), pp. 1673-80, ISSN 0021-9738

Bronke C, Palmer NM, Jansen CA, Westerlaken GH, Polstra AM, Reiss P, Bakker M, Miedema F, Tesselaar K, van Baarle D. (2005). Dynamics of cytomegalovirus (CMV)-specific T cells in HIV-1-infected individuals progressing to AIDS with CMV end-organ disease. *J Infect Dis.* Vol.191, No.6, (March 2005), pp. 873-80, ISSN 1553-6203

Campo M, Lewis RE, Kontoyiannis DP. (2010). Invasive fusariosis in patients with hematologic malignancies at a cancer center: 1998-2009. *J Infect.* Vol.60, No.5, (May 2010), pp. 331-7, ISSN 1553-6203

Canalejo Castrillero E, García Durán F, Cabello N, García Martínez J. (2010). Herpes esophagitis in healthy adults and adolescents: report of 3 cases and review of the literature. *Medicine (Baltimore).* Vol.89, No.4, (July 2010), pp. 204-10, ISSN 0025-7974

Cordes C, Tiemann M, Tiemann K, Knappe D, Hoffmann M, Gottschlich S. (2011). Epstein-Barr virus-associated diffuse large B-cell lymphoma of the hypopharynx. *B-ENT.* Vol.7, No.1, (2011), pp. 43-6, ISSN 1781-782X

Cortelezzi A, Viganò M, Zilioli VR, Fantini NN, Pasquini MC, Deliliers GL, Colombo M, Lampertico P. (2006). Adefovir added to lamivudine for hepatitis B recurrent infection in refractory B-cell chronic lymphocytic leukemia on prolonged therapy with Campath-1H. *J Clin Virol.*Vol.35, No.4, (April 2006), pp. 467-9, ISSN 1386-6532

Dearden C. (2008). Disease-specific complications of chronic lymphocytic leukemia. *Hematology Am Soc Hematol Educ Program.* ( 2008), pp.450-6, ISSN 1520-4391

Dordević H. (2006). Serological response to herpes simplex virus type 1 and 2 infection among women of reproductive age. *Med Pregl.* Vol.59, No.11-12, (November-December 2006), pp. 591-7, ISSN 0025-8105

Eid AJ, Razonable RR. (2010). New developments in the management of cytomegalovirus infection after solid organ transplantation. *Drugs.* Vol.70, No.8, (Fall 2009), pp. 965-81, ISSN 0012-6667

Elter T, Vehreschild JJ, Gribben J, Cornely OA, Engert A & Hallek M. (2009). Management of infections in patients with chronic lymphocytic leukemia treated with alemtuzumab. *Ann Hematol.* Vol.88, No.2, (February 2009), pp.121-32, ISSN 0939-5555

Emery VC.( 2001). Investigation of CMV disease in immunocompromised patients. *J Clin Pathol.* Vol.54, No.2, (February 2001), pp. 84-8, ISSN 0021-9746

Fätkenheuer G, Salzberger B, Diehl V. (1998). Disseminated infection with Mycobacterium avium complex (MAC) in HIV infection. *Med Klin (Munich).* Vol.93, No.6, (Jun 1998), pp. 360-4, ISSN 0723-5003

Gal AA, Plummer AL, Langston AA, Mansour KA. Gal AA, Plummer AL, Langston AA, Mansour KA. *Pathol Res Pract.* Vol.198, No.8, (2002), pp. 553-8, ISSN 0344-0338

Gamm H, Huber C, Chapel H, Lee M, Ries F, Dicato MA. (19994). Intravenous immune globulin in chronic lymphocytic leukaemia. *Clin Exp Immunol.* Vol.97, No. Suppl 1, (July 1994), pp. 17-20, ISSN 0009-9104

Gavin PJ, Katz BZ. (2002). Intravenous ribavirin treatment for severe adenovirus disease in immunocompromised children. *Pediatrics.* Vol.110, No.1, (July 2002), pp.9, ISSN 0031-4005

Haas WH, Amthor B, Engelmann G, Rimek D, Bremer HJ. (1998). Preoperative diagnosis of Mycobacterium avium lymphadenitis in two immunocompetent children by polymerase chain reaction of gastric aspirates. *Pediatr Infect Dis J.* Vol.17, No.11, (November 1998), pp. 1016-20, ISSN 0891-3668

Hamblin AD & Hamblin TJ. (2008). The immunodeficiency of chronic lymphocytic leukaemia. *Br Med Bull.* Vol.47, No.1, (2008), pp. 49-62, ISSN 0007-1420

Hartkamp A, Mulder AH, Rijkers GT, van Velzen-Blad H, Biesma DH. (2001). Antibody responses to pneumococcal and haemophilus vaccinations in patients with B-cell chronic lymphocytic leukaemia. *Vaccine.* Vol.19, No. (13-14), (February 2001), pp. 1671-7, ISSN 0264-410X

Heath ME, Cheson BD. (1985). Defective complement activity in chronic lymphocytic leukemia. *Am J Hematol.* Vol.19, No.1, (May 1985), pp. 63-73, ISSN 0361-8609.

Heider U, Fleissner C, Zavrski I, Jakob C, Dietzel T, Eucker J, Ockenga J, Possinger K, Sezer O. (2004). Treatment of refractory chronic lymphocytic leukemia with Campath-1H in combination with lamivudine in chronic hepatitis B infection. *Eur J Haematol.* Vol.72, No.1, (January 2004), pp. 64-6, ISSN 0902-4441

Herrero M, Cabrera JR, Briz M, Forés R, Díez JL, Regidor C, Sanjuán I, Fernández MN. (1995). Treatment with fludarabine of chronic refractory lymphoid leukemia. *Sangre (Barc).* Vol.40, No.2, (April 1995), pp. 115-9, ISSN 0036-3634

Higgins JP, Warnke RA. (1999). Herpes lymphadenitis in association with chronic lymphocytic leukemia. *Cancer.* Vol.86, No.7, (October 1999), pp. 1210-5. ISSN 0008-5472.

Hollander AA, Kluin-Nelemans HC, Haak HR, Stern AC, Willemze R, Fibbe WE. (1991). Correction of neutropenia associated with chronic lymphocytic leukaemia following treatment with granulocyte-macrophage colony-stimulating factor. Ann Hematol. Vol.62, No. 1, (February 1991), pp. 32-4, ISSN 0939-5555

Itälä M, Vainio O, Remes K.(1996). Functional abnormalities in granulocytes predict susceptibility to bacterial infections in chronic lymphocytic leukaemia. Eur J Haematol. Vol.57, No.1, (July 1996), pp. 46-53, ISSN 0902-4441

Itälä M, Pelliniemi TT, Remes K, Vanhatalo S, Vainio O. (1998). Long-term treatment with GM-CSF in patients with chronic lymphocytic leukemia and recurrent neutropenic infections. Leuk Lymphoma. Vol.32, No. (1-2), (December 1998), pp. 165-74. ISSN 1042-8194

Juliusson G, Liliemark J. (1996). Long-term survival following cladribine (2-chlorodeoxyadenosine) therapy in previously treated patients with chronic lymphocytic leukemia. Ann Oncol. Vol.7, No. 4, (April 1996), pp. 373-9, ISSN 0923-7534

Jurlander J, Geisler CH, Hansen MM. (1994). Treatment of hypogammaglobulinaemia in chronic lymphocytic leukaemia by low-dose intravenous gammaglobulin. Eur J Haematol. Vol.53, No. 2, (August 1994), pp. 114-8, ISSN 0902-4441

Jurlander J, de Nully Brown P, Skov PS, Henrichsen J, Heron I, Obel N, Mortensen BT, Hansen MM, Geisler CH, Nielsen HJ. (1995). Improved vaccination response during ranitidine treatment, and increased plasma histamine concentrations, in patients with B cell chronic lymphocytic leukaemia. Leukemia. Vol.9, No. 11, (November 1995), pp. 1902-9, ISSN 0887-6924

Khalil M, Enzinger C, Wallner-Blazek M, Scarpatetti M, Barth A, Horn S, Reiter G. (2008). Epstein-Barr virus encephalitis presenting with a tumor-like lesion in an immunosuppressed transplant recipient. J Neurovirol. Vol.14, No.6, (October 2008), pp. 574-8, ISSN 1355-0284

Kovacs JA, Masur H. Evolving health effects of Pneumocystis: one hundred years of progress in diagnosis and treatment. Schweiz Med Wochenschr. Vol.124, No.(1-2), (Jun 1994), pp. 73-8, ISSN 0036-7672

Krebs T, Zimmerli S, Bodmer T, Lämmle B. (2000). Mycobacterium genavense infection in a patient with long-standing chronic lymphocytic leukaemia. J Intern Med. Vol.248, No. 4, (October 2000), pp. 343-8, ISSN 0954-6820

Kusne S, Shapiro R, Fung J. (1999). Prevention and treatment of cytomegalovirus infection in organ transplant recipients. Transpl Infect Dis. Vol.1, No.3, (September 1999), pp. 187-203, ISSN 1398-2273

Li ZY, Lou JG, Chen J. (2004). Analysis of primary symptoms and disease spectrum in Epstein-Barr virus infected children. Zhonghua Er Ke Za Zhi. Vol.42, No.1, (Jane 2004), pp. 20-2, ISSN 0578-1310

Longerich T, Eisenbach C, Penzel R, Kremer T, Flechtenmacher C, Helmke B, Encke J, Kraus T, Schirmacher P. (2005).Recurrent herpes simplex virus hepatitis after liver retransplantation despite acyclovir therapy. Liver Transpl. Vol.11, No.10, (October 2005), pp. 1289-94. ISSN 1527-6465

Martin SI, Marty FM, Fiumara K, Treon SP, Gribben JG, Baden LR. (2006). Infectious complications associated with alemtuzumab use for lymphoproliferative disorders. Clin Infect Dis. Vol.43, No.1, (July 2006), pp. 16-24, ISSN 1058-4838

Maschmeyer G, Haas A, Cornely OA. (2007). Invasive aspergillosis: epidemiology, diagnosis and management in immunocompromised patients. *Drugs.* Vol.67, No.11, (2007), pp. 1567-601, ISSN 0012-6667

Massler A, Kolodkin-Gal D, Meir K, Khalaileh A, Falk H, Izhar U, Shufaro Y, Panet A. (2011). Infant lungs are preferentially infected by adenovirus and herpes simplex virus type 1 vectors: role of the tissue mesenchymal cells. *J Gene Med.* Vol.13, No.2, (February 2011), pp.101-13, ISSN 1099-498X

Medlicott SA, Falck VG, Laupland KB, Akbari M, Beck PL. (2005). Herpes simplex virus type II infection of ileum mesothelium: a case report and review of the literature. *Can J Gastroenterol.* Vol.19, No.6, (Jun 2005), pp. 367-71. ISSN 0835-7900

Mehta J, Powles R, Singhal S, Riley U, Treleaven J, Catovsky D. (1997). Antimicrobial prophylaxis to prevent opportunistic infections in patients with chronic lymphocytic leukemia after allogeneic blood or marrow transplantation. *Leuk Lymphoma.* Vol.26, No. (1-2), (June 1997), pp. 83-8. ISSN 1042-8194

Mercadal S, Martinez A, Nomdedeu B, Rozman M, Gaya A, Salamero O, Campo E. (2011). Herpes simplex and Epstein-Barr virus lymphadenitis in a patient with chronic lymphocytic leukemia treated with fludarabine. *Eur J Haematol.* Vol.77, No.5, (November 2006), pp. 442-4, ISSN 0902-4441

Midak-Siewirska A, Karabin K, Chudzik E, Dzieciatkowski T, Przybylski M, Majewska A, Łuczak M, Młynarczyk G. (2010).Application of real-time PCR assay for investigating the presence of herpes simplex virus type 1 DNA. *Med Dosw Mikrobiol.* Vol.62, No.1, ( 2010), pp. 85-92, ISSN 0025-8601

Morra E, Nosari A& Montillo M. (2006). Infectious complications of chronic lymphocytic leukemia. *Hematol Cell Ther.* Vol.41, No.4, (Agust 2006), pp.145-51, ISSN 1269-3286

Morrison VA. (2009). Infectious complications in patients with chronic lymphocytic leukemia: pathogenesis, spectrum of infection, and approaches to prophylaxis. *Clin Lymphoma Myeloma.* Vol.9, No.5, (October 2009), pp. 365-70, ISSN 1938-0712

Mseddi F, Sellami A, Sellami H, Cheikhrouhou F, Makni F, Ayadi A. (2011). Two new media Pinus halepensis seed agar and blackberry agar for rapid identification of Cryptococcus neoformans. *Mycoses.* Vol.54, No.4, (July 2011), pp. 350-3, ISSN 0933-7407

Ndiaye M, Diagne NR, Seck LB, Sow AD, Sène MS, Diop AG, Sow HD, Ndiaye MM.(2011). Cryptococcal meningitis in children: description of 3 cases. *Med Trop (Mars).* Vol.71, No.2, (April 2011), pp. 176-8, ISSN 0025-682X

Nolan A. (209). Interventions for prevention and treatment of herpes simplex virus in cancer patients. *Evid Based Dent.* Vol.10, No.4, (2009), pp. 116-7, ISSN 1462-0049

Otahbachi M, Nugent K, Buscemi D. (2007). Granulomatous Pneumocystis jiroveci Pneumonia in a patient with chronic lymphocytic leukemia: a literature review and hypothesis on pathogenesis. *Am J Med Sci.* Vol.333, No.2, (February 2007), pp. 131-5. ISSN 0002-9629

Ozdemir E, St John LS, Gillespie G, Rowland-Jones S, Champlin RE, Molldrem JJ, Komanduri KV. (2002). Cytomegalovirus reactivation following allogeneic stem cell transplantation is associated with the presence of dysfunctional antigen-specific CD8+ T cells. *Blood.* Vol.100, No.1, (November 2002), pp. 3690-7, ISSN 0006-4971

Pagano L, Fianchi L, Mele L, Girmenia C, Offidani M, Ricci P, Mitra ME, Picardi M, Caramatti C, Piccaluga P, Nosari A, Buelli M, Allione B, Cortelezzi A, Fabbiano F, Milone G, Invernizzi R, Martino B, Masini L, Todeschini G, Cappucci MA, Russo D, Corvatta L, Martino P, Del Favero A. (2002). Pneumocystis carinii pneumonia in patients with malignant haematological diseases: 10 years' experience of infection in GIMEMA centres. *Br J Haematol.* Vol.117, No.2, (May 2002), pp. 379-86, ISSN 1365-2141

Perkins JG, Flynn JM, Howard RS, Byrd JC. (2002). Frequency and type of serious infections in fludarabine-refractory B-cell chronic lymphocytic leukemia and small lymphocytic lymphoma: implications for clinical trials in this patient population. *Cancer.* Vol.94, No.7, (April 2002), pp. 2033-9, ISSN 0008-5472.

Price MS, Betancourt-Quiroz M, Price JL, Toffaletti DL, Vora H, Hu G, Kronstad JW, Perfect JR. (2007) . Cryptococcus neoformans Requires a Functional Glycolytic Pathway for Disease but Not Persistence in the Host. *MBio.* Vol.2, No.3, (Jun 2011), pp. 103-11, ISSN 2150-7511

Ravandi F & O'Brien S. (2006). Immune defects in patients with chronic lymphocytic leukemia. *Cancer Immunol Immunother.* Vol.55, No.2, (February 2006), pp. 197-209, ISSN 0340-7004

Reeves M, Sissons P, Sinclair J. (2005). Reactivation of human cytomegalovirus in dendritic cells. *Discov Med.* Vol.5, No.26, (April 2005), pp. 170-4, ISSN 1539-6509

Rodrigues L, Sampaio D, Couto I, Machado D, Kern WV, Amaral L, Viveiros M. (2009). The role of efflux pumps in macrolide resistance in Mycobacterium avium complex. *Int J Antimicrob Agents.* Vol.34, No.6, (December 2009), pp. 529-33, ISSN 0924-8579

Rossi D, Sala L, Minisini R, Fabris C, Falleti E, Cerri M, Burlone ME, Toniutto P, Gaidano G, Pirisi M. (2009). Occult hepatitis B virus infection of peripheral blood mononuclear cells among treatment-naive patients with chronic lymphocytic leukemia. *Leuk Lymphoma.* Vol.50, No.4, (April 2009), pp.604-11, ISSN 1042-8194

Ruhnke M, Rickerts V, Cornely OA, Buchheidt D, Glöckner A, Heinz W, Höhl R, Horré R, Karthaus M, Kujath P, Willinger B, Presterl E, Rath P, Ritter J, Glasmacher A, Lass-Flörl C, Groll AH. (2011). Diagnosis and therapy of Candida infections: joint recommendations of the German Speaking Mycological Society and the Paul-Ehrlich-Society for Chemotherapy. *Mycoses.* Vol.54, No.4, (July 2011), pp. 279-310, ISSN 0933-7407

Saadeh CE, Srkalovic G. (2008). Mycobacterium avium complex infection after alemtuzumab therapy for chronic lymphocytic leukemia. *Pharmacotherapy.* Vol.28, No.2, (February 2008), pp. 281-4, ISSN 0277-0008

Saritsiri S, Udomsantisook N, Suankratay C. (2006). Nontuberculous mycobacterial infections in King Chulalongkorn Memorial Hospital. J Med Assoc Thai. Vol.89, No.12, (December 2006), pp. 2035-46, ISSN 0125-2208

Sester M, Sester U, Gärtner BC, Girndt M, Meyerhans A, Köhler H.( 2002). Dominance of virus-specific CD8 T cells in human primary cytomegalovirus infection. *J Am Soc Nephrol.* Vol.13, No.10, (October 2002), pp. 2577-84, ISSN 1046-6673

Shiota T, Lixin W, Takayama-Ito M, Iizuka I, Ogata M, Tsuji M, Nishimura H, Taniguchi S, Morikawa S, Kurane I, Mizuguchi M, Saijo M. (2011). Expression of herpes simplex virus type 1 recombinant thymidine kinase and its application to a rapid antiviral sensitivity assay. *Antiviral Res.* Vol.91, No.2, (Jun 2011), pp. 142-149, ISSN 0166-3542

Sidrim JJ, Costa AK, Cordeiro RA, Brilhante RS, Moura FE, Castelo-Branco DS, Neto MP, Rocha MF. (2010). Molecular methods for the diagnosis and characterization of Cryptococcus: a review. *Can J Microbiol*. Vol.56, No.6, (Jun 2010), pp. 445-58, ISSN 0008-4166

Sinisalo M, Aittoniemi J, Käyhty H, Vilpo J. (2003). Vaccination against infections in chronic lymphocytic leukemia. *Leuk Lymphoma*. Vol.44, No. 4, (April 2003), pp. 649-52. ISSN 1042-8194

Sinisalo M, Aittoniemi J, Käyhty H, Vilpo J. (2002). Haemophilus influenzae type b (Hib) antibody concentrations and vaccination responses in patients with chronic lymphocytic leukaemia: predicting factors for response. *Leuk Lymphoma*. Vol.43, No. 10, (October 2002), pp. 1967-9. ISSN 1042-8194

Sinisalo M, Vilpo J, Taurio J, Aittoniemi J. (2007). Antibody response to 7-valent conjugated pneumococcal vaccine in patients with chronic lymphocytic leukaemia. *Vaccine*. Vol.26, No.1, (December 2007), pp. 82-7, ISSN **0264-410X**

Südhoff T, Arning M, Schneider W. (1997). Prophylactic strategies to meet infectious complications in fludarabine-treated CLL. *Leukemia*. Vol.11, No. Suppl 2, (April 1997), pp. 38-41, ISSN 0887-6924

Tafreshi NK, Sadeghizadeh M, Amini-Bavil-Olyaee S, Ahadi AM, Jahanzad I, Roostaee MH. (2005). Development of a multiplex nested consensus PCR for detection and identification of major human herpesviruses in CNS infections. *J Clin Virol*. Vol.32, No.4, (April 2005), pp. 318-24, ISSN1386-6532

Thalla R, Kim D, Venkat KK, Parasuraman R. (2009). Sequestration of active Cryptococcus neoformans infection in the parathyroid gland despite prolonged therapy in a renal transplant recipient. *Transpl Infect Dis*. Vol.11, No.4, (August 2009), pp. 349-52, ISSN 1398-2273

Thursky KA, Worth LJ, Seymour JF, Miles Prince H, Slavin MA. (2006). Spectrum of infection, risk and recommendations for prophylaxis and screening among patients with lymphoproliferative disorders treated with alemtuzumab. *Br J Haematol*. Vol.132, No. 1, (January 2006), pp. 3-12, ISSN 0902-4441

Todisco M. (2009). Chronic lymphocytic leukemia: long-lasting remission with combination of cyclophosphamide, somatostatin, bromocriptine, retinoids, melatonin, and ACTH. *Cancer Biother Radiopharm*. Vol.24, No. 3, (June 2009), pp. 353-5, ISSN 1084-9785

Travade P, Dusart JD, Cavaroc M, Beytout J, Rey M. (1986). Severe infections associated with chronic lymphoid leukemia. 159 infectious episodes in 60 patients. *Presse Med*. Vol.15, No.34, (October 1986), pp. 1715-8, ISSN **0755-4982**

Turkulov V, Madle-Samardzija N, Brkić S. (1999). Meningoencephalitis as the only manifestation of Epstein-Barr virus infection. *Med Pregl*. Vol.52, No.(9-10), (September 1999), pp. 391-3, ISSN 0025-8105

Vancíková Z, Dvorák P.( 2001). Cytomegalovirus infection in immunocompetent and immunocompromised individuals-a review. *Curr Drug Targets Immune Endocr Metabol Disord*. 2001 Vol.1, No.2, (February 2001), pp. 179-87, ISSN 1568-0088

Van der Velden AM, Mulder AH, Hartkamp A, Diepersloot RJ, van Velzen-Blad H, Biesma DH. (1995). Influenza virus vaccination and booster in B-cell chronic lymphocytic leukaemia patients. *Eur J Intern Med*. Vol.12, No. 5, (September 1995), pp. 420-424, ISSN 0953-6205

Van Koeveringe MP, Brouwer RE. (2010). Histoplasma capsulatum reactivation with haemophagocytic syndrome in a patient with chronic lymphocytic leukaemia. *Neth J Med.* Vol.68, No.12, (December 2010), pp. 418-21, ISSN 0300-2977

Vavricka SR, Halter J, Hechelhammer L, Himmelmann A. (2004). Pneumocystis carinii pneumonia in chronic lymphocytic leukaemia. *Postgrad Med J.* Vol.80, No.942, (April 2004), pp. 236-8, ISSN 0022-3859

Wadhwa PD & Morrison VA. (2006). Infectious complications of chronic lymphocytic leukemia. *Semin Oncol.* Vol.33, No.2, (April 2006), pp. 240-9, ISSN 0093-7754

Wierda WG.(2003). Immunologic monitoring in chronic lymphocytic leukemia. *Curr Oncol Rep.* Vol.5, No.5, (September 2003), pp. 419-25, ISSN 1523-3790

Yadegarynia D, Abbasi F, Haghighi M, Korooni Fardkhani S, Yadegarynia S. Pneumonitis due to cytomegalovirus in an immunocompromised patient. *Iranian Journal of Clinical Infectious Disease* Vol.4, No.4, (Fall 2009), pp. 238-240, ISSN 1735-5109

Yağci M, Acar K, Sucak GT, Aki Z, Bozdayi G, Haznedar R. (2006). A prospective study on chemotherapy-induced hepatitis B virus reactivation in chronic HBs Ag carriers with hematologic malignancies and pre-emptive therapy with nucleoside analogues. *Leuk Lymphoma.* Vol.47, No.8, (August 2006), pp. 1608-12, ISSN 1042-8194

Young JA. (2011). Epidemiology and management of infectious complications of contemporary management of chronic leukemias. (2011). *Infect Disord Drug Targets.* Vol.11, No.1, (February 2011), pp. 3-10, ISSN 1871-5265

Zahorodnia SD, Nesterova NV, Danylenko VP, Bukhtiarova TA, Baranova HV, Holovan' AV. (2011). Effect of isonicotinic acid derivates on reproduction of Epstein-Barr virus. *Mikrobiol Z.* Vol.73, No.2, (March-April 2011), pp. 65-72, ISSN 1028-0987

# 6

# *In Vitro* Sensitivity Testing in the Assessment of Anti-CLL Drug Candidates

Günter Krause, Mirjam Kuckertz, Susan Kerwien,
Michaela Patz and Michael Hallek
*Department I of Internal Medicine, University of Cologne,*
*Center of Integrated Oncology Köln Bonn,*
*Germany*

## 1. Introduction

Chronic lymphocytic leukemia (CLL) is characterized by the accumulation of morphologically mature, but immuno-incompetent B-lymphocytes in the bone marrow, peripheral blood, spleen and lymphoid organs. With an annual incidence of about 2-3/ 100000 in the general population (Hamblin, 2009), CLL represents a frequent leukemia type. Since CLL mostly affects persons of advanced age, the incidence among persons above 65 years reaches ten times this frequency (Eichhorst et al., 2009). Moreover CLL follows a remarkably heterogeneous course, emphasizing the need for personalized treatment approaches. Despite recent advances in CLL therapy, the disease still remains incurable and new treatment options need to be developed (Hallek et al., 2008). New insights into CLL biology have started to result in new targeted, sometimes patient group-specific treatment approaches (Pleyer et al., 2009; Zenz et al., 2010). Candidate substances for pre-clincial assays are mostly molecularly targeted drugs, i.e. either small molecules interfering with intracellular signaling (Wickremasinghe et al., 2011) or mononoclonal antibodies (Jaglowski et al., 2010). As examples we will discuss in this chapter the pre-clinical assessment of protein and lipid kinase inhibitors and of monoclonal antibodies.

Since candidate substances with a potential for treating CLL become available at an increasing pace, there is a growing need for comprehensive laboratory assessment of these substances. For this purpose the effects of these drug candidates on fresh CLL lymphocytes are compared by means of viability and cytotoxicity assays with the aim of selecting suitable candidates for further development. In addition viability and cytotoxicity assays on CLL cells serve to prepare candidate substances for clinical trials and to determine, which subgroups of patients respond best, in the sense of personalized medicine. This endeavor constitutes the small excerpt of the drug discovery process immediately preceding clinical trials (Collins & Workman, 2006). Since it links laboratory investigation and clinical application it can be understood as translational research, which is further underscored by patient samples being subjected to cultivation and observation in the laboratory.

B lymphocytes freshly isolated from peripheral blood of CLL patients constitute a readily available source for the pre-clinical *in vitro* assessment of drugs and combinations with therapeutic potential for treating CLL. Due to the epidemiological features of CLL as a frequent chronic leukemia, with many patients living with the disease for extended periods, a continuous supply of blood samples can be made available and used in a meaningful manner by performing pre-clinical assays, which, according to the concept of translational medicine, in turn could lead to improved therapies. Drug assessment on fresh CLL samples can be performed rapidly and relatively conveniently by comparing untreated and treated *in vitro* cultures.

On the other hand, primary cultures of B cells freshly isolated from the peripheral blood of CLL patients often may represent an insufficient model for predicting clinical drug efficacy, since they are known to behave differently from CLL lymphocytes in their *in vivo* environment. This is evident from the obviously contrasting behavior of CLL cells *in vivo* and during *in vitro* culture. Whereas accumulation of CLL cells *in vivo* is thought to occur due to resistance towards apoptosis and a certain degree of cell proliferation, *in vitro* cultures spontaneously undergo apoptosis and show low viability and almost completely absent proliferation. Because this contrasting behaviour of CLL cells *in vitro* and *in vivo* can be attributed to a lack of the appropriate micro-environment during laboratory culture, the value of drug assessment on CLL lymphocytes *ex vivo* can be greatly enhanced by mimicking certain micro-environmental stimuli.

Commonly used cytotoxicity and viability assays are compiled in this chapter and will be discussed in the context of the assessment of potential anti-CLL drugs. On the level of individual susceptibility it is well established for chemotherapeutic agents that sensitivity of tumor cells *in vitro* corresponds to the probability of clinical response (Bosanquet et al., 2009). Therefore one would expect also for targeted drugs that *in vitro* assays enable to some degree the comparison of the efficacies of different agents and the prediction of the response of molecularly defined subgroups of CLL patients. As examples for correlations of molecularly defined patient subgroups with treatment susceptibility *in vitro* we name here the clearly higher dasatinib sensitivity of CLL samples with unmutated IgHV genes as compared to mutated ones (Veldurthy et al., 2008) or the correlation of the B cell depletion induced by CD20 antibodies with antigen expression on the surface of CLL cells (Patz et al., 2011).

In this chapter we review the pros and cons of pre-clinical drug assessment in comparatively simple *ex vivo* assays. The predictability of treatment out-come from *in vitro* cultures of CLL lymphocytes must be considered, since there are known limitations of the assay system, which can, however, be overcome to a certain degree by linking the results to investigations of target and cell type specificity.

## 2. Performing cytotoxicity assays on CLL samples

In the course of the pre-clinical assessment of anti-CLL drug candidates, *in vitro* cultures of CLL lymphocytes are treated with test substances. Subsequently dose-dependent treatment effects on the viability of CLL cells are recorded by means of established proliferation and cytotoxicity assays. These assays yield a first measure of drug potency for CLL lymphocytes, but certainly need to be rigidly controlled and standardized. Moreover they should be accompanied by biochemical assays in order to assure cell type and target specificity. Such comprehensive approaches will allow the design of meaningful drug combinations, which then are to be subjected to another round of *in vitro* sensitivity assays.

Cytotoxicity assays play a pivotal role in pre-clinical drug testing (Kepp et al., 2011) and many of them are suitable for assessing treatment effects on fresh CLL cells (*Table 1*). Some of these assays are based on absolute cell counts or less laborious surrogate parameters determining total cellular activities e.g. in colorimetric or fluorimetric non-clonogenic microculture assays (Lindhagen et al., 2008). In contrast, flow cytometric assays usually yield percentages of cells with certain properties within the investigated cell population unless they are standardized for the examined volume, e.g. by absolute counting beads.

| Method | Technological platform | parameters |
|---|---|---|
| cell counting | light microscope | trypan blue exclusion |
| metabolic activity | absorbance reader | tetrazolium salt reduction |
| ATP consumption | luminometer | luciferase activity |
| intracellular esterase activity | fluorimeter | conversion of non-fluorescent fluorescein diacetate |
| DNA replication | absorbance reader flow cytometry | bromo-deoxyuridine incorporation |
| phosphatidylserine exposure | flow cytometry | annexin V-binding |
| membrane disintegration | flow cytometry | staining with DNA intercalating dye |
| Δψm dissipation | flow cytometry | fluorescent dye, e.g. DiOC6 |
| morphology | flow cytometry | forward scatter / side scatter |
| production of reactive oxygen species | flow cytometry | fluorigenic substrate, e.g. CM-H2-DCF-DA |
| caspase activation | flow cytometry immunoblotting | fluorescent substrates detection of cleaved fragments |

Table 1. Selected cytotoxicity and viability assays commonly used with CLL samples.

## 2.1 Flow cytometric cell death and viability assays

Flow cytometric assessment of phosphatidylserine exposure and membrane disintegration is among the viability and cytotoxicity assays most frequently applied for monitoring drug effects on CLL cells. Percentages of cell populations undergoing cell death can be determined by monitoring the loss of membrane asymmetry in early phases of apoptosis and subsequent membrane disruption (*Fig. 1*). This can be achieved by staining cells, e.g. B lymphocytes, with fluorescently labeled annexin V, which binds to phosphatidylserine with high affinity (Koopman et al., 1994). Phosphatidylserine exposure accompanies early phases of apoptosis, before membrane disintegration of the cytoplasma membrane allows access of DNA intercalating dies to the nucleus. Counter-staining with DNA intercalating dyes originally served the distinction of apoptotic from necrotic cells. Analysis of annexin V binding or DNA staining can be replaced for staining with dyes indicating mitochondrial membrane potential, e.g. 3,3′-dihexyloxacarbocyanine iodide (DiOC6) (Stanglmaier et al.,

2004; Veldurthy et al., 2008), or reactive oxygen species, e.g. the fluorogenic chloromethyl-2,7-dichlorodihydrofluorescein-diacetate (CM-$H_2$-DCF-DA) (Lilienthal et al., 2011). Usually populations of CLL cells with phosphatidylserine exposure coincide with those showing typical morphological signs of apoptosis, i.e. reduced size and increased granularity as indicated by forward-scatter (FSC) and side-scatter (SSC) in the flow cytometer. Concerns have been raised about a possible over-estimation of drug effects due to flow cytometry artefacts. For instance, the widely used determination of phosphatidylserine exposure was claimed to over-estimate apoptosis induction in the extraordinarily fragile CLL cells due to *in vitro* handling during sample preparation for flow cytometry (Groves et al., 2009). Similarly antibody effects on CLL samples determined by flow cytometry were suspected of being misinterpreted owing to cell aggregation (Golay et al., 2010). These concerns can be overcome by parallel biological effect monitoring in several different assay systems as controls.

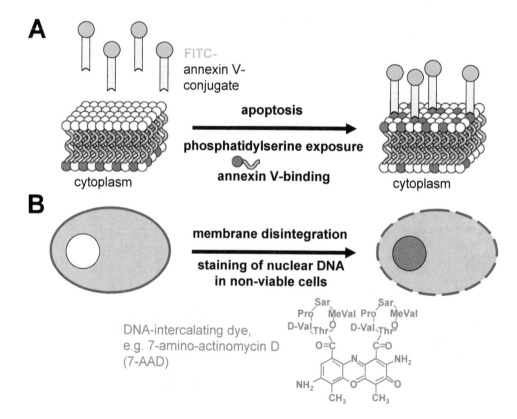

Fig. 1. Principle of a widely used assay for the determination of the percentages of apoptotic cells. The flow cytometric assessment of phosphatidylserine exposure (A) and membrane disintegration (B) can be performed simultaneously.
Part (A) adapted from Zhang et al., 1997 and Pharmingen, 1998.

## 2.2 Concentration dependence

Investigation of the dose-dependency of drug effects is an important confirmation of any observations that by far surpasses the importance of repeated measurements. In addition, the shape of dose response curves sometimes can provide mechanistic clues, e.g. in the case of saturation effects. When drugs are investigated for CLL that previously have been pre-clinically developed or admitted for the treatment of other cancers, it is possible to consider achievable plasma concentrations for the *in vitro* assessment. Biological effect measurements obtained at multiple concentrations can be conveniently summarized by concentrations inhibiting 50 % ($IC_{50}$). These $IC_{50}$ concentrations can be a useful manner of comparing the effects of different drugs or diverging sensitivities of different samples. In the case of saturation effects, as in the dose response of CLL lymphocytes to dasatinib (Veldurthy et al., 2008), it might be more appropriate to indicate the individual saturation levels of response rather than extrapolating $IC_{50}$ concentrations. Moreover, investigators must not be misled by the convenience of such tabulated values to regard them as sample-specific constants and therefore to apply them to different assay types, since $IC_{50}$ concentrations strictly depend on the type of assay performed (Krause & Hallek, 2011).

## 3. Mimicking micro-environmental interactions

Considering the micro-environment of CLL cells may improve predictions of clinical drug efficacy from *in vitro* assays on fresh CLL samples. Regarding their resistance to apoptosis CLL cells in culture behave entirely differently from the situation *in vivo*, owing to dependence on their micro-environment. Therefore it is necessary to simulate certain micro-environmental stimuli for drug assessment *in vitro*, for instance following the approaches described in the following subchapters. A number of ligand/receptor pairs have been identified that activate CLL cells (*Fig. 2*) (Munk Pedersen & Reed, 2004), among them the chemokine stroma-derived factor 1, nowadays referred to as CXCL12 and its receptor CXCR4 on CLL cells, that belongs to the class of G-protein-coupled 7-transmembrane domain receptors (Burger & Kipps, 2006) and VCAM-1 (CD106) expressed on the surface of stroma cells that interacts with the integrin VAL-4 (CD49a) on CLL cells (Burger et al., 2009). The strict dependence of CLL cells on the interactions with their environment is also apparent from the absence of good cell line models for CLL.

### 3.1 B cell receptor stimulation

Like for normal lymphocytes, also the fate of CLL cells is to a high degree determined by B cell receptor (BCR) stimulation (Stevenson & Caligaris-Cappio, 2004). According to the degree of somatic hypermutation in rearranged antigen receptor genes, subgroups of CLL clones with immunoglobulin heavy chain variable region (IgHV) genes can be distinguished that reflect progressing B cell development stages corresponding to naïve or memory B cells. Usually the threshold separating these molecularly defined prognostic subgroups is set at 2 % sequence divergence of rearranged IgHV genes from the closest germline sequences. The CLL subgroups with unmutated or mutated IgHV genes have a widely different prognosis indicated by 24 versus 8 years median overall survival after diagnosis (Hamblin et al., 1999). High expression of zeta-assoziated protein 70 (ZAP-70) and of CD38 serve as surrogate markers of unmutated IgHV genes (Crespo et al., 2003; Hamblin et al., 2002).

Antigen contact for CLL cells can be mimicked *in vitro* by crosslinking surface IgM by means of anti-IgM antibodies. Long lasting stimulation of the BCR leads to prolonged survival of CLL cells (Deglesne et al., 2006). This can be achieved by using soluble anti-IgM or anti-IgM-coated surfaces.

## 3.2 CD40 stimulation

The CD40 molecule expressed on the surface of CLL cells belongs to the tumor necrosis factor family and participates in antigen recognition as a co-receptor. Its cognate ligand, CD40 ligand (CD40L), also known as CD154, is expressed on the surface of activated T lymphocytes. Engagement of CD40 on CLL lymphocytes mimics the micro-environment inside lymph nodes and leads to protection against DNA damaging substances, e.g. chemotherapeutic agents. CD40L stimulation of CLL cells can be provided by co-culture with fibroblasts expressing recombinant CD154. For instance co-culture with CD40L expressing fibroblasts protects CLL cells from DNA damaging agents, but this effect can be partly reversed by the kinase inhibitor dasatinib (Hallaert et al., 2008). The sensitivity of CLL cells for the Bcl-2 antagonist ABT737 is decreased by a factor of 1000, if the CLL cells are co-cultivated with fibroblasts expressing CD40L (Vogler et al., 2009).

## 3.3 Stroma cell-derived soluble factors and cell surface interactions

The soluble factors produced by bone marrow stromal cells include the chemokine CXCL12, which despite its original designation as stroma-cell derived factor is shown in *Fig. 2* as a micro-environmental factor occurring in peripheral blood, owing to its alternate origin from nurse-like cells. Stimulation by purified recombinant CXCL12 induced the raf-dependent mitogen activated protein (MAP) kinase cascades in CLL cells, which augmented their survival and was targeted by the raf inhibitor sorafenib (Messmer et al., 2011).

*In vivo*, inhibition of apoptosis may occur preferentially in pseudofollicles containing CLL and accessory cells, due to cell contact and mutual paracrine and autocrine stimulation. *In vitro*, co-culture with bone-marrow-derived stromal cells, e.g. the cell line HS-5, may provide stimuli for long-term survival of CLL cells. In co-cultures of primary CLL cells with HS-5 cells, various chemokines attracting T lymphocytes, most prominently CCL4 and CCL3, were detected, which are not produced by HS-5 control cultures (Seiffert et al., 2010). The proteins found in the supernatant of HS-5 co-cultures included factors, which are commonly secreted by monocytes, e.g. soluble CD14. Among the soluble factors provided to CLL cells by co-culture with the bone marrow stromal cell line HS5, vascular endothelial growth factor (VEGF) is partly responsible for the increase in viability of co-cultivated CLL cells (Gehrke et al., 2011).

## 3.4 Oligonucleotides containing CpG dinucleotides

Toll like receptor 9 (TLR9) has been identified as a part of the innate immune response recognizing unmethylated foreign DNA that can be mimicked by phosphothioate oligodeoxynucleotides containing CpG dinucleotides (CpG-ODN) (Krieg, 2006). Survival and proliferation of CLL cells can be considerably enhanced by class B CpG-ODN, e.g. DSPN-30 (Decker et al., 2000). Like CD40 ligation, activation of CLL cells through TLR9 occupation by CpG-ODN was exploited as a mitogenic signal in order to obtain metaphase chromosomes for cytogenetic analysis by fluorescent in situ hybridization (Mayr et al., 2006). The importance of activated CLL cells in drug assessment is demonstrated by the example of mTOR inhibitors. In untreated CLL cells rapamycin showed an $IC_{50}$ of 10 µM for apoptosis induction (Aleskog et al., 2008). In contrast less than one thousandth of this concentration of RAD001 or 10 nM rapamycin was sufficient for complete inhibition of the cell proliferation induced by CpG-ODN (Decker et al., 2003).

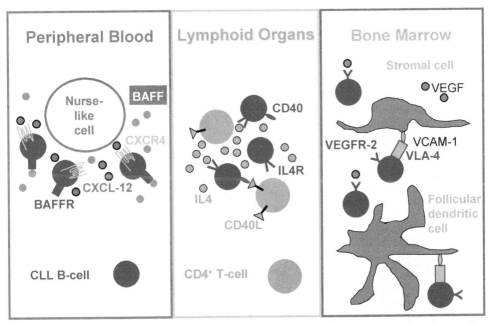

Fig. 2. Microenvironment interactions of CLL cells. The survival of CLL lymphocytes can be prolonged by contact with different accessory cells in the peripheral blood, lymphoid system and bone marrow. Some prominent interactions of CLL cells with soluble factors and cell surface molecules supplied by accessory cells are shown. On the surface of CLL cells receptors for various soluble factors are expressed, e.g. for the chemokine CXCL12, formerly designated as stroma-derived factor 1 (SDF-1), for the cytokine interleukin-4 (IL-4), and for vascular endothelial growth factor (VEGF). CD40 or the integrin VAL-4 on the surface of CLL cells interact with CD40 ligand (CD40L) on T cells or VCAM-1 on follicular dendritic cells and other stromal cells, respectively. Adapted from Munk Pedersen *et al.*, 2004.

In addition to activating CLL cells CpG-ODN were found to increase surface expression levels of co-stimulatory molecules including CD20 (Jahrsdorfer et al., 2001). Consequently, the same CpG-ODN DSPN-30 that is commonly used for activating CLL cells, increased CD20 expression on freshly isolated CLL cells, which in turn led to higher B cell depletion by the type II CD20 antibody GA101 (Patz et al., 2011).

## 3.5 B cell depletion from whole blood samples

Monoclonal antibodies (MABs) induce direct cell death (DCD) of tumor cells via signal transduction and additional Fc-mediated cytotoxic effects, namely antibody-dependent cell-mediated cytotoxicity (ADCC) and complement-dependent cytotoxicity (CDC) (*Fig. 3*). In order to include ADCC and CDC in measurements of overall MAB effects, the extent of tumor cell depletion by MABs from individual blood samples can be determined by multi-color flow cytometry comparing treated and untreated whole blood cultures.

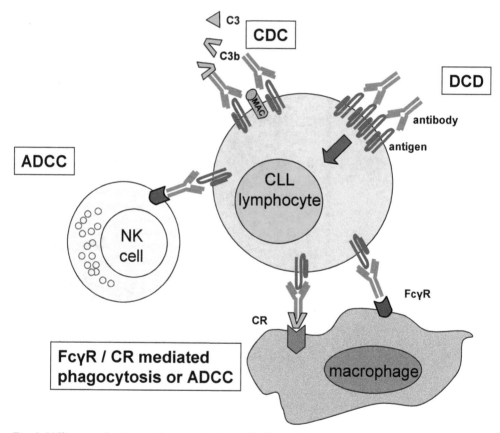

Fig. 3. Killing mechanisms of monoclonal antibodies and their assessment. Apart from direct cell death (DCD) induction in tumor cells, monoclonal antibodies exert their action via Fc-mediated functions, namely complement-mediated cytotoxicity (CDC) and antibody-dependent cell-mediated cytotoxicity (ADCC) and phagocytosis. Due to the importance of CD20 antibodies in CLL therapy, a structure crossing the cell membrane four times is shown as the surface antigen on CLL cells. This overall structural organization is shared by another emerging target for immunotherapy, the tetraspanin CD37. Ways to examine the above mechanisms on isolated CLL cells and whole blood samples are compiled in *Table* 2 and described in the text. Adapted from Olszewski & Grossbard, 2004 and Jaglowski et al., 2010.

## 4. Pre-clinical assessment of kinase inhibitors

Prototypic targeted therapy by the tyrosine kinase inhibitor imatinib was developed for Bcr-Abl positive leukemias, in which deregulated Abl activity is a predominant driving force (Druker et al., 2001). In contrast, the pathogenesis of CLL appears to be multi-factorial. The second generation of Abl inhibitors for treatment of imatinib-resistant Bcr-Abl positive leukemias achieves greater efficacy against mutant forms of the Abl kinase (Weisberg et al., 2007). Some of these inhibitors, e.g. dasatinib (Shah et al., 2004) and bosutinib (Puttini et al., 2006) are dual-specific and target Abl and additionally Src kinases. Since members of the latter tyrosine kinase family, e.g. Lyn (Contri et al., 2005) and Lck (Majolini et al., 1999) have been suggested to be involved in CLL pathogenesis, we conducted an assessment of dasatinib on CLL cells (Veldurthy et al., 2008). This pre-clinical investigation indicated an influence of Src kinase inhibition on the cellular survival of CLL cells with preference for the subgroups with unmutated immunoglobulin heavy chain genes or with high ZAP70 expression and thus indicated patient groups that might profit most from Src kinase inhibition. Since the fate of CLL B lymphocytes critically depends on BCR signaling (Stevenson & Caligaris-Cappio, 2004), inhibition by kinase inhibitors of survival pathways emanating from the BCR or from micro-environmental stimuli (Burger et al., 2009) represents a promising strategy for treating CLL (Gandhi, 2010).

Drug assessment on primary CLL cells serves as preparation for clinical trials and to some degree enables comparison of the efficacies of different agents and the prediction of the response of molecularly defined subgroups of CLL patients. The clearly higher dasatinib sensitivity of CLL samples with unmutated $IgV_H$ genes as compared to mutated ones is an example for this type of correlation (Veldurthy et al., 2008). Signaling analysis revealed that treatment of primary CLL cells with dasatinib drastically reduces the level of activated SFK in CLL cells, but inhibits downstream BCR signaling pathways and induces apoptosis more strongly in the patient subgroup with aggressive disease. The extent of dasatinib-induced apoptosis in CLL cells corresponds to the concomitant decrease in the phosphorylation of the direct SFK substrates Syk and phospholipase C-γ (Song et al., 2010). Signaling analysis during SFK inhibition thus contributed to the rationale for pre-clinical assessment of Syk inhibitors on CLL cells (Baudot et al., 2009; Buchner et al., 2009). For another second generation dual Abl/Src inhibitor, bosutinib, inhibition of the receptor tyrosine kinase Axl was found to be partially responsible for its apoptosis induction in CLL cells (Ghosh et al., 2010).

Inhibition of Abl does not reduce viability of CLL cells on its own, but can sensitize CLL cells for chemotherapeutic agents, e.g. chlorambucil, by interfering with DNA repair (Aloyz et al., 2004). Inhibitors of the delta isoform of the catalytic p110 subunit of phosphatidylinositol-3-kinase (PI3K) show moderate efficiencies on primary CLL lymphocytes without activation that contrast the promising effects in clinical trials. The observed pre-clinical efficiency of the PI3K-delta inhibitor CAL-101 is not abrogated by micro-environmental stimulation and other cell types, while other cell types, e.g. natural killer cells are not influenced by CAL-101 (Herman et al., 2010).

## 5. Pre-clinical assessment of monoclonal antibodies

Apart from small molecules, monoclonal antibodies constitute another group of targeted therapeutics for the treatment of CLL. This group includes the first biological anti-tumor agent, namely the CD20 antibody rituximab. As a common cell surface antigen of all B cells except stem or plasma cells, CD20 has become a very effective antibody target for the treatment of B cell malignancies (Molina, 2008) including CLL despite variable surface expression on CLL cells. Together with the monoclonal anti-CD52 antibody alemtuzumab, rituximab thus may be counted among the most efficient targeted treatment options for CLL achieved so far. In a recent phase III trial inclusion of rituximab was shown to substantially improve the established fludarabine / cyclophosphamide chemotherapy regimen (Hallek et al., 2010).

Apart from DCD induction in tumor cells, monoclonal antibodies exert their action via Fc-mediated functions, namely CDC, ADCC and phagocytosis (Jaglowski et al., 2010; Olszewski & Grossbard, 2004) (*Fig. 3*). Therefore an assessment of antibody effects on CLL cells *ex vivo* can either be performed on freshly isolated CLL cells in separate dedicated assays for each mentioned mechanisms, or in a comprehensive assay from whole (*Table 2*). For assessing antibody effects on isolated CLL cells, the same procedures as for other anti-CLL agents can only be applied for the determination of DCD. For instance DCD induction by rituximab in freshly isolated CLL cells was assessed according to viable cell counts, metabolic activity and phosphatidylserine exposure and was found variable among individual samples and considerably smaller than in lymphoma cell lines (Patz et al., 2011; Stanglmaier et al., 2004). Since DCD induction in primary CLL cells may constitute only a minor fraction of overall B cell depletion as in the case of rituximab (Voso et al., 2002), it is indispensable to additionally assess Fc-mediated mechanisms. For performing ADCC assays on isolated CLL lymphocytes, effector cells need to be externally added, e.g. autologous or heterologous peripheral blood mononuclear cells or a natural killer cell line (Weitzman et al., 2009). Similarly, CDC can be assessed by monitoring changes in the membrane integrity of CLL cells after incubation in medium containing high concentrations of complete as compared to heat-inactivated serum (Golay et al., 2000; Patz et al., 2011).

| Mechanism | Isolated CLL cells | Whole blood |
|---|---|---|
| DCD | Cytotoxicity or viability assays | Requires distinction of CLL lymphocytes from other cell populations |
| CDC | Comparison of effects with complete or heat-inactivated serum | Complement inhibition by cobra venom factor |
| ADCC | Externally added effector cells | Blocking antibodies for Fc receptors |

Table 2. Determination and dissection of different mechanisms of antibody-induced cytotoxicity.

As an alternative to these separate assays, we applied a B cell depletion assay from whole blood encompassing Fc-mediated antibody-induced cytotoxicity. This assay is based on the enumeration of B lymphocytes in differentially treated whole blood samples after staining the general, B- and T- lymphocyte antigens CD45, CD19 and CD3 using three color flow cytometry and commercially available fluorescently labeled immunoreagents. B cell depletion can be calculated from the B cell counts in antibody-treated versus untreated control samples. B/T cell ratios with the T cell population as an internal standard can be used for this calculation, if T cell counts are proven to be unaffected by the antibody treatment. Alternatively absolute B cell counts can be determined using externally added fluorescent counting beads. In part the contributions of DCD, CDC and ADCC to the observed B cell depletion from whole blood samples can be dissected. Thus, we were able to show a substantial contribution of ADCC to the B cell depletion by the novel type II CD20 antibody GA101 (Moessner et al., 2010) by blocking the interaction of FcγIIIa on NK cells and macrophages and the Fc exposed on antibody-coated target cells by incubation with anti-CD16 antibody in whole blood from healthy donors but not CLL patients (Patz et al., 2011). In summary, flow cytometric determination of B cell depletion from whole blood has the potential of comparing antibody effects on individual CLL samples and of predicting clinical responses.

Resistance mechanisms to anti-CLL antibodies have been unraveled by pre-clinical models and some of the influences interfering with antibody efficacy may be recapitulated in the the present B cell depletion from whole blood samples (*Table 3*) (Reslan et al., 2009). Thus the shape of the dose response curves of GA101 or mAb37.1 observed in the B cell depletion assay (Krause et al., 2011; Patz et al., 2011) is of saturation type and suggests an influence on antibody effects of individually different levels of endogenous human IgG in the assay matrix (Preithner et al., 2006). Similarly, varying ratios of effector to target cells, the Phe158Val polymorphism of FcγIIIa (Cartron et al., 2002) as well as complement depletion (Kennedy et al., 2004) will influence B cell depletion from whole blood samples. Thus, the assay described here has the advantage of reflecting both, the efficiency of antibody-induced B cell depletion and the potential to supply host-dependent immune functions and thus should be able to predict at the individual level the clinical efficiency of therapeutics assayed *in vitro*.

| Influence | References |
|---|---|
| Antigen density on target cells | Golay et al., 2001, Patz et al., 2011 |
| Complement depletion | Kennedy et al., 2004 |
| Complement inhibitors CD59 and CD55 | Golay et al., 2001 |
| Ratio of effector to target cells | |
| Plasma levels of IgG | Preithner et al., 2006 |
| Fc receptor polymorphisms | Cartron et al., 2002 |

Table 3. Influences on antibody efficacy in a whole blood matrix.

## 6. Conclusions

Due to the dependence of CLL lymphocytes on their micro-environment, the predictive value of simple cytotoxicity assays on freshly isolated CLL cells can be enhanced by activating CLL cells using procedures that mimic certain micro-environmental stimuli. In the case of monoclonal antibodies, effector cells and complement system need to be included in order to comprise indirect antibody-mediated mechanisms. For arriving at valid predictions, results of the individualized *in vitro* sensitivity testing should be linked to mechanistic and biochemical target validation studies, ideally involving genetically defined systems. Remarkably three major topics addressed in this chapter, namely the importance of accompanying signaling analysis, consideration of the micro-environment of CLL cells and combination with chemotherapeutic agents conceptually strongly overlap with general targeting strategies in contemporary pre-clinical anticancer drug discovery (Caponigro & Sellers, 2011).

## 7. Acknowledgements

Work in our laboratory has been supported by grants from the German Cancer Aid, German José Carreras Leukemia Foundation and CLL Global Research Foundation.

## 8. References

Aleskog, A., Norberg, M., Nygren, P., Rickardson, L., Kanduri, M., Tobin, G., Aberg, M., Gustafsson, M.G., Rosenquist, R. & Lindhagen, E. (2008). Rapamycin shows anticancer activity in primary chronic lymphocytic leukemia cells in vitro, as single agent and in drug combination *Leuk Lymphoma* , 49, 2333-43.

Aloyz, R., Grzywacz, K., Xu, Z.Y., Loignon, M., Alaoui-Jamali, M.A. & Panasci, L. (2004). Imatinib sensitizes CLL lymphocytes to chlorambucil *Leukemia* , 18, 409-14.

Baudot, A.D., Jeandel, P.Y., Mouska, X., Maurer, U., Tartare-Deckert, S., Raynaud, S.D., Cassuto, J.P., Ticchioni, M. & Deckert, M. (2009). The tyrosine kinase Syk regulates the survival of chronic lymphocytic leukemia B cells through PKCdelta and proteasome-dependent regulation of Mcl-1 expression *Oncogene* , 28, 3261-73.

Bosanquet, A.G., Richards, S.M., Wade, R., Else, M., Matutes, E., Dyer, M.J., Rassam, S.M., Durant, J., Scadding, S.M., Raper, S.L., Dearden, C.E. & Catovsky, D. (2009). Drug cross-resistance and therapy-induced resistance in chronic lymphocytic leukaemia by an enhanced method of individualised tumour response testing *Br J Haematol* , 146, 384-95.

Buchner, M., Fuchs, S., Prinz, G., Pfeifer, D., Bartholome, K., Burger, M., Chevalier, N., Vallat, L., Timmer, J., Gribben, J.G., Jumaa, H., Veelken, H., Dierks, C. & Zirlik, K. (2009). Spleen tyrosine kinase is overexpressed and represents a potential therapeutic target in chronic lymphocytic leukemia *Cancer Res* , 69, 5424-32.

Burger, J.A., Ghia, P., Rosenwald, A. & Caligaris-Cappio, F. (2009). The microenvironment in mature B-cell malignancies: a target for new treatment strategies *Blood* , 114, 3367-75.

Burger, J.A. & Kipps, T.J. (2006). CXCR4: a key receptor in the crosstalk between tumor cells and their microenvironment *Blood* , 107, 1761-7.

Caponigro, G. & Sellers, W.R. (2011). Advances in the preclinical testing of cancer therapeutic hypotheses *Nat Rev Drug Discov* , 10, 179-87.

Cartron, G., Dacheux, L., Salles, G., Solal-Celigny, P., Bardos, P., Colombat, P. & Watier, H. (2002). Therapeutic activity of humanized anti-CD20 monoclonal antibody and polymorphism in IgG Fc receptor FcgammaRIIIa gene *Blood* , 99, 754-8.

Collins, I. & Workman, P. (2006). New approaches to molecular cancer therapeutics *Nat Chem Biol* , 2, 689-700.

Contri, A., Brunati, A.M., Trentin, L., Cabrelle, A., Miorin, M., Cesaro, L., Pinna, L.A., Zambello, R., Semenzato, G. & Donella-Deana, A. (2005). Chronic lymphocytic leukemia B cells contain anomalous Lyn tyrosine kinase, a putative contribution to defective apoptosis *J Clin Invest* , 115, 369-78.

Crespo, M., Bosch, F., Villamor, N., Bellosillo, B., Colomer, D., Rozman, M., Marce, S., Lopez-Guillermo, A., Campo, E. & Montserrat, E. (2003). ZAP-70 expression as a surrogate for immunoglobulin-variable-region mutations in chronic lymphocytic leukemia *N Engl J Med* , 348, 1764-75.

Decker, T., Hipp, S., Ringshausen, I., Bogner, C., Oelsner, M., Schneller, F. & Peschel, C. (2003). Rapamycin-induced G1 arrest in cycling B-CLL cells is associated with reduced expression of cyclin D3, cyclin E, cyclin A, and survivin *Blood* , 101, 278-85.

Decker, T., Schneller, F., Sparwasser, T., Tretter, T., Lipford, G.B., Wagner, H. & Peschel, C. (2000). Immunostimulatory CpG-oligonucleotides cause proliferation, cytokine production, and an immunogenic phenotype in chronic lymphocytic leukemia B cells *Blood* , 95, 999-1006.

Deglesne, P.A., Chevallier, N., Letestu, R., Baran-Marszak, F., Beitar, T., Salanoubat, C., Sanhes, L., Nataf, J., Roger, C., Varin-Blank, N. & Ajchenbaum-Cymbalista, F. (2006). Survival response to B-cell receptor ligation is restricted to progressive chronic lymphocytic leukemia cells irrespective of Zap70 expression *Cancer Res* , 66, 7158-66.

Druker, B.J., Talpaz, M., Resta, D.J., Peng, B., Buchdunger, E., Ford, J.M., Lydon, N.B., Kantarjian, H., Capdeville, R., Ohno-Jones, S. & Sawyers, C.L. (2001). Efficacy and safety of a specific inhibitor of the BCR-ABL tyrosine kinase in chronic myeloid leukemia *N Engl J Med* , 344, 1031-7.

Eichhorst, B., Goede, V. & Hallek, M. (2009). Treatment of elderly patients with chronic lymphocytic leukemia *Leuk Lymphoma* , 50, 171-8.

Gandhi, V. (2010). Targeting kinases in CML CLL *Blood* , 116, 1999-2000.

Gehrke, I., Gandhirajan, R.K., Poll-Wolbeck, S.J., Hallek, M. & Kreuzer, K.A. (2011). Bone marrow stromal cell-derived VEGF rather than CLL cell-derived VEGF is essential for the apoptotic resistance of cultured CLL cells *Mol Med* .

Ghosh, A.K., Secreto, C., Boysen, J., Sassoon, T., Shanafelt, T.D., Mukhopadhyay, D. & Kay, N.E. (2010). The novel receptor tyrosine kinase Axl is constitutively active in B-cell chronic lymphocytic leukemia and acts as a docking site of nonreceptor kinases: implications for therapy *Blood* , 117, 1928-37.

Golay, J., Bologna, L., Andre, P.A., Buchegger, F., Mach, J.P., Boumsell, L. & Introna, M. (2010). Possible misinterpretation of the mode of action of therapeutic antibodies in vitro: homotypic adhesion and flow cytometry result in artefactual direct cell death *Blood* , 116, 3372-3; author reply 3373-4.

Golay, J., Zaffaroni, L., Vaccari, T., Lazzari, M., Borleri, G.M., Bernasconi, S., Tedesco, F., Rambaldi, A. & Introna, M. (2000). Biologic response of B lymphoma cells to anti-CD20 monoclonal antibody rituximab in vitro: CD55 and CD59 regulate complement-mediated cell lysis *Blood* , 95, 3900-8.

Groves, M.J., Maccallum, S., Boylan, M.T., Coates, P.J. & Tauro, S. (2009). The annexin-V assay reflects susceptibility to in vitro membrane damage in chronic lymphocytic leukemia and may overestimate cell death *Am J Hematol* , 84, 196-7.

Hallaert, D.Y., Jaspers, A., van Noesel, C.J., van Oers, M.H., Kater, A.P. & Eldering, E. (2008). c-Abl kinase inhibitors overcome CD40-mediated drug resistance in CLL: implications for therapeutic targeting of chemoresistant niches *Blood* , 112, 5141-9.

Hallek, M., Cheson, B.D., Catovsky, D., Caligaris-Cappio, F., Dighiero, G., Dohner, H., Hillmen, P., Keating, M.J., Montserrat, E., Rai, K.R. & Kipps, T.J. (2008). Guidelines for the diagnosis and treatment of chronic lymphocytic leukemia: a report from the International Workshop on Chronic Lymphocytic Leukemia updating the National Cancer Institute-Working Group 1996 guidelines *Blood* , 111, 5446-56.

Hallek, M., Fischer, K., Fingerle-Rowson, G., Fink, A.M., Busch, R., Mayer, J., Hensel, M., Hopfinger, G., Hess, G., von Grunhagen, U., Bergmann, M., Catalano, J., Zinzani, P.L., Caligaris-Cappio, F., Seymour, J.F., Berrebi, A., Jager, U., Cazin, B., Trneny, M., Westermann, A., Wendtner, C.M., Eichhorst, B.F., Staib, P., Buhler, A., Winkler, D., Zenz, T., Bottcher, S., Ritgen, M., Mendila, M., Kneba, M., Dohner, H. & Stilgenbauer, S. (2010). Addition of rituximab to fludarabine and cyclophosphamide in patients with chronic lymphocytic leukaemia: a randomised, open-label, phase 3 trial *Lancet* , 376, 1164-74.

Hamblin, T.J. (2009). Just exactly how common is CLL? *Leuk Res* , 33, 1452-3.

Hamblin, T.J., Davis, Z., Gardiner, A., Oscier, D.G. & Stevenson, F.K. (1999). Unmutated Ig V(H) genes are associated with a more aggressive form of chronic lymphocytic leukemia *Blood* , 94, 1848-54.

Hamblin, T.J., Orchard, J.A., Ibbotson, R.E., Davis, Z., Thomas, P.W., Stevenson, F.K. & Oscier, D.G. (2002). CD38 expression and immunoglobulin variable region mutations are independent prognostic variables in chronic lymphocytic leukemia, but CD38 expression may vary during the course of the disease *Blood* , 99, 1023-9.

Herman, S.E., Gordon, A.L., Wagner, A.J., Heerema, N.A., Zhao, W., Flynn, J.M., Jones, J., Andritsos, L., Puri, K.D., Lannutti, B.J., Giese, N.A., Zhang, X., Wei, L., Byrd, J.C. & Johnson, A.J. (2010). Phosphatidylinositol 3-kinase-delta inhibitor CAL-101 shows promising preclinical activity in chronic lymphocytic leukemia by antagonizing intrinsic and extrinsic cellular survival signals *Blood* , 116, 2078-88.

Jaglowski, S.M., Alinari, L., Lapalombella, R., Muthusamy, N. & Byrd, J.C. (2010). The clinical application of monoclonal antibodies in chronic lymphocytic leukemia *Blood* , 116, 3705-14.

Jahrsdorfer, B., Hartmann, G., Racila, E., Jackson, W., Muhlenhoff, L., Meinhardt, G., Endres, S., Link, B.K., Krieg, A.M. & Weiner, G.J. (2001). CpG DNA increases primary malignant B cell expression of costimulatory molecules and target antigens *J Leukoc Biol* , 69, 81-8.

Kennedy, A.D., Beum, P.V., Solga, M.D., DiLillo, D.J., Lindorfer, M.A., Hess, C.E., Densmore, J.J., Williams, M.E. & Taylor, R.P. (2004). Rituximab infusion promotes rapid complement depletion and acute CD20 loss in chronic lymphocytic leukemia *J Immunol* , 172, 3280-8.

Kepp, O., Galluzzi, L., Lipinski, M., Yuan, J. & Kroemer, G. (2011). Cell death assays for drug discovery *Nat Rev Drug Discov* , 10, 221-37.

Koopman, G., Reutelingsperger, C.P., Kuijten, G.A., Keehnen, R.M., Pals, S.T. & van Oers, M.H. (1994). Annexin V for flow cytometric detection of phosphatidylserine expression on B cells undergoing apoptosis *Blood* , 84, 1415-20.

Krause, G. & Hallek, M. (2011). On the assessment of dasatinib-induced autophagy in CLL *Leuk Res* , 35, 137-8.

Krause, G., Patz, M., Isaeva, P., Wigger, M., Baki, I., Vondey, V., Kerwien, S., Kuckertz, M., Brinker, R., Claasen, J., Frenzel, L.P., Wendtner, C.M., Heider, K.H. & Hallek, M. (2011). Action of novel CD37 antibodies on chronic lymphocytic leukemia cells *Leukemia* , in press.

Krieg, A.M. (2006). Therapeutic potential of Toll-like receptor 9 activation *Nat Rev Drug Discov* , 5, 471-84.

Lindhagen E, Nygren P, Larsson R (2008) The fluorometric microculture cyto-toxicity assay. *Nat Protoc* , 3 (8): 1364–9.

Lilienthal, N., Prinz, C., Peer-Zada, A.A., Doering, M., Ba, L.A., Hallek, M., Jacob, C. & Herling, M. (2011). Targeting the disturbed redox equilibrium in chronic lymphocytic leukemia by novel reactive oxygen species-catalytic 'sensor/effector' compounds *Leuk Lymphoma* , 52, 1407-11.

Majolini, M.B., Boncristiano, M. & Baldari, C.T. (1999). Dysregulation of the protein tyrosine kinase LCK in lymphoproliferative disorders and in other neoplasias. *Leuk Lymphoma* , 35, 245-54.

Mayr, C., Speicher, M.R., Kofler, D.M., Buhmann, R., Strehl, J., Busch, R., Hallek, M. & Wendtner, C.M. (2006). Chromosomal translocations are associated with poor prognosis in chronic lymphocytic leukemia *Blood* , 107, 742-51.

Messmer, D., Fecteau, J.F., O'Hayre, M., Bharati, I.S., Handel, T.M. & Kipps, T.J. (2011). Chronic lymphocytic leukemia cells receive RAF-dependent survival signals in response to CXCL12 that are sensitive to inhibition by sorafenib *Blood* , 117, 882-9.

Moessner, E., Brunker, P., Moser, S., Puntener, U., Schmidt, C., Herter, S., Grau, R., Gerdes, C., Nopora, A., van Puijenbroek, E., Ferrara, C., Sondermann, P., Jäger, C., Strein, P., Fertig, G., Friess, T., Schuell, C., Bauer, S., Dal Porto, J., Del Nagro, C., Dabbagh, K., Dyer, M.J.S., Poppema, S., Klein, C. & Umana, P. (2010). Increasing the efficacy of CD20 antibody therapy through the engineering of a new type II anti-CD20 antibody with enhanced direct and immune effector cell-mediated B-cell cytotoxicity *Blood* , 115, 4393-4402.

Molina, A. (2008). A decade of rituximab: improving survival outcomes in non-Hodgkin's lymphoma *Annu Rev Med* , 59, 237-50.

Munk Pedersen, I. & Reed, J. (2004). Microenvironmental interactions and survival of CLL B-cells *Leuk Lymphoma* , 45, 2365-72.

Olszewski, A.J. & Grossbard, M.L. (2004). Empowering targeted therapy: lessons from rituximab *Sci STKE* , 2004, pe30.

Patz, M., Isaeva, P., Forcob, N., Muller, B., Frenzel, L.P., Wendtner, C.M., Klein, C., Umana, P., Hallek, M. & Krause, G. (2011). Comparison of the in vitro effects of the anti-CD20 antibodies rituximab and GA101 on chronic lymphocytic leukaemia cells *Br J Haematol* , 152, 295-306.

Pharmingen. (1998). Apoptosis. Applied reagents and technologies. 2nd edition.

Pleyer, L., Egle, A., Hartmann, T.N. & Greil, R. (2009). Molecular and cellular mechanisms of CLL: novel therapeutic approaches *Nat Rev Clin Oncol* , 6, 405-18.

Preithner, S., Elm, S., Lippold, S., Locher, M., Wolf, A., da Silva, A.J., Baeuerle, P.A. & Prang, N.S. (2006). High concentrations of therapeutic IgG1 antibodies are needed to compensate for inhibition of antibody-dependent cellular cytotoxicity by excess endogenous immunoglobulin G *Mol Immunol* , 43, 1183-93.

Puttini, M., Coluccia, A.M., Boschelli, F., Cleris, L., Marchesi, E., Donella-Deana, A., Ahmed, S., Redaelli, S., Piazza, R., Magistroni, V., Andreoni, F., Scapozza, L., Formelli, F. & Gambacorti-Passerini, C. (2006). In vitro and in vivo activity of SKI-606, a novel Src-Abl inhibitor, against imatinib-resistant Bcr-Abl+ neoplastic cells *Cancer Res* , 66, 11314-22.

Reslan, L., Dalle, S. & Dumontet, C. (2009). Understanding and circumventing resistance to anticancer monoclonal antibodies *MAbs* , 1, 222-9.

Seiffert, M., Schulz, A., Ohl, S., Dohner, H., Stilgenbauer, S. & Lichter, P. (2010). Soluble CD14 is a novel monocyte-derived survival factor for chronic lymphocytic leukemia cells, which is induced by CLL cells in vitro and present at abnormally high levels in vivo *Blood* , 116, 4223-30.

Shah, N.P., Tran, C., Lee, F.Y., Chen, P., Norris, D. & Sawyers, C.L. (2004). Overriding imatinib resistance with a novel ABL kinase inhibitor *Science* , 305, 399-401.

Song, Z., Lu, P., Furman, R.R., Leonard, J.P., Martin, P., Tyrell, L., Lee, F.Y., Knowles, D.M., Coleman, M. & Wang, Y.L. (2010). Activities of SYK and PLCgamma2 predict apoptotic response of CLL cells to SRC tyrosine kinase inhibitor dasatinib *Clin Cancer Res* , 16, 587-99.

Stanglmaier, M., Reis, S. & Hallek, M. (2004). Rituximab and alemtuzumab induce a nonclassic, caspase-independent apoptotic pathway in B-lymphoid cell lines and in chronic lymphocytic leukemia cells *Ann Hematol* , 83, 634-45.

Stevenson, F.K. & Caligaris-Cappio, F. (2004). Chronic lymphocytic leukemia: revelations from the B-cell receptor *Blood* , 103, 4389-95.

Veldurthy, A., Patz, M., Hagist, S., Pallasch, C.P., Wendtner, C.M., Hallek, M. & Krause, G. (2008). The kinase inhibitor dasatinib induces apoptosis in chronic lymphocytic leukemia cells in vitro with preference for a subgroup of patients with unmutated IgVH genes *Blood* , 112, 1443-52.

Vogler, M., Butterworth, M., Majid, A., Walewska, R.J., Sun, X.M., Dyer, M.J. & Cohen, G.M. (2009). Concurrent up-regulation of BCL-XL and BCL2A1 induces approximately 1000-fold resistance to ABT-737 in chronic lymphocytic leukemia *Blood* , 113, 4403-13.

Voso, M.T., Pantel, G., Rutella, S., Weis, M., D'Alo, F., Urbano, R., Leone, G., Haas, R. & Hohaus, S. (2002). Rituximab reduces the number of peripheral blood B-cells in vitro mainly by effector cell-mediated mechanisms *Haematologica* , 87, 918-25.

Weisberg, E., Manley, P.W., Cowan-Jacob, S.W., Hochhaus, A. & Griffin, J.D. (2007). Second generation inhibitors of BCR-ABL for the treatment of imatinib-resistant chronic myeloid leukaemia *Nat Rev Cancer* , 7, 345-56.

Weitzman, J., Betancur, M., Boissel, L., Rabinowitz, A.P., Klein, A. & Klingemann, H. (2009). Variable Contribution of Monoclonal Antibodies to ADCC in patients with chronic lymphocytic leukemia *Leuk Lymphoma*, 1-8.

Wickremasinghe, R.G., Prentice, A.G. & Steele, A.J. (2011). Aberrantly activated anti-apoptotic signalling mechanisms in chronic lymphocytic leukaemia cells: clues to the identification of novel therapeutic targets *Br J Haematol* , 153, 545-56.

Zenz, T., Mertens, D., Kuppers, R., Dohner, H. & Stilgenbauer, S. (2010). From pathogenesis to treatment of chronic lymphocytic leukaemia *Nat Rev Cancer* , 10, 37-50.

Zhang G, Gurtu V, Kain SR& Yan G. (1997) Early detection of apoptosis using a fluorescent conjugate of annexin V. *Biotechniques* , 23, 525-31.

# 7

# Heat Shock Proteins in Chronic Lymphocytic Leukaemia

Nina C. Dempsey-Hibbert, Christine Hoyle and John H.H. Williams
*Chester Centre for Stress Research, University of Chester*
*United Kingdom*

## 1. Introduction

Over the last decade, research has implicated a group of molecular chaperones termed Heat Shock Proteins (HSPs) as major contributors to cancer progression and the development of chemo-resistance. HSPs were initially discovered as a group of proteins that were strongly induced in response to heat shock and other cellular stresses. Under non-stress conditions, they have a wide variety of roles within many sub-cellular compartments where they facilitate protein folding, prevent protein unfolding and assist protein transport across membranes. Due to their roles in maintaining protein conformation, HSPs are vital when other cellular proteins start to unfold due to cellular stress such as high temperature, exposure to cytotoxic chemicals or oxidative stress and are up-regulated rapidly in these situations (Ciocca and Calderwood, 2005). Under these stressful conditions, HSPs prevent protein aggregation, stabilise cell membranes and inhibit many of the key steps in cell death pathways (Beere & Green, 2001), thereby enabling cell survival in conditions that would otherwise be lethal. Importantly, in normal cells, once the stress has passed, HSP levels return to baseline and these proteins return to their regular house-keeping duties. However, a growing body of research shows that in tumour cells, including Chronic Lymphocytic Leukaemia (CLL) cells, HSPs remain elevated and may contribute to prolonged tumour cell survival via several mechanisms that remain to be fully revealed.

Human HSPs were originally identified as stress-induced proteins and were traditionally split into five families based on their molecular weight. These five families were the HSP27, HSP60, HSP90, HSP70 and HSP110 families. However, the sequencing of the human genome led to the identification of additional members of well established HSP families. Furthermore, the expansion of these HSP families resulted in many HSPs being referred to by several different names. Therefore, attempts to draw comparisons between studies examining specific HSPs has proved challenging. Consequently, Kampinga et al. (2009) recently introduced guidelines for the nomenclature of human HSPs which ensures that the genes and proteins are named in a consistent manner (Table 1). Readers are referred to Kampinga et al. (2009) for a complete listing of human HSP nomenclature. This chapter will focus on the involvement of the major HSPs, HSPB1 (Hsp27) HSPA1A (Hsp72) and HSPC1 (Hsp90) in the development and progression of CLL.

| Gene Name | New Protein Name | Old Names |
|-----------|------------------|-----------|
| HSPB1 | HSPB1 | Hsp27, Hsp28; Hsp25 |
| DNAJB1 | DNAJB1 | Hsp40 |
| HSPD1 | HSPD1 | Hsp60 |
| HSPA8 | HSPA8 | HSC70, Hsp71, Hsp73 |
| HSPA9 | HSPA9 | Mortalin, mtHsp70, GRP75 |
| HSPA1A | HSPA1A | Hsp72, Hsp70-1, HSPA1 |
| HSPC1 | HSPC1 | Hsp90, HSP90A, Hsp89, HSP90AA |
| HSPH2 | HSPH2 | Hsp110 |

(Adapted from Kampinga et al. 2009)

Table 1. New nomenclature for human HSPs referred to in this chapter

The up-regulation of a number of HSPs in response to stress stimuli is regulated by the transcription factor Heat Shock Factor-1 (HSF1) (Wu, 1995). Under non-stress conditions, members of the DNAJ and HSPA families along with HSPC1 are bound to monomeric HSF1 within the cytosol. However, under stress conditions these HSPs dissociate from HSF1 and bind misfolded proteins, suggesting that these HSPs have a higher affinity for misfolded proteins compared to HSF1. As a consequence HSF1 trimerises and migrates to the nucleus where, in this state, it has a high binding affinity for cis-acting DNA sequence elements known as Heat Shock Elements (HSEs) in the promoter region of the HSP genes resulting in transcription of HSP genes (Sorger , 1991). Once the stress is discontinued, the trimeric forms of HSF1 dissociate from the HSEs and are converted back to HSF1 monomers with the inability to bind DNA. It is believed that the increase in HSPs within the cell following the heat shock response are themselves negative regulators of HSF, binding to HSF and preventing further trimerisation (Wu, 1995). HSPC1 has been shown to be a negative regulator of HSF1, as immunodepletion of HSPC1 results in enhanced HSF1 activity (Zou et al. 1998).

## 2. HSPs in cancer

The potential importance of HSPs in tumour biology is clear when considering their activities in light of the Hanahan & Weinberg concept of the hallmarks of cancer (Hanahan & Weinberg 2000; Hanahan & Weinberg 2011), where the development of a malignant phenotype requires six modifications:

- self-sufficiency with respect to growth signals
- limitless replicative potential
- insensitivity to anti-growth signals
- sustained angiogenesis
- capacity for tissue invasion and metastasis
- evasion of apoptosis

HSPs have the potential to contribute to each of these modifications, and three HSPs (HSPB1, HSPA1A and HSPC1) can be shown to influence at least two of these modifications. Not surprisingly it is these three HSPs that feature most in tumour studies.

HSPB1 belongs to the family of small heat shock proteins. Besides its role as an ATP-independent molecular chaperone, it is involved in the regulation of cell differentiation, the acquisition of thermotolerance and the inhibition of apoptosis and cell senescence. HSPB1 is up-regulated in response to a wide variety of stress stimuli such as oxidative stress, exposure to anti-cancer agents and radiation (Lanneau et al. 2008). As a molecular chaperone, HSPB1 prevents protein aggregation and stabilises partially denatured proteins ensuring refolding by other chaperones such as HSPA1A and HSPC1.

HSPA1A is the main inducible member of the HSPA family and is not normally present in significant concentrations in non-stressed normal cells. HSPA1A mainly exists as a dimer, and similarly to HSPB1 is up-regulated in response to a wide variety of stress stimuli and promotes cell survival. HSPA1A has a high affinity for hydrophobic amino acids and will rapidly bind to partially denatured proteins in preparation for refolding or disposal.

HSPC1 is the most abundant member of the HSPC family, and is constitutively expressed in all eukaryotic cells where it binds a specific set of 'client proteins' including steroid receptors, non-receptor tyrosine kinases and cyclin-dependent kinases (McLaughlin et al. 2002). HSPC1 operates as part of a multimeric chaperone complex which includes members of the HSPA and DNAJ families, along with many other 'co-chaperones' and immunophillins (Holzbeierlein et al. 2010). It exists as a dimer, consisting of three major domains per monomer; A C-terminal homodimerisation domain, a middle ATP-hydrolysis-regulating domain, and an N-terminal, ATP binding domain (Krukenberg et al. 2011).

At one time HSPs were thought to be solely intracellular proteins (iHSPs). However certain HSPs have been found to be released from viable cells into the extracellular milieu (eHSPs) (Hightower & Guidon, 1989; Hunter-Lavin et al. 2004) and have also been found expressed on the tumour cell surface (sHSPs). The exact mechanism involved in the transport of these HSPs from the cytosol to the cell surface and extracellular environment have not been fully determined, but evidence suggests that HSPs may employ a number of methods including lipid-raft transport (Hunter-Lavin et al. 2004; Gastpar et al 2005; Vega et al. 2008), exosomal transport (Clayton et al. 2005) and ABC transporters (Mambula & Calderwood 2006). Regardless of their route of exit, sHSPs and eHSPs have critical roles in a variety of processes ranging from cell invasion and metastasis to immunomodulation.

## 3. Intracellular HSPs

### 3.1 Intracellular HSPs and prognosis

The up-regulation of HSPs inside cancer cells compared to normal cells has been well documented and has led to numerous studies investigating their prognostic and therapeutic potential (Calderwood et al. 2006; Ciocca et al. 2005; Sherman & Multhoff. 2007). In many cases high levels of HSPs have been found to be advantageous to the cancer cell, which is hardly surprising when considering that HSPB1, HSPA1A and HSPC1 are all anti-apoptotic factors, and would suggest that these proteins should have prognostic potential. However, although elevated HSPA1A, HSPB1, and HSPC1 are associated with poor prognosis in leukaemia, this pattern is not repeated in other cancers (Table 2) (Jaattela, 1999; Ciocca & Calderwood, 2005). In a minority of cancer types, the over-expression of HSPs appears to correlate with a positive prognosis for the patient (Kawanishi et al. 1999; Sagol et al. 2002; Santarosa et al. 1997) and at present it is still unclear as to how HSP expression may influence cancer progression.

Increased levels of HSPB1 have been documented in various cancers including breast, liver and prostate (Cornford et al. 2000; Romani et al. 2007; Vargas-Roig et al. 1997) and high levels have been found to correlate with poor prognosis (Duval et al. 2006; Thomas et al. 2005). However, there are contradictions within the literature; In breast cancer, for example, increased levels of HSPB1 have been associated with prolonged survival in oestrogen receptor-negative cases (Love & King, 1994). Low levels of HSPB1 in ovarian cancer have also been found to correlate with decreased survival (Geisler et al. 2004). However, these contradictions may be attributed to HSPB1, (synonymous with p24 and p29), being an oestrogen-regulated protein (Adams & McGuire, 1985; Ciocca & Luque, 1991).

Increases in HSPA1A have been observed in breast cancer (Tauchi et al. 1991), colorectal cancer (Milicevic et al. 2007; Shotar, 2005), kidney cancer (Ramp et al. 2007) and leukaemia (Chant et al. 1995; Thomas et al. 2005). Additionally, elevated HSPA1A has been associated with resistance to cancer therapy and/or poor prognosis for the patient (Thomas et al. 2005; Vargas-Roig et al. 1998). However, the relationship between the presence of HSPs and prognosis cannot be extrapolated to all cancers, as high intracellular HSPA1A expression has been correlated with a positive prognosis in oesophageal (Kawanishi et al. 1999), pancreatic (Sagol et al. 2002) and renal cancer (Santarosa et al. 1997).

HSPC1 levels are elevated in a number of cancer types including oesophageal squamous cell carcinoma (Wu et al. 2009), invasive breast carcinoma (Zagouri et al. 2010) and leukaemia (Thomas et al. 2005). Furthermore, in some cases, elevated HSPC1 levels have been associated with decreased survival and adverse karyotypes (Pick et al. 2007; Thomas et al. 2005).

| Cancer type | HSPA1A | HSPB1 | HSPC1 |
|---|---|---|---|
| Breast | Poor | Variable | n/d |
| Endometrial | Poor | n/d | Good |
| Kidney | Good | n/d | n/d |
| Leukaemia | Poor | Poor | Poor |
| Lung | n/d | n/d | n/d |
| Osteosarcoma | Good | Poor | Variable |
| Ovary | n/d | Poor | n/d |

(Adapted from Jaattela, (1999) and Ciocca & Calderwood, (2005))

Table 2. Association of HSP over-expression with prognosis

It is clear that different HSPs have distinct roles in normal cells and therefore it is not inconceivable that they may also have a variety of roles in tumour development. Indeed, the over-expression of one particular HSP within a tumour cell does not necessarily signify elevated levels of other HSPs within the same patient; In CLL particularly, HSPB1, HSPA1A and HSPC1 increases have been observed amongst patients but not necessarily simultaneously (Dempsey et al. 2010a). Similarly there is little correlation between the expression of HSPB1, HSPA1A and HSPC1 in prostate cancer (Cornford et al. 2000) or AML (Thomas et al. 2005). It is therefore imperative to understand the individual roles of these proteins in cancer development by studying them together within a specific sample but also considering them as distinct entities.

### 3.2 Intracellular HSPs and resistance to apoptosis

Mechanistic investigations have shown that HSPB1 interferes with the apoptotic pathway in several ways including the prevention of cytochrome c and Smac/DIABLO release from the mitochondria (Chauhan et al. 2003a; Paul et al. 2002) and direct interaction with cytochrome c (Garrido et al. 2001; LeBlanc, 2003; Samali et al. 2001) and Daxx (Charrette et al. 2000) thereby inhibiting their function. There is clear evidence that HSPB1 levels correlate with chemo-resistance (Schepers et al. 2005; Vargas-Roig et al. 1998). Studies designed to explore the role of HSPB1 in the development of chemo-resistance have utilised various techniques including siRNA and gene transfection. Depletion of HSPB1 has been shown to overcome resistance to drug-induced apoptosis (Chauhan et al. 2003b) while transfection of full-length HSPB1 into cancer cells confers resistance to Cisplatin and Doxorubicin (Richards et al. 1996).

HSPA1A is involved in carcinogenesis at many different stages from the enhancement of activity of many different oncogenes and inhibition of tumour suppressor genes such as p53 (Yaglom et al. 2007), to promoting the survival of tumour cells through inhibition of apoptosis (Khaleque et al. 2005; Nylandsted et al. 2000). Similarly to HSPB1, HSPA1A interacts with several key proteins in cell death pathways (Beere & Green, 2001). Direct interaction with APAF-1 and mutated p53 (Iwaya et al. 1995; Lehman et al. 1991) has been documented as well as direct inhibition of procaspases. Several studies have shown that depletion of HSPA1A results in increased sensitivity to chemotherapeutic drugs (Zhao & Shen, 2005) and ultimately apoptosis of various cell lines including breast, colon and prostate (Nylandsted et al. 2000), highlighting the importance of this protein for cell survival.

A wide variety of client proteins are held by HSPC1 in both tumour and non-tumour cells, and as a result it is involved in several vital signalling pathways including PI3K/Akt, Erk1/2, JNK and NFĸB pathways. It is the chaperoning of a variety of oncoproteins such as mutant B-Raf (Grbovic et al. 2006), Bcr/Abl (An et al. 2000) and mutant p53 (Lin et al. 2008), as well as the signalling pathway components, that has sparked interest into HSPC1's potential role in tumour development and progression. HSPC1 also cooperates with HSPA1A in inhibiting apoptosome formation. Furthermore, HSPC1 interferes with death receptor mediated apoptosis by stabilising the anti-apoptotic protein Receptor Interacting Protein (RIP) thereby promoting cell survival.

Clearly HSPB1, HSPA1A and HSPC1 interfere with apoptotic signalling at multiple points (Figure 1).

## 4. Extracellular HSPs

### 4.1 Extracellular HSPs in immunomodulation

As a consequence of their molecular chaperoning role, HSPs exit the cell bound to a wide variety of antigenic peptides. These extracellular HSP-peptide complexes bind to surface receptors on Antigen Presenting Cells (APCs) in a process termed cross-presentation (Bolhassani & Rafati, 2008). During the process of necrosis, when cell stress is highest and the cellular components leak out of the cell, these HSP-peptide complexes are abundant and can signal stress to local APCs, which in-turn can induce a Cytotoxic T-Lymphocyte (CTL)

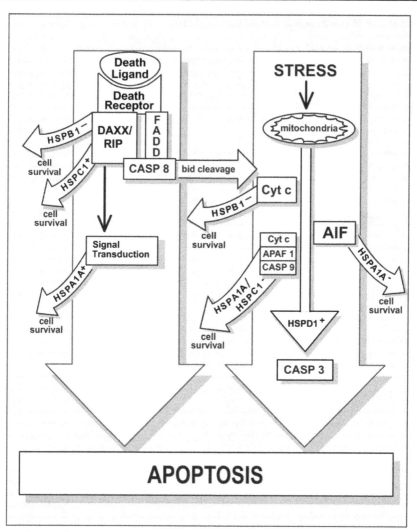

Fig. 1. Regulation of the Death Receptor and Mitochondrial Apoptosis Pathways by HSPs (Taken from Dempsey, 2009). Two main arrows represent the Death Receptor-mediated- and mitochondrial- apoptosis pathways. HSPB1 inhibits apoptosis by directly interacting with Daxx, and sequestering cytochrome c released from the mitochondria. HSPD1 has been shown to directly promote the proteolytic maturation of caspase-3, thereby displaying a pro-apoptotic role. HSPA1A inhibits apoptosis by inhibiting the activation of protein kinases involved in signal transduction pathways (e.g. JNK), binding to AIF thereby neutralising its effects and binding to Apaf-1 resulting in inhibition of apoptosome formation. HSPC1 has been shown to stabilise the anti-apoptotic protein, RIP and has also been shown to work synergistically with HSPA1A to inhibit apoptosome formation. Apoptosis induced by Death Receptors also results in activation of the mitochondrial pathway via cleavage of the pro-apoptotic protein Bid. A minus sign indicates negative regulation while a positive sign indicates positive regulation.

response. Similarly, viable tumour cells with high HSP levels may also actively release HSP-peptide complexes into the surrounding environment. Research investigating the HSP-APC interactions has revealed a number of APC receptors capable of binding HSPs; Scavenger receptors (SRs), Toll-like receptors (TLRs), CD40, CD14 and CD91 (Calderwood et al. 2007; Basu et al. 2001) allow HSP-peptide complexes to interact with a number of different immune cell types including Dendritic cells, Macrophages, Monocytes and NK-cells (Murshid et al. 2008).

The binding of HSPA1A-peptide complexes to the SR LOX-1 on Dendritic cells, for example, results in the internalisation of the HSP-peptide complex (Arnold-Schild et al. 1999) via the phagocytic pathway, and re-presentation of the antigenic peptide on MHC-I on the Dendritic cell surface. Work by Kurotaki et al. (2007) has revealed the significance of HSPs in this antigen cross presentation process; Dendritic cells were found to bind and internalise HSPC1-peptide complexes and generate a T-cell response, while unconjugated peptide was unable to stimulate this same response. In order for APCs to effectively activate a T-cell response, they must undergo maturation to express appropriate co-stimulatory molecules. Indeed, HSPA1A has been shown to stimulate the expression of CD40, CD83 and CD86 on Dendritic cells (Bausero et al. 2005; Kuppner et al. 2001). Additionally, the expression and release of pro-inflammatory cytokines such as IL-1β, IL-6, IL-12 and TNF-α is stimulated by HSPs (Asea et al. 2000; Baretto et al. 2003; Todryk et al. 1999). There appears to be a positive feedback system in which APC-released pro-inflammatory cytokines augment transcription and release of HSPA1A from tumour cells (Baretto et al. 2003). The immunomodulatory properties of extracellular HSPs have identified them as a potential 'danger signal', released by cells in order to signal stress to the immune system (Todryk et al. 2000; Williams & Ireland 2008). Furthermore, as HSP-peptide complexes can induce both innate and adaptive immunity, they have become attractive candidates for immunotherapy protocols. Clinical trials have investigated the use of HSP-based vaccines on solid tumours and lymphomas but results have been inconclusive (Murshid et al. 2008). The technique involves isolating and purifying HSP from the patient's tumour cells and re-applying this as a vaccine in order to stimulate an immune response. A critical advantage of using such treatments is that, by exploiting the chaperoning ability of HSPs, a broad range of tumour-specific peptides, unique to that specific tumour will be targeted.

## 4.2 Distinct roles of membrane bound HSPs

A number of HSPs are also present on the tumour cell surface, and have distinct roles dependent on the specific HSP. HSPA1A in particular has been found embedded in the cell membrane of a variety of tumour cell types (Kleinjung et al. 2003; Pfister et al. 2007) and work from our lab has shown sHSPA1A on CD5+/CD19+ cells from CLL patients (Dempsey et al. 2010a). To date, it appears that the membrane localisation of HSPA1A is specific to tumour cells and has attracted much attention as a potential therapeutic target (Gehrmann et al. 2008; Krause et al. 2004), the implications of which will be discussed later in this chapter.

sHSPA1A acts a recognition structure for activated NK-cells (Gehrmann et al. 2003; Gross et al. 2003; Multhoff et al. 1999) and is therefore detrimental for the tumour cell. The region of the HSPA1A molecule exposed to the extracellular milieu of tumours has been identified as the 14-mer peptide TKDNNLLGRFELSG (TKD peptide) (Multhoff et al. 2001). The stimulation of NK cells using the TKD peptide and low dose IL-2 results in up-regulation of CD94/CD56 on NK cells and initiates NK-cell killing of sHSPA1A+ tumour cells (Gross et al. 2003; Gross et al. 2008; Multhoff et al. 1999). Interestingly, purified (perforin-free) granzyme B from NK-cells was shown to bind to HSPA1A and result in granzyme B internalisation into sHSPA1A+ tumour cells (Gross et al. 2003). Stimulation of NK-cells was also observed following incubation with sHSPA1A+ tumour-cell derived exosomes (Gastpar et al. 2005). Wei et al. (1996) demonstrated that sHSPA1A is also a target for δγT-cells. Furthermore, the induced *in-vivo* expression of sHSPA1A on tumour cells increases their immunogenicity, resulting in both a CTL-mediated and NK-cell mediated response and rejection of the tumour (Chen et al. 2002a). The expression of sHSPA1A, therefore, overcomes many of the characteristics that tumour cells develop to evade immune recognition, including down-regulation of MHC molecules, and down-regulation of co-stimulatory and adhesion molecules (Bausero et al, 2005; Chen et al. 2002a). The literature to date, suggests that the cellular location of HSPA1A is crucial in determining disease outcome as iHSPA1A is advantageous to the tumour, while sHSPA1A appears to be detrimental.

In contrast to this theory, the small number of studies to date, investigating the presence of sHSPA1A in primary cells from leukaemic patients suggest that its presence may in fact be detrimental for the patient. The study by Gehrmann et al. (2003) demonstrated that although sHSPA1A acted as a recognition structure for NK cells, sHSPA1A expression could be correlated with unfavourable or intermediate cytogenetics. Similarly, sHSPA1A levels were found to be higher in AML patients with treatment-refractory disease and active disease than patients in complete remission, suggesting a correlation with poor prognosis (Steiner et al. 2006). Furthermore, AML patients continuing to express moderately high levels of sHSPA1A after achieving remission were shown to have a shorter relapse-free survival time than remission patients with lower levels of sHSPA1A (Steiner et al. 2006). No correlation between sHSPA1A expression and stage of AML or resistance to chemotherapy could be determined by Steiner et al. (2006), suggesting that surface localisation of HSPA1A cannot be investigated in isolation. Schilling et al. (2007) demonstrated co-expression of HSPA1A with phosphatidylserine (PS) on the surface of hypoxic tumour cell lines. Additionally, exogenously added HSPA1A was shown to bind to PS on the cell surface and enhance the response to radiation. The results indicate that the radiotherapy-resistance observed in many hypoxic tumours may be overcome by prior treatment with HSPA1A.

In addition to HSPA1A, cell surface expression of HSPC1 and HSPB1 on tumour cells has been reported (Becker et al. 2004; Brameshuber et al. 2010; Ferrarini et al. 1992; Shin et al. 2003). sHSPC1 has been shown to be involved in tissue invasion and metastasis (Eustace et al. 2004), while the role of sHSPB1 is still unclear. Indeed, inhibiting cell surface expression of HSPC1, both *in-vitro* and *in-vivo*, reduces cell motility and invasiveness (Eustace et al. 2004; Tsutsumi et al. 2008). Work by Sidera et al. (2008) proposes that in some cancer cell types, sHSPC1 interacts with and activates HER-2, resulting in homodimerisation with ErbB-3, signal transduction pathway activation and ultimately actin rearrangement. Secretion of HSPC1 in exosomes has also been discovered, and has been shown to contribute to cancer cell invasiveness (McCready et al. 2010).

It is clear that extracellular HSPs have critical roles in tumour development and immune responses and we therefore suggest that mechanistic investigations of tumour biology should include analysis of extracellular, as well as intracellular, HSPs.

## 5. HSPs in leukaemia

Although a large amount of data exists regarding the expression of HSPs in cancer, the majority of studies have focused on solid tumours. Cells within a solid tumour mass are subjected to high levels of stress; the tumour microenvironment is often hypoxic and nutrient deficient and there may be infiltration by large numbers of immune cells. Therefore it is not surprising that HSP levels are elevated in many solid tumour types. Leukaemia cells however, are not subjected to these same stresses and as a result may not necessarily show elevated levels of HSPs.

Of the limited number of studies investigating HSP expression in leukaemia, a number have focused on correlating HSP expression with prognosis and clinical outcome, while others have directed research towards HSP expression and susceptibility to apoptosis. One study by Thomas et al. (2005) explored the expression of intracellular HSPB1, HSPD1, HSPA1A, HSPC1 and HSPH2 in both peripheral blood and bone marrow from patients with Acute Myeloid Leukaemia (AML). It was noted that complete remission rates were higher in patients with lower HSP expression and that overall survival was also significantly longer in these patients. Similarly, overall survival was found to be significantly greater in Myelodysplastic Syndrome (MDS) patients with lower HSPB1, HSPD1, HSPC1 and HSPH2 expression (Duval et al. 2006). A study exploring the expression of surface HSPA1A (sHSPA1A) in bone marrow aspirates from AML patients demonstrated that patients in complete remission express significantly lower levels of sHSPA1A when compared to patients with active AML (Steiner et al. 2006). Taken together these results suggest that higher levels of HSP expression both internally and on the surface of the leukaemic cell are advantageous to the cancer cell and therefore an adverse factor for the patient. This is in contrast to studies that have demonstrated the involvement of sHSPA1A in immune recognition and tumour regression (Chen et al. 2002; Multhoff et al. 1999; Gross et al. 2003; Gross et al. 2008).

HSP expression in AML and MDS has also been found to correlate with expression of the myeloblast surface antigen CD34, a well established poor prognostic factor (Duval et al. 2006; Thomas et al. 2005). Moreover, AML and MDS patients with intermediate or unfavourable karyotypes display a higher level of HSP expression than patients with favourable karyotypes. In contrast, Steiner et al. (2006) did not establish a correlation between sHSPA1A expression and cytogenetic risk group or FAB subtype. A study into expression of HSPD1, HSPA1A, HSPA8 (constitutive and heat-inducible forms) and HSPC1 in AML cells showed a heterogeneous expression of all three HSPs and no correlation was found between this extensive range of HSP expression and clinical outcome (Chant et al. 1995). However, a more recent study by the same group demonstrated that although AML cells show a broad range of HSPA1A expression, this expression correlates with susceptibility to apoptosis (Chant et al. 1996). Surprisingly, the correlation between HSPA1A expression and apoptosis was positive, indicating that cells with higher levels of the protein are more susceptible to apoptosis. This finding is contradictory to the theory that HSPA1A protects cells from apoptosis. In spite of this correlation between HSPA1A and apoptosis, none was found between expression of HSPC1 and susceptibility to apoptosis. In contrast, levels of HSPA1A in MDS did not correlate with either pro- or anti-apoptotic protein levels (Duval et al. 2006). However, levels of HSPB1, HSPD1, HSPC1 and HSPH2 negatively correlated with the expression of the pro-apoptotic proteins Bad and Bak, while correlating positively with the anti-apoptotic proteins Bcl-2 and Bcl-Xl.

Research into acute lymphoblastic leukaemia (ALL) has shown decreased expression of HSPA1A and HSPB1 in bone marrow aspirates from patients who achieved complete remission when compared to those patients who did not achieve complete remission (Campos et al. 1999). Additionally, ALL cells displaying the Bcr/Abl fusion protein contained high levels of HSPA1A (Nimmanapalli et al. 2002). Further studies have demonstrated that HSPA1A contributes to the Bcr-Abl–mediated resistance to apoptosis by chemotherapeutic agents such as etoposide. Moreover, down-regulation of HSPA1A can sensitise these Bcr/Abl ALL cells to cytotoxic drugs (Guo et al. 2005). The Bcr/Abl fusion protein was shown to be a client protein of HSPC1. Furthermore, inhibition of HSPC1, but not HSPA1A, in myeloid cells was found to result in degradation of Bcr/Abl (Peng et al. 2007).

## 6. HSPs in chronic lymphocytic leukaemia

An extensive study by our group analysed the levels of HSPB1, HSPA1A and HSPC1 in CD5+/CD19+ and CD5-/CD19+ cells from CLL patients and normal lymphocytes from control subjects (Dempsey et al. 2010a). At first glance, it would appear that levels of both iHSPC1 and iHSPB1 are significantly higher in CLL patients overall than normal age-matched control subjects. An initial analysis of our data would also support the hypothesis that elevated intracellular HSP leads to tumour cells being resistant to apoptosis (Khaleque et al. 2005; Nylandsted et al. 2000; Thomas et al. 2005; Vargas-Roig et al. 1998); Caspase-3, a marker of apoptosis, was found to be lower in CLL patients compared to age-matched control subjects, while levels of iHSPB1 and iHSPC1 were higher in CLL patients. We also observed a negative correlation between levels of caspase-3 and iHSPB1. An observed difference in caspase-3 levels between CLL and control subjects is not surprising since the underlying basis of CLL is an inability for B-lymphocytes to commit to apoptosis. There was, however, no difference in caspase-3 levels between patients at different stages of the disease which suggests that the progression of CLL is more likely to be a result of an increased cellular clonal replication rather than an increased resistance to apoptosis from the same cells. A more detailed analysis of the data has demonstrated that CLL patients in different Binet stages express distinct levels of iHSPC1; Levels of iHSPC1 in Binet stage A patients are significantly higher than levels observed in Binet stage B and C patients. This is surprising, as the anti-apoptotic nature of these proteins would suggest they may be elevated in patients with a more advanced disease. However, the elevated levels of HSPC1 in patients with a less severe disease could be interpreted as a stress response in the early stages of the disease, which aids CLL cells in surviving immune destruction. As the disease progresses and CLL cells replicate uncontrollably, these very high HSPC1 levels are no longer required for cell survival and therefore begin to decrease.

Our data has also revealed that CLL patients can be divided into two groups based on their expression of iHSPA1A in CD5+/CD19+ cells; one group of patients presents very low levels of iHSPA1A while the other group expresses levels up to 1000-fold higher. This is also the case for sHSPA1A, although the difference is less pronounced. It should be noted that patients expressing very low levels of iHSPA1A are not necessarily the same patients that express low levels of sHSPA1A as no correlation between sHSPA1A and iHSPA1A could be found. Interestingly these CLL patients classified into the 'low sHSPA1A or iHSPA1A expressing' groups display HSPA1A levels similar to levels in non-malignant CD5-/CD19+ cells from the same patients and also lymphocytes from control subjects. In spite of this differential expression of HSPA1A amongst CLL patients, neither sHSPA1A nor iHSPA1A can be correlated with stage of disease or cytogenetic abnormality. Our data supports the work by Chant et al. (1995) who have demonstrated a wide range of HSP expression amongst AML patients. We have also determined that CLL patients with stable disease (not requiring treatment) possess significantly higher levels of iHSPA1A than patients with progressive disease (requiring treatment), which is in line with the decrease in HSPC1 seen as the disease progresses.

There is also considerable variation in the levels of extracellular HSPA1A (eHSPA1A) present in the serum of CLL patients. When considered as a group, levels of eHSPA1A in CLL patients are not significantly different from levels in control subjects. However, a more detailed analysis of the data reveals a correlation between the levels of extracellular and intracellular HSPA1A in CLL patients. Interestingly patients receiving corticosteroid treatment display significantly lower levels of HSPA1A in serum when compared to patients not receiving corticosteroid treatment, with some steroid-treated patients showing near-undetectable levels of eHSPA1A. This suggests that steroid treatment may totally inhibit the secretion of HSPA1A, although this remains to be confirmed. However, in addition to their negative effects on lymphocyte proliferation, T-cell activation and NK-cell function, corticosteroids have been shown to regulate transcription factors. As eHSPA1A and iHSPA1A levels correlate and eHSPA1A levels are lower in steroid-treated patients, it could be deduced that the transcription of HSPA1A has been inhibited. This conclusion is supported by the decrease in HSPA1A release observed following commencement of glucocorticoid treatment in CLL patients.

CLL patients often display resistance to corticosteroid therapy which is attributed to the imbalanced expression of glucocorticoid receptor (GR) isoforms. Indeed, higher expression of the transcriptionally inactive glucocorticoid receptor-beta (GR-beta) in relation to the hormone-activated transcription factor GR-alpha has been observed in CLL cells (Shahidi et al. 1999). However, as the GR is a client protein of HSPC1, variation in HSPC1 concentration may result in defective ligand binding, which may also contribute to resistance (Bailey et al. 2001). Indeed it has been demonstrated that the ratio of HSPC1 to GR expression is significantly higher in steroid-resistant compared to steroid-sensitive multiple sclerosis patients (Matysiak et al. 2008). This suggests that CLL patients in Binet stage A, whose HSPC1 expression is high, may have a reduced sensitivity for the steroid.

In summary although HSPs appear to be elevated in CLL patients compared to control subjects, closer examination of the data reveals that this is not the case in all CLL patients and in fact, there is a large variability in HSPB1, HSPA1A and HSPC1 amongst patients which can be associated with disease stage and also treatment regime. The results indicate that the concept of HSPs being over-expressed in cancer may in fact be oversimplified. Indeed, it is now becoming apparent that there is also great variability in HSP expression in solid tumours such as breast cancer (Zagouri et al. 2010). These findings are crucial in helping to determine whether future treatments targeting HSPs maybe considered as a universal option.

## 7. Heat shock proteins as therapeutic targets

Many of the most recently developed anti-cancer treatments are targeted towards a single specific oncoprotein. Although in many cases, this has been largely successful (Flaherty et al. 2010; Kantarjian et al. 2003) cancer cells may acquire resistance to these treatments via a number of mechanisms including secondary mutations in the target binding domain and activation of alternative signalling pathways (Nazarian et al. 2010; Shah et al. 2002). Indeed, by their very nature, cancers accumulate oncogenic mutations as they progress and therefore a treatment strategy that involves the selective targeting of a specific protein kinase, for example, is unlikely to show continued success. As stated earlier, HSPs contribute to each of the six hallmarks of cancer and as a result have multiple molecular targets. In particular, HSPC1 appears to play a fundamental role in the development and maintenance of several tumour characteristics (Neckers, 2007). HSPC1 binds and stabilises a broad array of mutated oncoproteins (An et al. 2000; Minami et al. 2002; Pashtan et al. 2008), so the targeting of this single chaperone, should in theory, destabilise and degrade a wide variety of signalling kinases, therefore simultaneously targeting a number of cell signalling pathways. Furthermore, by selectively inhibiting HSPC1, all six 'hallmarks of cancer' (Hanahan & Weinberg, 2001; Hanahan & Weinberg, 2011) can be targeted in parallel, thereby dramatically reducing the probability that a resistant clone will develop. Since the identification of the first HSPC1 inhibitors 25 years ago, interest into these novel therapies has expanded considerably and the development of newer inhibitors has focussed on increasing efficacy and reducing side effects. Indeed a large body of data now exists documenting their anti-cancer effects on a wide variety of tumour cell types (Kim et al. 2009) both in isolation and in combination with common chemotherapeutic agents. HSPC1 inhibitors are currently grouped according to their site of action; N-terminal inhibitors and C-terminal inhibitors.

### 7.1 N-terminal HSPC1 inhibitors

The original N-terminal inhibitors, geldanamycin (GA) and radicicol were naturally occurring antibacterial products discovered in *Streptomyces hygroscopicus*. Initial experiments using these compounds revealed binding to HSPC1 and consequent degradation of the HSPC1 client protein v-src (Whitesell et al. 1994). Although subsequent experiments proved that these natural HSPC1 inhibitors were able to cause the degradation of a wide range of client proteins, the non-specific toxicity of these compounds prevented their clinical use. However, these experiments led to the development of the first clinically applicable HSPC1 inhibitor, 17-AAG (17-allylamino-17-demethoxygeldanamycin, also known as tanespimycin) (Holzbeierlein et al. 2010). As a derivative of GA, 17-AAG resulted in the degradation of a variety of oncogenic proteins in a number of tumour cell types, while displaying reduced toxicity. This compound was entered into clinical trials and tested on a broad array of cancers including a large variety of haematological malignancies such as AML, ALL, CML and CLL. Detailed reviews of clinical trial data can be found in Kim et al. (2009), Taldone et al. (2008) and Holzbeierlein et al. (2010). In addition to showing initial promise as a novel therapy in isolation, 17-AAG also demonstrated synergism with a number of chemotherapeutic agents such as Bortezomib (Richardson et al. 2010), Trastuzumab (Modi et al. 2007) and Paclitaxel (Ramalingam et al. 2008). An alternative derivative of GA, 17-DMAG (17-dimethylaminoethylamino-17-demethoxygeldanamycin, also known as alvespimycin) was subsequently produced, with greater solubility and showed similar initial success in phase I and II clinical trials. Based on the results using 17-AAG and 17-DMAG, interest into the development of alternative HSPC1 inhibitors has increased greatly and has produced a number of N-terminal inhibitors including IPI-504 (Retaspimycin hydrochloride), AUY922, BIIB021 and SNX-2112 (Eccles et al. 2009; Hanson & Vesole, 2009; Lundgren et al. 2009; Okawa et al. 2008). In spite of these promising results and continuous research and development, clinical trials involving N-terminal inhibitors have not been without limitations. Hepatotoxicity and poor solubility of the drugs have been frequently reported. Furthermore, despite the idea of targeting the six 'hallmarks of cancer' through the inhibition of HSPC1, drug resistance has become an issue. This has been attributed to the increase in HSPB1 and HSPA1A following HSPC1 inhibition (Dakappagari et al. 2010; Ravagnan et al. 2001) due to enhanced activity of HSF-1, thereby increasing cellular resistance to apoptosis. This increase in HSPB1 and HSPA1A appears to be a complication related to the use of all N-terminal inhibitors (Taldone et al. 2008). A review by Holzbeierlein et al. (2010) highlights three significant clinical trials involving 17-AAG in which no anti-cancer response was observed and recruitment into the trials was terminated prematurely. Similarly, unexpected problems have been encountered using 17-DMAG. Another issue with HSPC1 inhibition is that, in addition to chaperoning many oncogenic proteins, HSPC1 also chaperones many other proteins with anti-tumour activities. The tumour suppressor proteins LKB1 (Boudeau et al. 2003), LATS1, LATS2 (Huntoon et al. 2010) and wild-type p53 (Walerych et al. 2004) are all down-regulated following treatment with HSPC1 inhibitors. These results highlight the potential disadvantages of HSPC1 inhibitor therapies.

## 7.2 C-terminal HSPC1 inhibitors

Research into HSPC1 inhibitors has primarily focused on N-terminal inhibition, however a small number of C-terminal inhibitors have been identified. Novobiocin was the first C-terminal HSPC1 inhibitor to be identified, and similarly to GA, is a naturally occurring antibiotic produced in *Streptomyces niveu*. However, novobiocin was found to have a weak affinity for its target and as a result was not therapeutically applicable. Subsequently, research has focused on the synthesis of novobiocin analogues with a stronger affinity for HSPC1. According to a review by Holzbeierlein et al. (2010), over 300 analogues have been screened resulting in the identification of compounds with improved activity and selectivity of tumour over non-tumour cells. It has also been noted that the anti-cancer agent cisplatin and the polyphenolic flavanoid Epigallocatechin-3-gallate (EGCG) can inhibit HSPC1 activity via C-terminal inhibition (Soti et al. 2002; Yin et al. 2009). Cisplatin has been used as a conventional chemotherapy for decades due to its ability to form DNA adducts and therefore prevent DNA transcription. By binding to the C-terminal, cisplatin hinders nucleotide binding. Treatment of a human ovarian cell line with EGCG was found to inhibit HSPC1 activity and therefore result in the degradation of several client proteins including ErbB2, Raf-1, and phosphorylated Akt (Yin et al. 2009).

C-terminal inhibitors appear to have many non-specific effects and as a result have not been entered into clinical trials (Sreedhar et al. 2004). However, recent research has revealed that C-terminal inhibition, unlike N-terminal inhibition, does not result in the enhanced activity of HSF-1 (Conde et al. 2009; Holzbeierlein et al. 2010). Indeed, treatment of Xenopus oocytes with heat shock in the presence of novobiocin results in a dose dependent decrease in HSF-1 transcriptional activity (Conde et al. 2009). In contrast similar treatment of these cells in the presence of GA resulted in a dose-dependent increase in HSF-1 activity. This lack of HSF-1 induction is a very attractive attribute of C-terminal inhibitors and therefore research and development into synthetic C-terminal inhibitors continues.

## 7.3 Important HSPC1 client proteins in CLL

Research into the involvement of HSPC1 in cancer progression has identified a wide variety of client proteins that may contribute to the progression of both solid tumours and haematological malignancies. There are a number of HSPC1 clients that have been implicated in the development and progression of CLL in particular (Johnson et al. 2007) and therefore the use of HSPC1 inhibitors as a treatment option appears attractive. The list of HSPC1 client proteins is continually expanding suggesting that novel therapeutic targets in CLL may present themselves in the future.

The tyrosine kinase Zeta-associated Protein-70 (ZAP-70) is a well established poor prognostic factor and an HSPC1 client (Bartis et al. 2007). In normal T-cells, ZAP-70 is associated with the TCR where it functions in downstream TCR signalling (Cruse et al. 2007). However, although ZAP-70 is present in normal pre-B-cells, its expression should be lost on maturation of the cell. Hence, the presence of ZAP-70 in CLL cells is indicative of an immature clone. A study by Crespo et al. (2003) found that ZAP-70 expression in CLL correlates with disease progression and survival, and also correlates with another well established CLL prognostic factor, IgV$_H$ mutational status. Castro et al. (2005) demonstrated that ZAP-70 in CLL cells co-immunoprecipitates with HSPC1, while ZAP-70 from normal T-cells does not. In addition, treatment of ZAP-70$^+$ CLL cells with HSPC1 inhibitors resulted in degradation of ZAP-70, while treatment of T-cells from CLL and control patients with HSPC1 inhibitors did not affect the expression of ZAP-70. Manipulation of ZAP-70$^-$ CLL cells to express ZAP-70 was shown to activate HSPC1 and induce sensitivity to 17-AAG.

The tumour suppressor protein p53, encoded by the TP53 gene is frequently mutated in CLL, and other cancer types. Mutant p53$^+$ CLL patients show increased resistance to a wide range of chemotherapeutic agents (Sturm et al. 2003) and therefore are often treated as a distinct sub-group of patients. Indeed agents that act independently of the p53 pathway, such as the monoclonal antibodies rituximab and alemtuzumab and other agents such as lenalidomide, are often used as alternative first-line treatments for patients with a 17p deletion (mutated p53 status). HSPC1 inhibitor treatment of CLL cells results in a dose-dependent reduction in mutant p53 levels, a simultaneous up-regulation of wild type p53 and consequent cytotoxicity (Lin et al. 2007). This treatment also results in an increase in p21, an inducer of cell cycle arrest.

It should be noted that this same study showed that CLL cells without a p53 mutation were also sensitive to HSPC1 inhibitor treatment. However, this could be due to activation of wild-type p53 and consequent p53-dependent apoptosis. Further research has shown a synergistic effect between 17-DMAG and Doxorubicin, demonstrating a sensitisation of p53 mutated cells to Doxorubicin-induced cell death (Robles et al. 2006).

HSPC1 chaperones a broad array of protein kinases involved in signal transduction pathways including phosphorylated Akt, Lyn, B-Raf and I$\kappa$K (Broemer et al. 2004; da Rocha Dias et al. 2005; Sato et al. 2000; Trentin et al. 2011). The interaction of HSPC1 with these phosphorylated kinases prevents dephosphorylation of the kinase and its subsequent inactivation, therefore maintaining its activity. The over-activity of Akt (Ringshausen et al. 2002), Lyn (Contri et al. 2005), and implied elevation of I$\kappa$K (Hertlein et al. 2010) in CLL cells has been previously observed and thought to contribute to cell survival and activation of downstream kinases. Indeed, as I$\kappa$K regulates the activation of the NF-$\kappa$B family of transcription factors, its over-activity has implications for a large number of NF-$\kappa$B target genes including Bcl-2, X-IAP, c-FLIP and Mcl-1 (Hertlein et al. 2010). In fact, a number of these proteins have been implicated in the progression of CLL and have been found to correlate with poor prognosis (Pepper et al. 2008; Pepper et al. 2009) which may suggest a clear link to over-activity of NF-$\kappa$B. Nevertheless, HSPC1 inhibitor treatment has been shown to destabilise Akt, Lyn and I$\kappa$K (Hertlein et al. 2010; Johnson et al. 2007; Jones et al. 2004; Lin et al. 2007; Trentin et al. 2008), in CLL cells resulting in proteosomal degradation of these HSPC1 clients and ultimately apoptosis. A study by McCraig et al. (2011) showed that CD40 stimulation of CLL cells *in-vitro* increased the expression of the anti-apoptotic protein Mcl-1 and enhanced cell survival, suggesting that Mcl-1 may be responsible for *in-vivo* survival of CLL cells following CD40 stimulation by T-cells. 17-DMAG treatment of CLL cells was found to result in down-regulation of Mcl-1 even in the presence of CD40 stimulation and inhibit *in-vitro* survival (Hertlein et al. 2010; McCraig et al. 2011) suggesting that *in-vivo* treatment with 17-DMAG may prevent CLL survival associated with T-cell stimulation in lymph nodes.

The B-cell restricted enzyme, Activation-Induced Cytidine Deaminase (AID) has been shown to have prognostic significance in CLL (Heintel et al. 2004; Palacios et al. 2010). This enzyme is required in normal B-cells for somatic hypermutation and class switch recombination (CSR) and is induced following interaction of CD40 with CD40L on T-cells in germinal centres. However, AID expression has been found in CLL cells circulating in peripheral blood and has been found to correlate with unmutated IgV$_H$ status and unfavourable cytogenetics (Heintel et al. 2004). AID expressing CLL cells were also shown to expresses high levels of anti-apoptotic proteins and proliferation factors (Palacios et al. 2010). It was proposed that these high levels of AID and ongoing CSR are a consequence of recent contact with the proliferation centres and provides further evidence that the microenvironment plays a critical role in CLL cell survival and disease progression. Interestingly, AID is an HSPC1 client and chemical inhibition of HSPC1 activity results in destabilisation and proteosomal degradation of AID and reduced antibody diversification (Orthwein et al. 2010).

It would appear that HSPC1 inhibitor treatment of CLL cells targets a wide variety of client proteins, many of which have been implicated in the progression of the disease.

Furthermore, HSPC1 inhibitor-induced cell death appears to be p53 independent suggesting that it may also be useful in the treatment of patients with a mutated p53 status. However, it is well established that CLL has an extremely heterogeneous clinical course and as a result patients show great variation in their responses to specific treatments. Results from our lab have shown that CLL patients also show great heterogeneity in HSP levels with some patients expressing very high levels of a particular HSP and some patients expressing extremely low levels (Dempsey et al. 2010a). These results indicate that although targeting HSPs may appear an attractive strategy, it may not be successful in all patients. Therefore, HSP analysis may prove useful in providing a personalised treatment.

### 7.4 Effect of HSPC1 inhibition on normal cells

As HSPC1 is abundant in non-tumour cells, the use of HSPC1 inhibitors as anti-cancer therapies may seem impractical. Indeed, the survival of normal cells following exposure to stressors such as ionising radiation or cytotoxic drugs is dependent upon activation of signal transduction pathways, the components of which are HSPC1 client proteins. This is important as in the clinical setting, both tumour and non-tumour cells may have been pre-exposed to cytotoxic drugs or ionising radiation as part of previous therapy. Little is known about the effects of HSPC1 inhibition on signal transduction pathways in stressed non-tumour cells and whether the response to HSPC1 inhibitors depends upon the pre-existing levels of HSPA1A and HSPB1 in target cells. Although HSPC1 inhibitors have been shown to be highly tumour-specific, this has recently been questioned (Gooljarsingh et al. 2006). If correct, introduction of these inhibitors into the systemic circulation, where they will have access to both tumour and non-tumour cells, may introduce complications and this issue warrants further investigation.

### 7.5 Targeting HSPA1A

At present, the modulation of HSPA1A activity using chemical inhibitors does not appear to be achievable in the clinical setting. Although, several compounds are able to inhibit the activity of HSF-1 and therefore regulate HSPA1A, the associated toxicity with HSF-1 and HSPA1A inhibitors is too severe. Furthermore, the inhibition of HSF-1 appears to have a number of associated effects such as the up-regulation of Hsp32, which itself is anti-apoptotic (Lin et al. 2004; Yao et al. 2007). The flavanoid quercetin and the benzylidene lactam KNK-437 have both been shown to inhibit HSPA1A and HSPB1 and sensitise cells to chemotherapeutic drugs or hyperthermia (Taba et al. 2011; Sahin et al. 2011; Zanini et al. 2007). Furthermore, the ability of KNK-437 to enhance the anti-tumour activity of HSPC1 inhibitors has been demonstrated (Guo et al. 2005), although as yet, this has not been tested on primary cells. These data suggest that if the solubility issues and non-specific effects of these inhibitors can be resolved, HSF-1 and/or HSPA1A may prove effective therapeutic targets. Recent work by Zaarur et al. (2006) used a high throughput screening programme to identify chemicals with the capacity to inhibit the heat shock response. Although a number of compounds were identified, one in particular, Emunin, showed very low levels of toxicity while sensitising cells to HSPC1 inhibitors and proteosome inhibitors. Interestingly, this compound appeared to have a novel mode of action as it did not affect HSF-1 activity. Although its exact mechanism remains to be determined, it appears to possess a specific regulatory affect on HSP protein translation. A further benefit of using this type of compound is that if, as in some cases, the over-expression of HSPs in a tumour is HSF-1 independent (Zaarur et al. 2006), manipulating the stress response in this way may still prove advantageous.

The surface expression of HSPA1A on tumour cells provides a novel focus for anti-cancer therapies. The ability of membrane embedded HSPA1A to bind and stimulate NK-cells and induce killing of sHSPA1A+ tumour cells (Gross et al. 2003; Gross et al. 2008; Multhoff et al. 1999) has led to trials involving *ex-vivo* stimulation of autologous NK-cells with TKD peptide and low dose IL-2. This patient-specific technique involves obtaining leukocyte concentrates from the patient by leukapheresis, purifying PBMCs and stimulating them with TKD peptide/low dose IL-2 for four days. Following stimulation, the activated PBMC preparation is re-infused into the patient. Re-infusion is repeated every fortnight for a maximum of five doses (Krause et al. 2004). This technique has been shown to eliminate the primary tumour, prevent metastasis and significantly increase life expectancy in tumour mouse models (Mutlhoff et al. 2000; Stangl et al. 2006). Furthermore, use of this technique in patients with lower rectal carcinoma and non-small cell lung carcinoma was found to increase NK-cell cytotoxicity against sHSPA1A+ tumour cells (Krause et al. 2004) and was found to be well tolerated. However, it should be noted that patients included in this study did not show complete remission following treatment but these were patients with advanced disease and were refractory to standard chemotherapy. A subsequent case study using another advanced disease patient was unsuccessful in attaining remission, but did demonstrate the maintenance of NK-cell cytolytic activity following TKD-IL-2 stimulation (Milani et al. 2009). These data suggest that *ex-vivo* TKD/IL-2 stimulation of autologous NK-cells may have therapeutic potential.

As an alternative strategy to inhibiting the activity of HSPs, recent work from our lab attempted to manipulate the cellular location of HSPs in order to sensitise CLL cells to chemotherapeutic agents (Dempsey et al. 2010b). As mentioned earlier, a number of HSPs associate with lipid rafts and incorporate into the plasma membrane (Gastpar et al. 2005; Nagy et al. 2007; Vega et al. 2008) where they may remain or may be released into the extracellular environment. Vigh et al. (2007b) have proposed a 'membrane sensor model' in which cell stress may be detected at the membrane level and the cell is able to produce a stress response. It is proposed that stress signals originating from the cell membrane result in activation of specific HSP genes and movement of these newly synthesised HSPs to the membrane where they facilitate in stabilising the cell membrane (Vigh et al. 2007a) and therefore facilitating cell survival (Figure 2). It is proposed that a change in membrane fluidity and microdomain organisation (Torok et al. 2003; Vigh et al. 2007a) may be sufficient to result in such membrane stress signals. Our group used several membrane fluidising treatments including aliphatic alcohol, local anaesthetic or mild hyperthermia to fluidise the cell membrane and induce movement of HSPs to the cell surface (Dempsey et al. 2010b). The result was a change in the cellular localisation of HSPA1A, HSPD1, and to a lesser extent, HSPB1 and HSPC1. We found that this movement to the cell surface resulted in a transient decrease in internal levels of HSPs. This temporary decrease in anti-apoptotic HSPs allowed a number of chemotherapeutic agents including Doxorubicin, Cyclophosphamide and TRAIL to act on the cells resulting in significant cytotoxicity of CLL cells. Interestingly, by combining membrane fluidising treatments with chemotherapeutic agents, low doses of drugs were able to cause considerable apoptosis. These low doses were unable to cause cytotoxicity in isolation. We found that inhibiting the movement of HSPs using methyl-β-cyclodextrin (mβcd), a cholesterol sequestering agent, and inhibitor of lipid raft transport, prior to combination treatment, prevented the synergistic effect of fluidising treatment and chemotherapeutic drug. The results suggest that manipulation of HSP cellular location may be an attractive strategy for enhancing the chemotherapeutic treatment of CLL. Furthermore, this method does not rely on CLL patients expressing similar levels of internal HSPs and therefore is an attractive therapeutic approach for a heterogeneous disease. Furthermore, the data may point to a revival of targeted hyperthermia to induce HSP translocation in combination with other therapeutic agents.

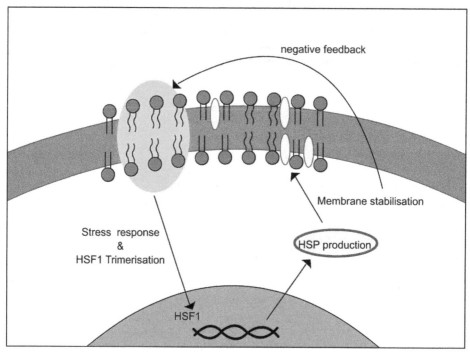

Fig. 2. Induction of an HSP Response via Alteration in Membrane Fluidity (Taken from Dempsey, 2009). Change in membrane fluidity is detected at the membrane, activating a membrane signal which results in the transcription of HSP genes. Newly synthesised HSPs then move to the membrane resulting in membrane stabilisation and re-established membrane-lipid order. This stabilisation effect may itself be a negative feedback regulator to turn off HSP transcription.

## 8. Conclusion

The up-regulation of HSPs in cancer has led to a large variety of studies investigating their prognostic and therapeutic potential. Due to the stressful nature of tumour development, it is not surprising that these anti-apoptotic proteins remain elevated in cancer cells. The anti-apoptotic characteristics of these proteins enable tumour cells to survive in otherwise lethal conditions and hence have been associated with a poor prognosis and resistance to therapy.

These elements alone suggest HSPs may be suitable targets for therapy. However after considering that a number of HSPs are involved in the modifications required for cancer development (the six 'hallmarks of cancer'), they become particularly attractive. Further work on inhibiting HSP activity is required before such compounds can be considered as routine therapies. Extracellular HSPs have been shown to have critical roles in cancer progression with surface-bound HSPC1 in particular contributing to cell invasion and metastasis. Conversely, sHSPA1A has been shown to be detrimental to the tumour, stimulating NK-cell responses and resulting in tumour regression, while a number of extracellular HSPs present tumour-derived peptides to APCs resulting in antigen cross-presentation and T-cell responses. The beneficial effects of these extracellular HSPs have also formed the basis of research into HSP-based therapies focusing on increasing the immune response against tumours. Increasing HSP translocation via cell membrane fluidisation may therefore have the double benefit of increasing the susceptibility of tumours to chemotherapeutic agents and stimulating the immune response. Our work on CLL has found that HSPA1A, HSPB1 and HSPC1 are located inside CLL cells, on the cell surface and also in the serum of CLL patients. However, the pattern of patient variability within and between specific HSPs suggests that analysis of patient HSP profile would be beneficial in directing therapy.

## 9. References

Adams, D.J. & McGuire, W.L. (1983). Quantitative Enzyme-linked Immunosorbent Assay for the Estrogen-regulated Mr 24,000 Protein in Human Breast Tumors: Correlation with Estrogen and Progesterone Receptors. *Cancer Research.* 45(6):2445-2449

An, W.G., Schulte, T.W. & Neckers, L.M. (2000). The heat shock protein 90 antagonist geldanamycin alters chaperone association with p210(bcr-abl) and v-src proteins before their degradation by the proteasome. *Cell Growth & Differentiation.* 11(7):355-360

Arnold-Schild, D., Hanau, D., Spehner, D., Schmid, C., Rammensee, H.G., de la Salle, H. & Schild, H. (1999). Cutting Edge: Receptor-Mediated Endocytosis of Heat Shock Proteins by Professional Antigen-Presenting Cells. *The American Association of Immunologists.* 162(7):3757-3760

Asea, A., Kraeft, S.K., Kurt-Jones, E.A., Stevenson, M.A., Chen, L.B., Finberg, R.W., Koo, G.C. & Calderwood, S.K. (2000). HSP70 stimulates cytokine production through a CD14-dependant pathway, demonstrating its dual role as a chaperone and cytokine. *Nature Medicine.* 6(4):435-442

Bailey, S., A. G. Hall, A. D. J. Pearson and C. P. F. Redfern (2001). The role of AP-1 in glucocorticoid resistance in leukaemia. *Leukaemia Research.* 15(3):391-397.

Barreto, A., Gonzalez, J.M., Kabingu, E.K., Asea, A. & Fiorentino, S. (2003). Stress-induced release of HSC70 from human tumors. *Cellular Immunology.* 222(2):97–104

Bartis, D., Boldizsar, F., Kvell, K., Szabo, M., Palinkas, L., Nemeth, P., Monostori, E. & Berki, T. (2007). Intermolecular relations between the glucocorticoid receptor, ZAP-70 kinase, and Hsp-90. *Biochemical and Biophysical Research Communications.* 354(1):253-258

Basu, S., Binder, R., Ramalingam, T. & Srivastava, P. (2001). CD91 is a common receptor for Heat Shock Proteins gp96, hsp90, hsp70, and calreticulin. *Immunity*. 14(3):303-313

Bausero,M.A., Gastpar, R., Multhoff, G. & Asea, A. (2005). Alternative Mechanism by which IFN-γ Enhances Tumor Recognition: Active Release of Heat Shock Protein 72. *Journal of Immunology*. 175(5):2900-2912

Becker, B., Multhoff, G., Farkas, B., Wild, P.J., Landthaler, M., Stolz, W. & Vogt, T. (2004). Induction of Hsp90 protein expression in malignant melanomas and melanoma metastases. *Experimental Dermatology*.13(1):27–32.

Beere, H.M. & Green, D.R. (2001). Stress management – heat shock protein-70 and the regulation of apoptosis. *Trends in Cell Biology*. 11(1):6-10

Bolhassani, A. & Rafati, S. (2008). Heat-shock proteins as powerful weapons in vaccine development. *Expert Review Vaccines*. 7(8):1185-1189

Boudeau, J., Deak, M., Lawlor, M.A., Morrice, N.A. & Alessi, D.R. (2003). Heat-shock protein 90 and Cdc37 interact with LKB1 and regulate its stability. *Journal of Biochemistry*. 370(3):849-857

Brameshuber, M., Weghuber, J., Ruprecht, V., Gombos, I., Horvath, I., Vigh, L., Eckerstorfer, P., Kiss, E., Stockinger, H. & Schutz, G.J. (2010). Imaging of Mobile Long-lived Nanoplatforms in the Live Cell Plasma Membrane. *The Journal of Biological Chemistry*. 285(53):41765-41771

Broemer, M., Krappmann, D. & Scheidereit, C. (2004). Requirment of Hsp90 acitvity for IκB kinase (IKK) biosynthesis and for constitutive and inducible IKK and NF-κB function. *Oncogene*. 23(31):5378-5386

Calderwood, S.K., Khaleque, M. A., Sawyer, D.B. & Ciocca, D.R. (2006). Heat shock proteins in cancer: chaperones of tumorigenesis. *Trends in Biochemical Sciences*. 31(3):164-172

Calderwood, S.K., Mambula, S.S., Gray Jr., P.J. & Theriault, J.R. (2007). Extracellular heat shock proteins in cell signalling. *FEBS Letters*. 581(19):3689-3694

Campos, L., Chautard, S., Viallet, A. & Guyotat, D. (1999). Expression of heat-shock proteins in acute leukaemia cells. *Haematologica*. 84:13.

Castro, J.E., Prada, C.E., Loria, O., Kamal, A., Chen, L., Burrows, F.J. & Kipps, T.J. (2005). ZAP-70 is a novel conditional heat shock protein 90 (Hsp90) client: inhibition of Hsp90 leads to ZAP-70 degradation, apoptosis, and impaired signaling in chronic lymphocytic leukemia. *Blood*. 106(7):2506-2512

Chant, I. D., Rose, P. E., & Morris, A. G. (1995). Analysis of Heat-Shock Protein Expression in Myeloid-Leukemia Cells by Flow-Cytometry. *British Journal of Haematology*. 90(1):163-168.

Chant, I. D., Rose, P. E., & Morris, A. G. (1996). Susceptability of AML cells to in vitro apoptosis correlates with heat shock protein 70 (hsp70) expression. *British Journal of Haematology*. 93(4):898-902.

Charette, S.J., Lavoie, J.N., Lambert, H. & Landry, J. (2000). Inhibition of Daxx-mediated apoptosis by heat shock protein 27. *Molecular and Cellular Biology*. 20(20):7602-7612

Chauhan, D., Li, G., Hideshima, T., Podar, K., Mitsiades, C., Mitsiades, N., Catley, L., Tai, Y.T., Hayashi, T., Shringarpure, R., Burger, R., Munshi, N., Ohtake, Y., Saxena, S. & Anderson, K.C. (2003a). Hsp27 inhibits release of mitochondrial protein Smac in multiple myeloma cells and confers dexamethasone resistance. *Blood*. 22(3):816-834

Chauhan D, Li GL, Shringarpure R, Podar K, Ohtake Y, Hideshima T, Anderson KC (2003b). Blockade of Hsp27 overcomes bortezomib/proteasome inhibitor PS-341 resistance in lymphoma cells. *Cancer Research*. 63(19):6174-6177

Chen, X., Tao, Q., Yu, H., Zhang, L. & Cao, X. (2002a). Tumor cell membrane-bound heat shock protein 70 elicits antitumor Immunity. *Immunology Letters*. 84(2):81-87

Chen, L.G., Widhopf, G., Huynh, L., Rassenti, L., Rai, K.R., Weiss, A. & Kipps, T.J. (2002b). Expression of ZAP-70 is associated with increased B-cell receptor signaling in chronic lymphocytic leukemia. *Blood*. 100(13):4609-4614

Ciocca, D.R. & Calderwood, S.K. (2005). Heat shock proteins in cancer: diagnostic, prognostic, predictive, and treatment implications. *Cell Stress & Chaperones*. 10(2):86-103

Ciocca, D.R. & Calderwood, S.K. (2005). Heat shock proteins in cancer: diagnostic, prognostic, predictive and treatment implications. *Cell Stress & Chaperones*. 10(2):86-103

Ciocca, D.R. & Luque, E.H. (1991). Immunological Evidence for the Identity Between the Hsp27 Estrogen-Regulated Heat-Shock Protein and the P29 Estrogen Receptor-Associated Protein in Breast and Endometrial Cancer. *Breast Cancer Research and Treatment*. 20(1):33-42

Clayton, A., Turkes, A., Navabi, H., Mason, M.D. & Tabi, Z. (2005). Induction of heat shock proteins in B-cell exosomes. *Journal of Cell Science*. 118(16):3631-3638

Conde, R., Belak, Z.R., Nair, M., O'Carroll, R.F. & Ovsenek, N. (2009). Modulation of Hsf1 activity by novobiocin and geldanamycin. *International journal of Biochemistry and Cell Biology*. 87(6):845-851

Contri, A. Brunati, A.M., Trentin, L., Cabrelle, A., Miorin, M., Cesaro, L., Pinna, L.A., Zambello, R., Semenzato, G. & Donella-Deana, A. (2005). Chronic lymphocytic leukaemia B Cells contain anomalous Lyn tyrosine kinase, a putative contribution to defective apoptosis. *The Journal of Clinical Investigation*. 115(2):369-378

Cornford, P.A., Dodson, A.R., Parsons, K.F., Desmond, A.D., Woolfenden, A., Fordham, M., Neoptolemos, J.P., Ke, Y. & Foster, C.S. (2000). Heat Shock Protein Expression Independently Predicts Clinical Outcome in Prostate Cancer. *Cancer Research*. 60(24):7099-7105

Crespo, M., Bosch, F., Villamor, N., Bellosillo, B., Colomer, D., Rozman, M., Marce, S., Lopez-Guillermo, A., Campo, E. & Montserrat, E. (2003). Zap-70 expression as a surrogate for immunoglobulin-variable-region mutations in chronic lymphocytic leukemia. *N. Engl. J. Med*. 348, 1764–1775

Cruse, J.M., Lewis, R.E., Webb, R.N., Sanders, C.M. & Suggs, J.L. (2007). Zap-70 and CD38 as predictors of IgVH mutation in CLL. *Experimental and Molecular Pathology*. 83(3):459-461

Dakappagari, N. Neely, L. Tangri, S. Lundgren, K. Hipolito, L. Estrellado, A. Burrows, F & Zhang, H. (2010). An investigation into the potential use of Hsp70 as a novel tumour biomarker for Hsp90 inhibitors. *Biomarkers*. 15(1):31-38

Dempsey, N.C. (2009). *Heat Shock Protein Localisation in Haematological Malignancies*. Doctoral Thesis. University of Liverpool. Liverpool, UK.

Dempsey, N.C., Leoni, F., Ireland, H.E., Hoyle, C., & Williams, J.H.H. (2010). Differential Heat Shock Protein Localization in Chronic Lymphocytic Leukemia. *Journal of Leukocyte Biology.* 87(2):467-476.

Dempsey, N.C., Ireland, H.E., Smith, C.M., Hoyle, C.F. & Williams, J.H.H. (2010). Heat Shock Protein translocation induced by membrane fluidization increases tumor-cell sensitivity to chemotherapeutic drugs. *Cancer Letters.* 296(2):256-267

Duval, A., Olaru, D., Campos, L., Flandrin, P., Nadal, N. & Guyotat, D. (2006). Expression and prognostic significance of heat-shock proteins in myelodysplastic Syndromes. *Haematologica.* 91(5):713-714

Eccles, S.A., Massey, A., Raynaud, F.I., Sharp, S.Y., Box, G., Valenti, M.V., et al. (2008). NVP-AUY922: A Novel Heat Shock Protein 90 Inhibitor Active against Xenograft Tumor Growth, Angiogenesis, and Metastasis. *Cancer Research.* 86(8):2850-2860

Eustace BK, Sakurai T, Stewart JK, Yimlamai D, Unger C, Zehetmeier C, Lain B, Torella C, Henning SW, Beste G, Scroggins BT, Neckers L, Ilag LL, Jay DG. (2004). Functional proteomic screens reveal an essential extracellular role for hsp90 alpha in cancer cell invasiveness. *Nature Cell Biology.* 3(9):1098-1100

Faried, A., Sohda, M., Nakajima, M., Miyazaki, T., Kato, H. & Kuwano, H. (2004). Expression of heat-shock protein Hsp60 correlated with the apoptotic index and patient prognosis in human oesophageal squamous cell carcinoma. *European Journal of Cancer.* 40(18):2804-2811

Ferrarini, M., Heltai, S., Zocchi, M.R. & Rugarli, C. (1992). Unusual Expression and Localisation of Heat-Shock Proteins in Human Tumor-Cells. *International Journal of Cancer.* 51(4):613-619

Flaherty, K.T., Puznov, I., Kim, K.B., Ribas, I., McArther, G.A., Sosman, J.A., O'Dwyer, P.J., Lee, R.J., Grippo, J.F., Nolop, K. &Chapman, P.B (2010). Inhibition of Mutated, Activated BRAF in Metastatic Melanoma. The New England Journal of Medicine. 363(9):809-819

Garrido, C., Gurbuxani, S., Ravagnan, L. & Kroemer, G. (2001). Heat Shock Proteins: Endogenous Modulators of Apoptotic Cell Death. *Biochemical & Biophysical Research Communications.* 286(3):433-442

Gastpar, R., Gehrmann, M., Bausero, M.A., Asea, A., Gross, C., Schroeder, J.A. & Multhoff, G. (2005). Heat Shock Protein 70 Surface-Positive Tumor Exosomes. *Cancer Research.* 5;65(12):5238-47.

Gehrmann, M., H. Schmetzer, G. Eissner, T. Haferlach, W. Hiddemann and G. Multhoff (2003). Membrane-bound heat shock protein 70 in acute myeloid leukemia: a tumor-specific recognition structure for the cytolytic activity of autologous natural killer cells. *Haematologica.* 88(4): 474-476.

Gehrmann, M., Radons, J., Molls, M. & Multhoff, G. (2008). The therapeutic implications of clinically applied modifiers of heat shock protein 70 (Hsp70) expression by tumor cells. *Cell Stress & Chaperones.* 13(1):1-10

Geisler, J.P., Tammela, J.E., Manahan, K.J., Geisler, H.E., Miller, G.A., Zhou, Z. & Wiemann, M.C. (2004). HSP27 in patients with ovarian carcinoma: still an independent prognostic indicator at 60 months follow-up. *European Journal of Gynaecological Oncology.* 25(2):165-168

Giaginis, C., Daskalopoulou, S.S., Vgenopoulou, S., Sfiniadakis, I., Kouraklis, G. & Theocharis, S.E. (2009). Heat Shock Protein-27, -60 and -90 expression in gastric cancer: association with clinicopathological variables and patient survival. *BMC Gastroenterology*. 9:1-10

Glaessgen, A., Jonmarker, S., Lindberg, A., Nilsson, B., Lewensohn, R., Ekman, P., Valdman, A. & Egevad, L. (2008). Heat shock proteins 27, 60 and 70 as prognostic markers of prostate cancer. *APMIS*. 116(10):888-895

Gooljarsingh, L.T. Fernandes, C. Yan, K. Zhang, H. Grooms, M. Johanson, K. Sinnamon, R.H. Kirkpatrick, R. B. Kerrigan, J. Lewis, T. Arnone, M. King, A.J. Lai, Z. Copeland, R.A. & Tummino, P.J. (2006). A Biochemical rationale for the anticancer effects of Hsp90 inhibitors: slow, tight binding inhibition by geldanamycin and its analogues. *PNAS*. 103(20):7625-7630

Gross, C., Hansch, D., Gastpar, R. & Multhoff, G. (2003). Interaction of Heat Shock Protein 70 Peptide with NK Cells Involves the NK Receptor CD94. *Biological Chemistry*. 384(2):267 – 279

Gross, C., Holler, E., Stangl, S., Dickinson, A., Pockley, A.G., Asea, A.A., Mallappa, N., & Multhoff, G. (2008). An Hsp70 peptide initiates NK cell killing of leukemic blasts after stem cell transplantation. *Leukemia Research*. 32(4):527-534

Guo, F., Sigua, C., Bali, P., George, P., Fiskus, W., Scuto, A. & Annavarapu, S. (2005). Mechanistic role of heat shock protein 70 in Bcr-Abl–mediated resistance to apoptosis in human acute leukemia cells. *Blood*. 105(3):1246-1255

Hanahan, D. & Weinberg, R.A. (2000). The Hallmarks of Cancer. *Cell*. 100(1):57–70

Hanahan, D. & Weinberg, R.A. (2011). Hallmarks of Cancer: The Next Generation. *Cell*. 144(5):646-674

Hanson, B.E. & Vesole, D.H. (2009). Retaspimycin hydrochloride (IPI-504): a novel heat shock protein inhibitor as an anti-cancer agent. *Expert Opinion on Investigational Drugs*. 18(9):1375-1383

Heintel, D., Kroemer, E., Kienle, D., Schwarzinger, I., Gleiss, a, Schwarzmeier, J., Marculescu, R., et al. (2004). High expression of activation-induced cytidine deaminase (AID) mRNA is associated with unmutated IGVH gene status and unfavourable cytogenetic aberrations in patients with chronic lymphocytic leukaemia. *Leukemia*. 18(4):756-62

Hertlein, E. Wagner, A.J. Jones, J. Lin, T.S. Maddocks, K.J. Towns, W.H. Goettl, V.M. Zhang, X. Jarjoura, D. Raymond, C.A. West, D.A. Croce, C.M. Byrd, J.C. & Johnson, A.J. (2010). 17-DMAG targets the Nuclear-Factor-{kappa}B family of proteins to induce apoptosis in Chronic Lymphocytic Leukaemia: clinical implications of Hsp90 inhibition. *Blood*. 116(1):45-53

Holzbeierlein, J.M., Windsperger, A. & Vielhauer, G. (2010). Hsp90: A Drug Target? *Current Oncology Reports*. 12:95-101

Hightower, L. E., Guidon, P. T. (1989) Selective release from cultured mammalian cells of heat-shock (stress) proteins that resemble glia-axon transfer proteins. *Journal Cellular Physiology*. 138:257–266.

Hunter-Lavin, C., Davies, E. L., Bacelar, M., Marshall, M. J., Andrew, S. M. and Williams, J. H. H. (2004). Hsp70 release from peripheral blood mononuclear cells. *Biochemical and Biophysical Research Communications.* 324(2):511-517.

Huntoon, C.J., Nye, M.D., Geng, L., Peterson, K.L., Flatten, K.S., Haluska, P., Kaufmann, S.H., Karnitz, L.M. (2010). Heat shock protein 90 inhibition depletes LATS1 and LATS2, two regulators of the mammalian hippo tumor suppressor pathway. *Cancer Research.* 70(21):8642-8650

Iwaya, K., Tsuda, H., Fujita, S., Suzuki, M. & Hirohashi, S. (1995). Natural State of Mutant P53 Protein and Heat-Shock Protein-70 in Breast-Cancer Tissues. *Laboratory Investigation.* 72(6):707-714

Jaattela, M. (1999). Escaping Cell Death: Survival Proteins in Cancer. *Experimental Cell Research.* 248:30-43

Johnson, A.J., Wagner, A.J., Cheney, C.M., Smith, L.L., Lucas, D.M., Guster, S.K., Grever, M.R., Lin, T.S. & Byrd, J.C. (2007). Rituximab and 17-allylamino-17-demethoxygeldanamycin induce synergistic apoptosis in B-cell chronic lymphocytic leukaemia. *British Journal of Haematology.* 139(5):837-844

Jones, D.T., Addison, E., North, J.M., Lowdell, M.W., Hoffbrand, A.V., Mehta, A.B., Ganeshaguru, K., Folarin, N.I. & Wickremasinghe, R.G. (2004). Geldanamycin and herbimycin A induce apoptotic killing of B chronic lymphocytic leukemia cells and augment the cells' sensitivity to cytotoxic drugs. *Blood.* 103(5):1855-1861

Kampinga, H.H., Hageman, J., Vos, M.J., Kubota, H., Tanguay, R.M., Bruford, E.A., Cheetham, M.E., Chen, B. & Hightower, L.E. (2009). Guidelines for the nomenclature of the human heat shock proteins. *Cell Stress and Chaperones.* 14(1):105-111

Kantarjian, H.M.,O'Brien, S.,Cortes, J., Giles, F.J.,Rios, M.B., Shan, J.Q., Faderl, S., Garcia-Manero, G., Ferrajoli, A., Verstovsek, S., Wierda, W., Keating, M. & Talpaz, M. (2003). Imatinib mesylate therapy improves survival in patients with newly diagnosed Philadelphia chromosome-positive chronic myelogenous leukemia in the chronic phase - Comparison with historic data. *Cancer.* 98(12):2636-2642

Kawanishi, K., Shiozaki, H., Doki, Y., Sakita, I., Inoue, M., Yano, M., Tsujinaka, T., Shamma, A. & Monden, M. (1999). Prognostic significance of heat shock proteins 27 and 70 in patients with squamous cell carcinoma of the esophagus. *Cancer.* 85(8):1649-1657

Khaleque, M.A., Bharti, A., Sawyer, D., Gong, J.L., Benjamin, I.J., Stevenson, M.A. & Calderwood, S.K. (2005). Induction of heat shock proteins by heregulin beta 1 leads to protection from apoptosis and anchorage-independent growth. *Oncogene.* 24(43): 6564-6573

Kim, Y. S. Alarcon, S. V. Lee, S. Lee, M.-J. Giaccone, G. Neckers, L. & Trepel, J. B. (2009). Update on Hsp90 inhibitors in clinical trial. *Current Topics in Medicinal Chemistry.* 9(15):1479-1492

Kleinjung, T., Arndt, O., Feldmann, H., Bockmühl, U., Gehrmann, M., Zilch, T., Pfister, K., Schönberger, J., Marienhagen, J. & Eilles, C. (2003). Heat shock protein 70 (Hsp70) membrane expression on head-and-neck cancer biopsy - a target for natural killer (NK) cells. *International Journal of Radiation Oncology Biology Physics.* 57(3):820-826

Krause, S.W., Gastpar, R., Andreesen, R., Gross, C., Ullrich, H., Thonigs, G., Pfister, K. & Multhoff, G. (2004). Treatment of colon and lung cancer patients with ex vivo heat shock protein 70-peptide-activated, autologous natural killer cells: a clinical phase I trial. *Clinical Cancer Research.* 10(11):3699-3707

Krukenberg, K.A., Street, T.O., Lavery, L.A. & Agard, D.A. (2011). Conformational dynamics of the molecular chaperone Hsp90. *Quarterly Reviews of Biophysics.* 44(2):229-255

Kuppner, M.C., Gastpar, R., Gelwer, S., Nossner, E., Ochmann, O., Scharner, A. & Issels, R.D. (2001). The role of heat shock protein (hsp70) in dendritic cell maturation: Hsp70 induces the maturation of immature dendritic cells but reduces DC differentiation from monocyte precursors. *European Journal of Immunology.* 31(5):1602-1609

Kurotaki, T., Tamura, Y., Ueda, G., Oura, J., Kutomi, G., Hirohashi, Y., Sahara, H., Torigoe, T., Hiratsuka, H., Sunakawa, H., Hirata, K. & Sato, N. (2007). Efficient cross-presentation by heat shock protein 90-peptide complex-loaded dendritic cells via an endosomal pathway. *Journal of Immunology.* 179(3):1803-1813

Lanneau, D., Brunet, M., Frisan, E., Solary, E., Fontenay, M., Garrido, C. (2008). Heat shock proteins: essential proteins for apoptosis regulation. *Journal of Cellular and Molecular Medicine.* 12(3):743-761

Le Blanc, A.C. (2003). Natural cellular inhibitors of caspases. *Progress in Neuro-Psychopharmacology & Biological Psychiatry.* 27:215-229

Lehman, T.A., Bennett, W.P., Metcalf, R.A., Welsh, J.A., Ecker, J., Modali, R.V., Ullrich, S., Romano, J.W., Appella, E., Testa, J.R., Gerwin, B.I. & Harris, C.C. (1991). P53 Mutations, Ras Mutations and P53-Heat Shock 70 Protein complexes in Human Lung-Carcinoma Cell-Lines. *Cancer Research.* 51(15):4090:4096

Li, Y., Zhang, T., Schwartz, S.J. & Sun, D. (2009). New developments in Hsp90 inhibitors as anti-cancer therapeutics: Mechanisms, clinical perspective and more potential. *Drug Resistance Updates.* 12(1-2)17-27

Lin, K., Rockliffe, N., Johnson, G.G., Sherrington, P.D. & Pettitt, A.R. (2007). Hsp90 inhibition has opposing effects on wild-type and mutant p53 and induces p21 expression and cytotoxicity irrespective of p53/ATM status in chronic lymphocytic leukaemia cells. *Oncogene.* 27(17): 2445-2455

Love, S. & King, R.J.B. (1994). A 27kDa Heat-Shock-Protein that has anomalous prognostic powers in early and advanced breast-cancer. *British Journal Of Cancer.* 69(4):743-748

Lundgren, K., Zhang, H., Brekken, J., Huser, N., Powell, R.E., Timple, N., Busch, D.J., Neely, L., Sensintaffar, J.L., Yang, Y.C., McKenzie, A., Friedman, J., Scannevin, R., Kamal, A., Hong, K., Kasibhatla, S.R., Boehm, M.F., Burrows, F.J. (2009). BIIB021, an orally available, fully synthetic small-molecule inhibitor of the heat shock protein Hsp90. *Molecular Cancer Therapeutics.* 8(4):921-929

Mambula, S.S. & Calderwood, S.K. (2006). Heat induced release of Hsp70 from prostate carcinoma cells involves both active secretion and passive release from necrotic cells. *International Journal of Hyperthermia.* 22(7):575-585

Matysiak, M., B. Makosa, A. Walczak and K. Selmaj (2008). Patients with multiple sclerosis resisted to glucocorticoid therapy: abnormal expression of heat-shock protein 90 in glucocorticoid receptor complex. *Multiple Sclerosis* 14(7): 919-926

McCraig, A.M., Cosimo, E., Leach, M.T. & Michie, A.M. (2011). Dasatinib inhibits B cell receptor signalling in chronic lymphocytic leukaemia but novel combination approaches are required to overcome additional pro-survival microenvironmental signals. *British Journal of Haematology*. 153:199-211

McCready, J., Sims, J.D., Chan, D. & Jay, D.J. (2010). Secretion of extracellular Hsp90α via exosomes increases cancer cell motility: a role for plasminogen activation. *BMC Cancer*. 10:294-304

McLaughlin, S.H., Smith, H.W. & Jackson, S.E. (2002). Stimulation of the Weak ATPase Activity of Human Hsp90 by a Client Protein. *Journal of Molecular Biology*. 315:787-798

Milicevic, Z. T., Petkovic, M. Z., Drndarevic, N. C., Pavlovic, M. D., & Todorovic, V. N. (2007). Expression of heat shock protein 70 (HSP70) in patients with colorectal adenocarcinoma - immunohistochemistry and Western blot analysis. *Neoplasma*. 54(1):37-45.

Minami, Y., Kiyoi, H., Yamamoto, Y., Ueda, R., Saito, H. & Naoe, T. (2002). Selective apoptosis of tandemly duplicated FLT3-transformed leukemia cells by Hsp90 inhibitors. *Leukemia*. 16(8): 1535-1540

Modi, S., Stopeck, A.T., Gordon, M.S., Mendelson, D., Solit, D.B., Bagatell, R., Ma, W., Wheler, J., Rosen, N., Norton, L., Cropp, G.F., Johnson, R.G., Hannah, A.L. & Hudis, C.A. (2007). Combination of Trastuzumab and Tanespimycin (17-AAG, KOS-953) Is Safe and Active in Trastuzumab-Refractory HER-2–Overexpressing Breast Cancer: A Phase I Dose-Escalation Study. *Journal of Clinical Oncology*. 25(34):5410-5417

Murshid, A., Gong, J. & Calderwood, S.K. (2008). Heat-shock proteins in cancer vaccines: agents of antigen cross presentation. *Expert Reviews in Vaccines*. 7(7):1019-1030

Nagy, E., Balogi, Z., Gombos, I., Akerfelt, M., Bjorkbom, A., Balogh, G., Torok, Z., Maslyanko, A., Fiszer-Kierzkowska, A., Lisowska, K., Slotte, P.J., Sistonen, L., Horvath, I. & Vigh, L. (2007). Hyperfluidisation-coupled membrane microdomain reorganisation is linked to activation of the heat shock response in a murine melanoma cell line. *PNAS*. 104(19):7945-7950

Nazarian, R., Shi, H., Wang, Q., Kong, X., Koya, R.C., Lee, H., Chen, Z., Lee, M.K., Attar, N., Sazegar, H., Chodon, T., Nelson, S.F., McArthur, G., Sosman, J.A., Ribas, A. & Lo, R.S. (2010). Melanomas acquire resistance to B-RAF(V600E) inhibition by RTK or N-RAS upregulation. *Nature*. 468(7326):973-977

Neckers, L. (2007). Heat shock protein 90: the cancer chaperone. *Journal of Bioscience*. 32(3):517-530

Nimmanapalli, R., O'Bryan, E., Huang, M., Bali, P., Burnette, P.K., Loughran, T., Tepperberg, J., Jove, R. & Bhalla, K. (2002). Molecular Characterization and Sensitivity of STI-571 (Imatinib Mesylate, Gleevec)- resistant, Bcr-Abl-positive, Human Acute Leukemia Cells to SRC Kinase Inhibitor PD180970 and 17-Allylamino-17-demethoxygeldanamycin. *Cancer Research*. 62:5761-5769,

Nylandsted, J., Brand, K., & Jaattela, M. (2000). Heat shock protein 70 is required for the survival of cancer cells. *Mechanisms of Cell Death*. 926:122-125.

Okawa, Y., Hideshima, T., Steed, P., Vallet, S., Hall, S., Huang, K., Rice, J., Barabasz, A., Foley, B., Ikeda, H., Raje, N., Kiziltepe, T., Yasui, H., Enatsu, S., Anderson, K.C. (2009). SNX-2112, a selective Hsp90 inhibitor, potently inhibits tumor cell growth, angiogenesis, and osteoclastogenesis in multiple myeloma and other hematologic tumors by abrogating signaling via Akt and ERK. *Blood*. 113(4):846-855

Orthwein, A., Patenaude, A.-M., Affar, E. B., Lamarre, A., Young, J. C., & Di Noia, J. M. (2010). Regulation of activation-induced deaminase stability and antibody gene diversification by Hsp90. *The Journal of experimental medicine*. 207(12):2751-65

Palacios, F., Moreno, P., Morande, P., Abreu, C., Correa, A., Porro, V., Landoni, A. I., et al. (2010). High expression of AID and active class switch recombination might account for a more aggressive disease in unmutated CLL patients: link with an activated microenvironment in CLL disease. *Blood*. 115(22):4488-96

Pashtan, I., Tsutsumi, S., Wang, S.Q., Xu, W.P., Neckers, L. (2008). Targeting Hsp90 prevents escape of breast cancer cells from tyrosine kinase inhibition. *Cell Cycle*. 7(18): 2936-2941

Paul, C., Manero, F., Gonin, S., Kretz-Remy, C., Virot, S. & Arrigo, A.P. (2002). Hsp27 as a negative regulator of cytochrome c release. *Molecular and Cellular Biology*. 22(3):816-834

Peng, C., Li, D. & Li, S. (2007). Heat Shock Protein 90. A Potential Therapeutic Target in Leukemic Progenitor and Stem Cells Harboring Mutant BCR-ABL Resistant to Kinase Inhibitors. *Cell Cycle*. 6(18):2227-2231

Pepper, C., Lin, T.T., Pratt, G., Hewamana, S., Brennan, P., Hiller, L., Hills, R., Ward, R., Starczynski, J., Austen, B., Hooper, L., Stankovic, T. & Fegan, C. (2008). Mcl-1 expression has in vitro and in vivo significance in chronic lymphocytic leukemia and is associated with other poor prognostic markers. *Blood*. 112(9):3807-3817

Pepper, C., Hewamana, S., Brennan, P. & Fegan, C. (2009). NF-kappaB as a prognostic marker and therapeutic target in chronic lymphocytic leukemia. *Future Oncology*. 5(7):1027-37

Pfister, K., Radons, J., Busch, R., Tidball, J.G., Pfeifer, M., Freitag, L., Feldmann, H.J., Milani, V., Issels, R. & Multhoff, G. (2007). Patient survival by Hsp70 membrane phenotype. *American Cancer Society*. 110(4):926-935

Pick, E., Kluger, Y., Giltnane, J.M., Moeder, C., Camp, R.L., Rimm, D.L. & Kluger, H.M. (2007). High HSP90 expression is associated with decreased survival in breast cancer. *Cancer Research*. 67(7): 2932-7.

Ramalingam, S.S., Egorin, M.J., Ramanathan, R.K., Remick, S.C., Sikorski, R.P., ...Lagattuta, T.F., Chatta, G.S., Friedland, D.M., Stoller, R.G., Potter, D.M., Ivy, S.P. & Belani, C.P. (2008). A phase I study of 17-allylamino-17-demethoxygeldanamycin combined with paclitaxel in patients with advanced solid malignancies. *Clinical Cancer Research*. 14(11): 3456-3461

Ramp, U., Mahotka, C., Heikaus, S., Shibata, T., Grimm, M.O., Willers, R. & Gabbert, H.E. (2007). Expression of heat shock protein 70 in renal cell carcinoma and its relation to tumor progression and prognosis. *Histology and Histopathology*. 22:1019-1107

Ravagnan, L., Gurbuxani, S., Susin, A., Maisse, C., Daugas, E., Zamzami, N., Mak, T., Jaatella, Penninger, J.M., Garrido, C. & Kroemer, G. (2001). Heat-shock protein 70 antagonizes apoptosis-inducing factor. *Nature Cell Biology*. 3(9): 839-843

Richards, E.H., Hickey, E., Weber, L., Masters, J.R.W. (1996). Effect of overexpression of the small heat shock protein HSP27 on the heat and drug sensitivities of human testis tumor cells. *Cancer Research*. 56(10):2446-2451

Richardson, P.G., Badros, A.Z., Jagannath, S., Tarantolo, S., Wolf, J.L., Albitar, M., Berman, D., Messina, M. & Anderson, K.C. (2010). Tanespimycin with bortezomib: activity in relapsed/refractory patients with multiple myeloma. *British Journal of Haematology*. 150(4):428-437

Ringshausen, I., Schneller, F., Bogner, C., Hipp, S., Duyster, J., Peschel, C., Decker, T. (2002). Constitutively activated phosphatidylinositol-3 kinase (PI-3K) is involved in the defect of apoptosis in B-CLL: association with protein kinase Cdelta. *Blood*. 100(10):3741-3748.

Robles, A.I., Wright, M.H., Gandhi, B., Feis, S.S., Hanigan, C.L., Wiestner, A. & Varticovski, L. (2006). Schedule-dependent synergy between the heat shock protein 90 inhibitor 17-(dimethylaminoethylamino)-17-demethoxygeldanamycin and doxorubicin restores apoptosis to p53-mutant lymphoma cell lines. *Clinical Cancer Research*. 12(21): 6547-6556

Romani, A.A., Crafa, P., Desenzani, S., Graiani, G., Lagrasta, C., Sianesi, M., Soliani, P. & Borghetti, A.F. (2007). The expression of HSP27 is associated with poor clinical outcome in intrahepatic cholangiocarcinoma. *BMC Cancer*. 7(232):232

Sagol, O., Tuna, B., Coker, A., Karademir, S., Obuz, F., Astarcioglu, H., Kupelioglu, A., Astarcioglu, I. & Topalak, O. (2002). Immunohistochemical detection of PS2 protein and heat shock protein-70 in pancreatic adenocarcinomas. relationship with disease extent and patient survival. *Pathology Research & Practice*.198(2):77-84.

Sahin, E., Sahin, M., Sanlioğlu, A.D. & Gümüslü, S. (2011). KNK437, a benzylidene lactam compound, sensitises prostate cancer cells to the apoptotic effect of hyperthermia. *International Journal of Hyperthermia*. 27(1):63-73

Samali, A., Cai, J., Zhivotovsky, B., Jones, D.P. & Orrenius, S. (1999). Presence of a pre-apoptotic complex of pro-caspase-3, Hsp60 and Hsp10 in the mitochondrial fraction of Jurkat cells. *EMBO Journal*. 18(8):2040-2048

Samali, A., Robertson, J.D., Peterson, E., Manero, F., van Zeijl, L., Paul, C., Cotgreave, I.A., Arrigo, A.P. & Orrenius, S. (2001). Hsp27 protects mitochondria of thermotolerant cells against apoptotic stimuli. *Cell Stress and Chaperones*. 6(1):49-58

Santarosa, M., Favaro, D., Quaia, M. & Galligioni, E. (1997). Expression of heat shock protein 72 in renal cell carcinoma: Possible role and prognostic implications in cancer patients. *European Journal of Cancer*. 33(6):873-877

Sato, S., Fujita, N. & Tsuruo, T. (2000). Modulation of Akt kinase activity by binding to Hsp90. *PNAS*. 97(20): 10832–10837

Schepers, H., Geugien, M., van der Toorn, M., Bryantsev, A.L., Kampinga, H.H., Eggen, B.J.L. & Vellenga, E. (2005). HSP27 protects AML cells against VP-16-induced apoptosis through modulation of p38 and c-Jun. *Experimental Haematology*. 33(6):660-670

Schilling, D., Gehrmann, M., Steinem, C., De Maio, A., Pockley, A.G., Abend, M., Molls, M. Multhoff, G. (2007). Binding of heat shock protein 70 to extracellular phosphatidylserine promotes killing of normoxic and hypoxic tumor cells. *FASEB Journal*. 23(8):2467-77

Schneider, J., Jimenez, E., Marenbach, K., Romero, H., Marx, D. & Meden, H. (1999). Immunohistochemical detection of HSP60-expression in human ovarian cancer. Correlation with survival in a series of 247 patients. *Anticancer Research*. 19(3A): 2141-2146

Shah, N.P., Nicoll, J.M., Nagar, B., Gorre, M.E., Paquette, R.L., Kuriyan, J. & Sawyers, C.L. (2002). Multiple BCR-ABL kinase mutations confer polyclonal resistance to the tyrosine kinase inhibitor Imatinib (STI571) in chronic phase and blast crisis chronic myeloid leukemia. *Cancer Cell*. 2:117-125

Shahidi, H., A. Vottero, C. A. Stratakis, S. E. Taymans, M. Karl, C. A. Longui, G. P. Chrousos, W. H. Daughaday, S. A. Gregory and J. M. D. Plate (1999). Imbalanced expression of the glucocorticoid receptor isoforms in cultured lymphocytes from a patient with systemic glucocorticoid resistance and chronic lymphocytic leukemia. *Biochemical and Biophysical Research Communications*. 254(3): 559-565.

Shan, Y.X., Liu, T.J., Su, H.F., Samsamshariat, A., Mestril, R. & Wang, P.H. (2003). Hsp10 and Hsp60 modulate Bcl-2 family and mitochondria apoptosis signaling induced by doxorubicin in cardiac muscle cells. *Journal of Molecular and Cellular Cardiology*. 35(9):1135-1143

Sherman, M. & Multhoff, G. (2007). Heat Shock Proteins in Cancer. *Annals of the New York Academy of Sciences*. 1113:192-201

Shotar, A. M. (2005). P53 and heat shock protein 70 expressions in colorectal adenocarcinoma. *Saudi Medical Journal*. 26(10):1602-1606.

Sidera, K., Gaitanou. M., Stellas, D., Matsas, R. & Patsavoudi, E. (2008). A Critical Role for HSP90 in Cancer Cell Invasion Involves Interaction with the Extracellular Domain of HER-2. *The Journal of Biological Chemistry*. 283(4):2031-2041

Shin BK, Wang H, Yim AM, Le Naour F, Brichory F, Jang JH, Zhao R, Puravs E, Tra J, Michael CW, Misek DE, Hanash SM. (2003). Global profiling of the cell surface proteome of cancer cells uncovers an abundance of proteins with chaperone function. *Journal of Biological Chemistry*. 278(9):7607-1

Sorger, P.K. (1991). Heat Shock Factor and the Heat Shock Response. *Cell*. 65(3):363-366

Soti, C., Racz, A. & Csermely, P. (2002). A Nucleotide-Dependent Molecular Switch Controls ATP Binding at the C-Terminal Domain of Hsp90. *The Journal of Biological Chemistry*. 277(9):7066-7075

Sreedhar, A.S., Soti, C. & Csermely, P. (2004). Inhibition of Hsp90: a new strategy for inhibiting protein kinases. *Biochemica & Biophysica Acta*. 1697:233-242

Steiner, K., Graf, M., Hecht, K., Reif, S., Rossbacher, L., Pfister, K., Kolb, H.J., Schmetzer, H.M. & Multhoff, G. (2006). High HSP70-membrane expression on leukemic cells from patients with acute myeloid leukemia is associated with a worse prognosis. *Leukemia*. 20:2076-2079

Sturm, I., Bosanquet, AG., Hermann, S., Guner, D., Dorken, B. & Daniel, P.T. (2003). Mutation of p53 and consecutive selective drug resistance in B-CLL occurs as a consequence of prior DNA-damaging chemotherapy. *Cell Death & Differentiation.* 10:477-484

Taba, K., Kuramitsu, Y., Ryozawa, S.,Yoshida, K., Tanaka, T., Mori-Iwamoto, S., Maehara, S., Maehara, Y., Sakaida, I., Nakamura, K. (2011). KNK437 Downregulates Heat Shock Protein 27 of Pancreatic Cancer Cells and Enhances the Cytotoxic Effect of Gemcitabine. *Chemotherapy.* 57(1):12-16

Taldone, T., Gozman, A., Maharaj, R. & Chiosis, G. (2008). Targeting Hsp90: small-molecule inhibitors and their clinical development. *Current Opinion in Pharmacology.* 8(4):370-4

Tauchi, K., Tsutsumi, Y., Hori, S., Yoshimura, S., Osamura, R.Y. & Watanabe, K. (1991). Expression of Heat-Shock Protein-70 and C-Myc Protein in Human Breast-Cancer – An Immunohistochemical Study. *Japanese Journal of Clinical Oncology.* 21(4):256-263

Thomas, X., Campos, L., Mounier, C., Cornillon, J., Flandrin, P., Le, Q.H., Piselli, S. & Guyotat, D. (2005). Expression of heat-shock proteins is associated with major adverse prognostic factors in acute myeloid leukemia. *Leukaemia Research.* 29:1049-1058

Todryk, S., Melcher, A.A., Harwick, N., Linardakis, E., Bateman, A., Colombo, M.P., Stoppacciaro, A. & Vile, R.G. (1999). Heat shock protein 70 induced during tumor cell killing induces Th1 cytokines and targets immature dendritic cell precursors to enhance antigen uptake. *Journal of Immunology.* 163(3):1398-1408

Todryk, S., Melcher, A.A., Dalgleish, A.G., Vile, R.G. (2000). Heat shock proteins refine the danger theory. *Immunology.* 99:334-337

Torok, Z., Tsvetkova, N.M., Balogh, G., Horvath, I., Nagy, E., Penzes, Z., Hargitai, J., Bensaude, O., Csermely, P., Crowe, J.H., Maresca, B. & Vigh, L. (2003). Heat shock protein coinducers with no effect on protein denaturation specifically modulate the membrane lipid phase. *PNAS.* 100(6):3131-3136

Trentin, L., Frasson, M., Donella-Deana, A., Frezzato, F., Pagano ,M.A., Tibaldi, E., Gattazzo, C., Zambello, R., Semenzato, G. & Brunati, A.M. (2008). Geldanamycin-induced Lyn dissociation from aberrant Hsp90-stabilized cytosolic complex is an early event in apoptotic mechanisms in B-chronic lymphocytic leukemia. *Blood.* 112(12):4665-74

Tsutsumi, S., Scroggins, B., Koga, F., Lee, M.J., Trepel, J., Felts, S., Carreras, C. & Neckers, L. (2008). A small molecule cell-impermeant Hsp90 antagonist inhibits tumor cell motility and invasion. *Oncogene.* 27: 2478-2487

Urushibara, M., Kageyama, Y., Akashi, T., Otsuka, Y., Takizawa, T,. Koike, M. & Kihara, K. (2007). HSP60 may predict good pathological response to neoadjuvant chemoradiotherapy in bladder cancer. *Japanese Journal of Clinical Oncology.* 37(1):56-61

Vargas-Roig, L.M., Gago, F.E., Tello, O., Anzar, J.C. & Ciocca, D.R. (1998). Heat Shock Protein Expression and Drug Resistance in breast cancer patients treated with induction chemotherapy. *International Journal of Cancer.* 79:468-475

Vega, V.L., Rodrıguez-Silva, M., Frey, T., Gehrmann, M., Diaz, J.C., Steinem, C., Multhoff, G., Arispe, N. & De Maio, A. (2008). Hsp70 Translocates into the Plasma Membrane after Stress and Is Released into the Extracellular Environment in a Membrane-

Associated Form that Activates Macrophages. *Journal of Immunology.* 180(6):4299-4307

Vigh, L., Horvath, I., Maresca, B. & Harwood, J.L. (2007a). Can the stress protein response be controlled by 'membrane-lipid therapy'? *Trends in Biochemical Sciences.* 32(8):357-363

Vigh, L., Nakamoto, H., Landry, J., Gomez-Munoz, A., Harwood, J.L. & Horvath, I. (2007b). Membrane Regulation of the Stress Response from Prokaryotic Models to Mammalian Cells. *Annals of the New York Academy of Sciences.* 1113:40–51

Walerych, D., Kudla, G., Gutkowska, M., Wawrzynow, B., Muller, L., King, F.W., Helwak, A., Boros, J., Zylicz, A., Zylicz, M. (2004). Hsp90 chaperones wild-type p53 tumor suppressor protein. *Journal of Biological Chemistry.* 279(47):48836-45

Wei, Y.Q., Zhao, X., Kariya, Y., Fukata, H., Teshigawara, K. & Uchida, A. (1996). Induction of autologous tumor killing by heat treatment of fresh human tumor cells: involvement of gamma delta T cells and heat shock protein 70. *Cancer Research.* 56(5):1104–1110.

Whitesell, L., Mimnaugh, E.G., De Costa, B., Myers, C.E. & Necker, L.M. (1994). Inhibition of heat shock protein HSP90-pp60 heteroprotein complex formation by benzoquinone ansamycins: Essential role for stress proteins in oncogenic transformation. *PNAS.* 91:8324-8328

Williams, J. H. H. and Ireland, H. E. (2008). Sensing danger - Hsp72 and HMGB1 as candidate signals. *Journal of Leukocyte Biology.* 83(3):489-492.

Wu, C. (1995). Heat Shock Treanscription Factors. Structure & Regulation. *Annual Review of Cell and Developmental Biology.* 11:441-469

Wu, X., Wanders, A., Wardega, P., Tinge, B., Gedda, L., Bergstrom, S., Sooman, L., Gullbo, J., Bergqvist, M., Hesselius, P., Lennartsson J. & kman, S. (2009). Hsp90 is expressed and represents a therapeutic target in human oesophageal cancer using the inhibitor 17-allylamino-17-demethoxygeldanamycin. *British Journal of Cancer.* 100, 334-343

Xanthoudakis, S., Roy, S., Rasper, D., Hennessey, T., Aubin, Y., Cassady, R., Tawa, P., Ruel, R., Rosen, A. & Nicholson, D.W. (1999). Hsp60 accelerates the maturation of pro-caspase-3 by upstream activator proteases during apoptosis. *EMBO Journal.* 18(8):2049-2056

Yaglom, J.A., Gabai, V.L. & Sherman, M.Y. (2007). High Levels of Heat Shock Protein Hsp72 in Cancer Cells Suppress Default Senescence Pathways. *Cancer Research.* 67(5):2373-2381

Yao, P., Nussler, A., Liu, L., Hao, L., Song, F., Schirmeier, A. & Nussler, N. (2007). Quercetin protects human hepatocytes from ethanol-derived oxidative stress by inducing heme oxygenase-1 via the MAPK/Nrf2 pathways. *Journal of Hepatology.* 47(2):253-61

Yin, Z., Henry, E.C. & Gasiewicz, T.A. (2009). (-)-Epigallocatechin-3-gallate is a novel Hsp90 inhibitor. *Biochemistry.* 48(2):336-45.

Zaarur, N., Gabai, V.L., Porco, J.A. Jr., Calderwood, S. & Sherman, M.Y. (2006). Targeting Heat Shock Response to Sensitise Cancer Cells to Proteosome and Hsp90 Inhibitors. *Cancer Research.* 66(3): 1783-1791

Zagouri, F., Sergentanis, T.N., Nonni, A., Papadimitriou, C.A., Michalopoulos, N.V., Domeyer, P., Theodoropoulos, G., Lazaris, A., Patsouris, E., Zogafos, E., Pazaiti, A. & Zografos

G.C. (2010). Hsp90 in the continuum of breast ductal carcinogenesis: Evaluation in precursors, preinvasive and ductal carcinoma lesions. *BMC Cancer.* 10:353-341

Zanini, C., Giribaldi, G., Mandili, G., Carta, F., Crescenzio, N., ...Bisaro, B., Doria, A., Foglia, L., Di Montezemolo, C., Timeus, F. & Turrini, F. (2007). Inhibition of heat shock proteins (HSP) expression by quercetin and differential doxorubicin sensitization in neuroblastoma and Ewing's sarcoma cell lines. *Journal of Neurochemistry.* 103(4):1344-1354

Zhao, Z.G. & Shen, W.L. (2005). Heat shock protein 70 antisense oligonucleotide inhibits cell growth and induces apoptosis in human gastric cancer cell line SGC-7901. *World Journal of Gastroenterology.* 11(1):73-78

Zou, J.Y., Guo, Y.L., Guettouche, T., Smith, D.F., Voellmy, R. (1998). Repression of heat shock transcription factor HSF1 activation by HSP90 (HSP90 complex) that forms a stress-sensitive complex with HSF1. *Cell.* 94(4):471-480

# 8

# Emerging Therapies in Chronic Lymphocytic Leukemia

Reslan Lina and Dumontet Charles
*Université Lyon 1, Lyon,*
*France*

## 1. Introduction

The introduction of new therapies has opened new therapeutic hopes in the field of treating Chronic Lymphocytic Leukemia (CLL). CLL is extremely heterogeneous in its clinical course; some patients live for decades with no need for treatment, whereas others develop aggressive clinical course with a survival of less than 2-3 years. The decision to treat CLL patients should be guided by clinical staging, the presence of symptoms and disease activity (Diehl et al. 1999).

Once the diagnosis of CLL has been made, the treating physician is faced with the decision of not only how to treat the patient, but when to initiate therapy. In general practice, newly diagnosed patients with asymptomatic early-stage disease (Rai 0, Binet A) are monitored without therapy until they have evidence of disease progression. Studies from the French Cooperative Group on CLL, (Dighiero et al. 1998) the Cancer and Leukemia Group B,(Shustik et al. 1988) the Spanish Group PETHEMA, (Montserrat et al. 1996) and the Medical Research Council (Catovsky et al. 1988) confirm that the use of alkylating agents in patients with early-stage disease does not prolong survival (Group. 1999). Patients at intermediate (I and II) or high-risk (III and IV) according to the modified Rai classification or Binet stage B or C usually require the initiation of treatment at presentation. Some of these patients (in particular Rai intermediate risk or Binet stage B) can still be monitored without therapy until they exhibit evidence of progressive or symptomatic disease.

During the past decade there have been major advances in understanding the pathogenesis of the disease and more efficient treatments have been developed. CLL treatments have seen the transition from single-agent alkyator-based therapies to nucleoside analogs, combination chemotherapy, and recently to monoclonal antibodies (MAbs) and chemoimmunotherapy.

The use of immunotherapy is emerging as an exciting modality with significant potential to advance the treatment of B-cell malignancies. In the field of lymphoproliferative diseases rituximab, followed by the anti-CD52 antibody alemtuzumab, has changed the therapeutic landscape of B-cell cancers, particularly in patients with non-Hodgkin's lymphoma (NHL) with more recent indications in the setting of CLL (Cheson 2006).

Novel therapies are being evaluated both in pre-clinical studies and in clinical trials. These treatments include new MAbs such as ofatumumab, GA101, veltuzumab, epratuzumab, lumiliximab, TRU-016 as well as agents targeting the anti-apoptotic Bcl-2 family of proteins, antisense oligonucleotides and other agents. This review attempts to summarize the current knowledge of these treatments and point to potential opportunities in the future with other targeted therapies currently being explored.

## 2. Best compounds of alkylating agents and purine analogs used in CLL

Chlorambucil, an alkylating agent, has been considered the "gold standard" for several decades. Due to its low toxicity and its oral administration, this drug remains the appropriate option for non-fit, elderly patients as well as for younger fit patients. Chlorambucil achieved higher remission rates (Overall response rates (ORR) 89%, Complete responses (CR) 59%) when administered at a fixed dose of 15 mg daily up to achievement of a CR or occurrence of grade 3 toxicity, for a maximum of six months (Jaksic et al. 1997). However, chlorambucil is no longer considered an appropriate option for younger or physically fit patients because of its low to non-existent CR rate (Catovsky et al. 2007).

Besides chlorambucil, cyclophosphamide (C) is another alkylating agent with activity in CLL patients. It is generally utilized in combination regimen. (Hansen et al. 1988; Raphael et al. 1991).

Fludarabine is the best purine analog studied in CLL. When used as single agent, it achieves superior ORR and longer progression-free survival (PFS) rates compared with other treatment regimens containing alkylating agents or corticosteroids (Anaissie et al. 1998; Plunkett et al. 1993; Rai et al. 2000). In phase III studies in naive CLL patients, fludarabine induced more CRs (7–40%) as well as longer duration of remission than other chemotherapies or chlorambucil. However, overall survival (OS) was not improved by this drug when used as a single agent (Johnson et al. 1996; Leporrier et al. 2001; Rai et al. 2000; Steurer et al. 2006).

Bendamustine, a hybrid of an alkylating nitrogen mustard group and a purine-like benzimidazole, has been used for more than 30 years in Germany. Results of a recent randomized trial, comparing bendamustine to chlorambucil, showed that more patients achieved CRs with bendamustine than with chlorambucil (31% vs. 2%). Moreover, the median PFS was 21.6 months and 8.3 months for bendamustine and chlorambucil, respectively (Knauf et al. 2009).

## 3. Rituximab: The first anti-CD20 MAb

Rituximab has revolutionized the therapeutic approach for patients with a wide variety of B-cell malignancies, including CLL. Rituximab is a chimeric human-mouse MAb with a high affinity for the CD20 surface antigen, a transmembrane protein that is expressed on pre-B cells and normal differentiated B lymphocytes. The predominant mechanism of action of rituximab-induced cell death is proposed to be primarily the result of antibody-dependent cell-mediated cytotoxicity (ADCC), complement-dependent cytotoxicity (CDC) and direct cell death (Di Gaetano et al. 2003; Golay et al. 2000; Manches et al. 2003).

Rituximab was first approved in the United States for the treatment of relapsed or refractory, low grade or follicular, B-cell NHL (Grillo-Lopez et al. 1999) then approved in Europe, for the treatment of relapsed stage III/IV follicular NHL (Gopal & Press 1999;

McLaughlin et al. 1998). In CLL, rituximab is less active as single agent than in other lymphomas, unless very high doses or denser dosing regimen are used. The objective response rates observed in CLL patients are ranged between 25% and 35% (Huhn et al. 2001; Itala et al. 2002).

In contrast, the greatest benefit of rituximab is demonstrated when used in combination with chemotherapy. Multiple combinations are currently in use and others are in investigational phases. Here, we will present some of these combinations to highlight the synergistic effect of rituximab with other agents.

The combination of fludarabine with rituximab prolonged the PFS and OS of CLL patients compared to fludarabine alone (Byrd et al. 2005).

A phase II study performed by the German CLL Study Group (GCLLSG) of fludarabine and rituximab in both refractory and previously untreated patients resulted in an ORR of 87% with a subset achieving CR (Schulz et al. 2002).

CALGB 9712 evaluated fludarabine in combination with rituximab given either concurrently or sequentially. Patients in the concurrent arm experienced more severe hematologic and infusion-related toxicity, but the ORR was 90% with a CR of 47% compared with an ORR of 78% and CR of 28% in the sequential arm (Byrd et al. 2003).

Likewise, rituximab induced a high ORR and complete remission rates when combined either with fludarabine/cyclophosphamide in refractory/relapsed CLL patients (73% and 25%, respectively) (Wierda et al. 2005) or in those with previously untreated CLL (95% and 72%, respectively) (Tam et al. 2008). The superiority of fludarabine, cyclophosphamide plus rituximab (FCR) compared to fludarabine and cyclophosphamide, alone was also confirmed in randomized phase III trials (Hallek 2008; Robak 2008; Tam et al. 2008).

In the CLL8 protocol of the German CLL Study Group (GCLLSG), 817 treatment-naive, physically fit patients (aged 30-81 years) were randomly assigned to receive either fludarabine, cyclophosphamide, and rituximab (FCR group) or fludarabine and cyclophosphamide (FC group). At 3 years after randomization, 65% of patients in the FCR group were free of progression compared with 45% in the FC group (P < 0.0001); The three-year survival rates were 87% and 83% for FCR-treatment and FC-treatment (p=0.012), respectively. FCR treatment was more frequently associated with hematologic adverse events, particularly neutropenia; these results suggest that the choice of FCR as first-line treatment prolongs OS of CLL patients (Hallek et al., 2010).

Furthermore, when combined with pentostatin and cyclophosphamide in previously untreated CLL patients, rituximab achieved a significant clinical activity despite poor risk-based prognoses, including achievement of minimal residual disease in some patients (Kay et al. 2007; Keating et al. 2005; Tam et al. 2006).

The German CLL Study Group initiated two studies to explore the combination of bendamustine plus rituximab in patients with relapsed CLL (Fischer 2008) and in previously untreated CLL patients (Fischer 2009). Results showed an ORR of 77%, CR rate of 15% for relapsed patients and an OR of 91%, CR of 33% for untreated ones. A retrospective Italian study was conducted in 109 relapsed/refractory CLL patients. Results showed that the combination of rituxmab plus bendamustine was an effective and well-tolerated treatment for these patients, producing a remarkable high CR rate and mild toxicity (Iannitto et al. 2011).

Investigations of the mechanism underlying the anti-tumor activity of rituximab as a single agent and in combination with chemotherapy are ongoing. By understanding these mechanisms, it might be possible to further enhance current cell killing strategies or develop novel agents and strategies.

## 4. Newer anti-CD20 antibodies for CLL

### 4.1 Ofatumumab

Ofatumumab is a fully humanized MAb targeting a small-loop CD20 epitope distinct from that of rituximab (Teeling et al. 2004). Compared to rituximab, it demonstrates an increased target-binding affinity to CD20 and slower dissociation rates. It exhibits stronger complement-mediated toxicity and shows potent lysis of rituximab-resistant cells.

In phase I/II study in relapsed/refractory CLL patients, ofatumumab achieved an ORR of 44%; however, these were almost exclusively partial responses (Coiffier et al. 2008). In a phase I/II dose-escalation trial, the efficacy and safety of single-agent ofatumumab (300-1000 mg) have been evaluated in 40 patients with relapsed or refractory Follicular Lymphoma (FL). Rapid, efficient and sustained peripheral B-cell depletion was observed in all dose groups. The ORR in evaluable patients (n=36) was 43% (Hagenbeek et al. 2008).

This antibody was recently approved by the Food and Drug Administration (FDA) for fludarabine and alemtuzumab refractory CLL patients and for fludarabine refractory patients with bulky disease. Ofatumumab was administered in these two groups with an ORR of 58% and 47%, respectively (Wierda G 2009). It is currently being combined with other agents in CLL, including bendamustine.

A recently completed phase II trial of ofatumumab in combination with fludarabine and cyclophosphamide demonstrated CRs in up to 50% of patients with previously untreated CLL, despite poor prognostic factors (Wierda G 2009). The median PFS has not been reached with the short median follow-up of 8 months.

Moreover, a randomized phase II study was conducted using two dose schedules of ofatumumab (500 mg and 1000 mg) in combination with fludarabine 25 mg/m2 and cyclophosphamide 250 mg/m2. The CR rate was 32% for the 500-mg and 50% for the 1000-mg cohort; the ORR was 77% and 73%, respectively (Wierda et al. 2010).

### 4.2 GA101

GA101 is the first humanized type II anti-CD20 MAb with glycolengineered Fc portion and a modified elbow hinge (Bello & Sotomayor 2007). The adapted Fc region gives GA101 a 50-fold higher binding affinity to FCγRIII (CD16) compared to a non-glycoengineered antibody, resulting in 10- to 100-fold increase in ADCC against CD20+ NHL cell lines via the activation of effector cells (Umana 2006). Moreover, the modified elbow hinge area also results in strong induction of direct cell death of several NHL cell lines and primary malignant B cells *in vitro* (Alduaij W & S. 2009; Bello & Sotomayor 2007; Umana 2006). However, these modifications result in reduced CDC activity (Umana 2007). In vitro B-cell depletion assays with whole blood from healthy and leukemic patients showed that the combined activity of ADCC, CDC, and apoptosis for GA101 was significantly superior to rituximab (Alduaij W & S. 2009; Patz M 2009; Umana 2006; Zenzl 2009).

The enhanced efficacy of GA101 has been also shown *in vivo*. In xenograft models of Diffuse large B-cell lymphoma (DLBCL ) and mantle cell lymphoma, treatment with GA101 resulted in CR and long-term survival compared with tumor stasis achieved with rituximab (Umana 2006). In cynomolgus monkeys, GA101 (10 and 30 mg/kg infused on days 0 and 7) showed significantly superior depletion of B cells compared to rituximab (10 mg/kg) from day 9 to day 35 and was more efficacious at clearing B cells from lymph nodes and the spleen (Umana 2007).

Initial phase I study of patients with relapsed/refractory CD20+ disease (n=21), including CLL, DLBCL, and other NHLs, for whom no therapy of higher priority was available (95% of patients had previously received rituximab), GA101 demonstrated a favorable safety profile with no dose-limiting toxicities (Salles 2009). The depletion of B-cell was rapid and sustained in the majority of patients. Nine of the evaluable patients responded to therapy (ORR, 43%; five CR/unconfirmed CR and four partial responses), with responses observed at all dose levels and across all FcγRIIIA genotypes.

The pharmacokinetics of GA101 are generally similar to those of rituximab and dose-dependent. However, significant inter- and intra-patient variabilities have been observed, the clinical relevance of which will need further investigation [86]. Results from a phase I study in patients with previously treated B-CLL (n=13) who were given single-agent GA101 (400–2000 mg; nine infusions) showed similar safety and pharmacokinetic profiles to those observed in the previously described patients with NHL, except for an increased incidence of neutropenia (Morschhauser 2009).

GA101 is currently being explored as a single agent in phase II studies in relapsed/refractory B-CLL and indolent/aggressive NHL, and in combination with chemotherapy in a phase Ib study.

### 4.3 Veltuzumab (IMMU-106)

Veltuzumab is a humanized CD20 MAb (type I) constructed recombinantly on the framework regions of epratuzumab, with complementarity-determining regions (CDRs) identical to rituximab, except for a single amino acid in CDR3 of the variable heavy chain. It showed anti-proliferative, apoptotic, and ADCC effects *in vitro* similar to rituximab, but with significantly slower off-rates and increased CDC in several human lymphoma cell lines. In addition, at very low doses, given either intravenously or subcutaneously, veltuzumab showed a potent anti-B cell activity in cynomolgus monkeys and controlled tumor growth in mice bearing human lymphomas (Goldenberg et al. 2009).

In a phase I/II dose-escalating clinical trial in patients with recurrent NHL, the ORR for veltuzumab-treatment was 41% (33/81), including 17 patients (21%) with CR or unconfirmed CR (Morschhauser et al. 2009). Veltuzumab caused B-cell depletion after the first infusion even at the lowest dose of 80 mg/m², which persisted after the fourth infusion, and was well tolerated, with no evidence of immunogenicity.

Veltuzumab is additionally being developed for subcutaneous administration, which may provide advantages for this agent versus other MAbs (Goldenberg et al. 2010). Veltuzumab is undergoing clinical trials using a low-dose subcutaneous formulation in patients with NHL and CLL.

## 5. Other MAbs for CLL

### 5.1 Alemtuzumab

Alemtuzumab is a recombinant, fully humanized, MAb targeting the CD52 antigen. CD52 is expressed on virtually all lymphocytes at various stages of differentiation, as well as monocytes, macrophages and eosinophils, whereas hematopoeitic stem cells, erythrocytes and platelets do not express it (Hale et al. 1990). A high level of CD52 is found on T-prolymphocytic leukemia, followed by B-CLL, with the lowest levels expressed on normal B cells. The mechanisms of action of alemtuzumab include CDC, ADCC and induction of apoptosis (Mone et al. 2006).

The use of alemtuzumab monotherapy is approved in the United States in the first-line treatment of patients with CLL. In a pivotal phase II study in 93 patients with fludarabine-refractory disease, alemtuzumab yielded an ORR of 33% with a median OS of 16 months (Keating et al. 2005).

Alemtuzumab has been approved for the initial treatment of CLL based on randomized trial conducted including 297 patients who received either alemtuzumab or chlorambucil. The antibody induced an ORR rate of 83.2% with 24.2% CRs compared with 55.4% and 2%, for alemtuzumab and chlorambucil, respectively (Hillmen et al. 2007). In addition, alemtuzumab has proven efficacy even in patients with poor prognostic factors, including high-risk genetic markers such as deletions of chromosome 11 or 17 and p53 mutations (Lozanski et al. 2004; Stilgenbauer & Dohner 2002). The combination of alemtuzumab with fludarabine was investigated in a phase II trial with relapsed CLL patients. The ORR was 83% including 30% CR (Elter et al. 2005). The combination of both alemtuzumab with rituximab has been also studied in patients with lymphoid malignancies including patients with refractory/relapsed CLL, producing an ORR of 52% with 8% CR (Faderl et al. 2003).

The combination of fludarabine, cyclophosphamide plus alemtuzumab (FCA) was recently compared to fludarabine, cyclophosphamide plus rituximab (FCR) in a phase III study by "the french Cooperative Group On CLL and WM" (FCGCLL/MW) and "the Groupe Ouest-est d'Etudes des Leucemies Aigues et Autres Maladies du Sang" (GOELAMS). Response rates of the first 100 patients were reported in a preliminary analysis with safety data presented for the entire cohort of 178 patients. The ORR in the first 100 patients was 96% for FCR compared to 85% in the FCA arm (p=0.086) with a CR rate of 78% in the FCR arm versus 58% in the FCA arm (p=0.072). Increased toxicity of FCA compared with FCR was found, preventing the use of the FCA combination outside of clinical trials (Lepretre 2009).

### 5.2 Lumiliximab

Lumiliximab is an anti-CD23 macque-human chimeric MAb with a strong similarity to the human antibody. The CD23 antigen is a low-affinity IgE receptor that is found in high levels in CLL patients (Fournier et al. 1992). Lumiliximab inhibits the IgE secretion *in vitro*, binds complement and mediates ADCC by binding FcγRI and RII receptors.

A phase I pilot study reported a limited single-agent activity in patients with refractory/relapsed CLL (Byrd et al. 2007b). Based on preclinical evidences of synergistic improvement of survival when lumiliximab was combined with fludarabine or rituximab, a phase I/II trial evaluated the safety and efficacy of lumiliximab in combination with FCR in 31 patients of relapsed CLL patients (Byrd J 2008). This combination regimen yielded an ORR of 65%, which was comparable to the results seen with FCR in the pivotal phase II study conducted by the M.D. Anderson Cancer Center (Byrd J 2008; Wierda et al. 2005). Lumiliximab/FCR appeared to double the CR rate compared to FCR alone (52% vs. 25%) without increasing the rate of toxicities.

## 5.3 Epratuzumab

Epratuzumab is a humanized anti-CD22 MAb currently in clinical trials for treatment of NHL and autoimmune disorders (Leonard & Goldenberg 2007). Epratuzumab is selectively active against normal and neoplastic B-cells. This MAb acts as an immunomodulatory agent in contrast to rituximab which is an actually cytotoxic therapeutic antibody. *In vitro*, epratuzumab has demonstrated the ability to elicit ADCC and induce CD22 phosphorylation and signaling, both of which may contribute as potential mechanisms of action (Carnahan et al. 2007; Carnahan et al. 2003).

Phase I/II studies demonstrated objective responses across various dose levels in both relapsed/refractory FL (24%) (Leonard et al. 2003) and DLBCL (15%) (Leonard et al. 2004).

Epratuzumab has also been combined with rituximab in phase II studies showing at least an additive benefit while toxicities of the combination were comparable with those of single-agent rituximab (Leonard et al. 2005). In a recent international, multicenter trial evaluating rituximab plus epratuzumab in patients with post-chemotherapy relapsed/refractory, indolent NHL, an objective response was seen in 54% FL patients including 24% with CR/unconfirmed CR (CRu) whereas 57% of Small Lymphocytic Lymphoma patients had ORs including 43% with CR/Cru (Leonard et al. 2008). Rituximab-naive patients had an ORR of 50%, whereas patients who previously responded to rituximab had an ORR of 64%.

Thus, the combination of epratuzumab and rituximab induced durable responses in patients with recurrent, indolent NHL. Epratuzumab is also being evaluated in combination with rituximab plus cyclophosphamide, doxorubicin, vincristine, and prednisone (CHOP) and as a therapy in other B-cell neoplasms (Micallef et al. 2006).

## 5.4 TRU-016

TRU-016 is a CD37-directed small modular immunopharmaceutical protein composed of IgG1 variable regions (VL and VH) and a small, engineered constant region. CD37 is expressed at high concentrations on the surface of B cells and mature B-cell lymphomas and leukemias. *In vitro* studies demonstrated that the chimeric version of TRU-016 induced apoptosis and ADCC-dependent cytotoxicity in CLL cells (Zhao, Lapalombella et al. 2007).

Interim results of a phase I study of TRU-016 reported a favorable toxicity profile and partial responses at higher doses (Andritsos 2009).

## 6. Emerging drugs

### 6.1 Bcl-2 inhibitors

The expression of high levels of anti-apoptotic Bcl-2 protein is characteristic of CLL cells (Hanada et al. 1993). Many studies have suggested that an increased ratio of anti- to pro-apoptotic proteins such as Bcl-2/Bax is correlated with poor response to chemotherapy, disease progression and shorter survival (Pepper et al. 1997; Robertson et al. 1996).

Modulation of anti-apoptotic proteins is a promising strategy to sensitize cells to antileukemic agents. Preclinical data have shown that inhibition of Bcl-2, inhibition of the interaction between Bcl-2 or Bcl-xL and partner proteins with compounds such as ABT-737 (Mason et al. 2009) or inhibition of Mcl-1 were associated with increased sensitivity to antileukemic agents (Hallaert et al. 2007).

Numerous novel agents have shown *in vitro* promise in overcoming the pro-apoptotic defects in CLL cells. These do not, however, always translate into a therapeutic *in vivo* effect.

### 6.2 Oblimersen sodium (G3139)

Oblimersen sodium is a phosphorothioate antisense oligodeoxynucleotide composed of 18 nucleotides targeting the first six codons of the open reading frame of the bcl-2 mRNA. Preclinical evaluation has demonstrated good antineoplastic effect in B-cell cancers; several clinical trials have confirmed its safety and efficacy both alone and in combination with other therapeutics.

A phase I/II clinical trial was conducted in patients with relapsed or refractory CLL to determine the maximum tolerated dose (MTD), efficacy, safety, and pharmacokinetics of oblimersen sodium. A total of 40 patients (who had received at least one prior chemotherapy regimen containing a purine analogue) were treated (14 in Phase I and 26 in Phase II) with single-agent oblimersen sodium in doses ranging from 3 to 7 mg/kg/day in the phase I portion of the study. The MTD for the phase II part of the study was determined to be 3 mg/kg/day with higher doses of oblimersen sodium being associated with a cytokine release reaction characterized by fever, rigors and hypotension. This was attributed to the release of large amounts of cytokines. Thus, oblimersen sodium has shown a modest single-agent activity in heavily pretreated patients with advanced CLL (O'Brien et al. 2005).

A phase II trial was conducted to evaluate the safety and efficacy of the combination of fludarabine, rituximab and oblimersen in previously untreated or relapsed/previously treated CLL patients. Preliminary results have been encouraging especially in the setting of CLL with poor prognostic markers (Marvromatis 2006; Mavromatis 2005).

A randomized phase III trial of fludarabine and cyclophosphamide (FC) with or without oblimersen sodium in 241 patients with relapsed or refractory CLL who had received at least one prior fludarabine-containing regimen has been conducted. The rate of CR/nodular PR was significantly higher for patients treated with FC plus oblimersen, 17% versus 7%, respectively. The oblimersen treated group was associated with a significant survival benefit (O'Brien et al. 2007).

Overall, oblimersen has shown new hope and potential in the management of CLL, enhancing the efficacy of other commonly used agents. Further studies with oblimersen should have a special focus on correlating response and survival outcomes with Bcl-2 overexpression and subsequent decrease in Bcl-2 protein.

## 6.3 Navitoclax (ABT-263)

Navitoclax (ABT-263), a novel, orally bioavailable, small molecule, binds with high affinity to anti-apoptotic proteins Bcl-2, Bcl-xL, and Bcl-w, promoting apoptosis. *In vitro*, navitoclax shows potent targeted cytotoxicity against T and B lymphoid malignancies that over-express Bcl-2. A phase I trial demonstrated oral navitoclax monotherapy to be well-tolerated and to have anti-tumor activity in CLL patients.

Phase II study was conducted in patients with heavily pretreated CLL, the drug attained an objective response rate of 33% (currently confirmed in 19% of patients); 58% of patients with baseline nodal enlargement showed shrinkage of greater than 50%.

The combination of navitoclax with bendamustine/rituximab was effective for patients with relapsed or refractory CLL and presented encouraging results in a phase II trial. Moreover, phase III studies showed that the combination of navitoclax with fludarabine/cyclophosphamide/rituximab combination improved outcomes in CLL patients (Kipps 2010).

## 6.4 Obatoclax (GX15-070)

Obatoclax is a hydrophobic molecule, developed as a Bcl-2 family antagonist. This agent inhibits several anti-apoptotic Bcl-2 family proteins including Bcl-$x_L$, Bcl-2, Bcl-w, BCL-B, A-1 and Mcl-1. It induces the release of Bak from Mcl-1, the liberation of Bim from both Bcl-2 and Mcl-1 as well as the formation of an active Bak/Bax complex. Moreover, it can promote the release of cytochrome c from mitochondria leading to apoptosis (Konopleva et al. 2008).

A phase I trial of obatoclax was conducted in heavily pretreated patients with advanced CLL. Obatoclax was administered at doses ranging from 3.5 to 14 mg/m$^2$ as a 1-hour infusion and from 20 to 40 mg/m$^2$ as a 3-hour infusion every 3 weeks. Obatoclax demonstrated biologic as well as modest clinical activity in these patients with one (4%) of 26 patients achieving a partial response (O'Brien et al. 2009).

# 7. Newer treatment options

## 7.1 Lenalidomide

The immunomodulatory agent lenalidomide has shown activity in CLL in the relapsed/refractory as well as in the untreated setting.

Activity in CLL was first demonstrated by Chanan-Khan *et al.* in a phase II study. 25 mg of lenalidomide was administered in this trial daily on days 1 through 21 of a 28-day cycle in 45 pretreated CLL patients (Chanan-Khan et al. 2006). This regimen was associated with a 47% ORR and a 9% CR rate.

Ferrajoli *et al.* adopted this dose escalation scheme in 45 patients with relapsed CLL. The dosing started at 10 mg daily for 28 days, with dose escalation to a maximum of 25 mg/day as tolerated. The ORR was 32% with 7% of patients achieving a CR (Ferrajoli et al. 2008). Moreover, lenalidomide therapy was well tolerated and induced durable remissions in elderly patients with CLL (Badoux et al. 2011).

The combination of lenalidomide plus rituximab is currently being investigated in 60 patients with relapsed CLL patients. 37 patients are to date evaluable for response. The ORR was 68%, no CR was achieved. The results obtained suggest that the combination of rituximab and lenalidomide is superior to the single agent lenalidomide.

Currently, a study is recruiting participants to evaluate the combination of fludarabine plus rituximab with or without lenalidomide or cyclophosphamide in treating patients with symptomatic CLL.

### 7.2 Flavopiridol (Alvocidib)

Flavopiridol, a synthetic flavon, induces apoptosis in CLL cell lines by targeting cyclin-dependent kinases.

It shows high activity in CLL patients with relapsed high-risk CLL (Byrd et al. 2007a; Phelps et al. 2009). A phase II trial on relapsed CLL patients with genetically high risk features achieved an ORR of 53%, including one CR (Lin et al. 2009). Currently, a registration trial for flavopiridol in relapsed CLL is conducted in the United States and Europe.

## 8. Conclusion

A refreshing change is taking place in CLL research. There is an increasing interest to fully understand all subsets of CLL patients in order to develop novel and specific agents which cater to individualized needs of each subset. Currently available therapies are only partially efficient in CLL; thus, obvious clinical and scientific needs to develop new therapeutic options are under investigation to circumvent the limitations of currently used therapies in CLL.

Further studies should elucidate the role of these new agents and their combinations in the management of CLL.

## 9. References

Alduaij W, P.S., Ivanov A, Honeychurch J, Beers & S. 2009, 'New-generation anti-CD20 monoclonal antibody (GA101) evokes homotypic adhesion and actin-dependent, lysosome-mediated cell death in B-cell lymphom [abstract]', *ASH Annual Meeting Abstracts*, vol. 114:725.

Anaissie, E.J. et al. 1998, 'Infections in patients with chronic lymphocytic leukemia treated with fludarabine', *Ann Intern Med*, vol. 129, no. 7, pp. 559-66.

Andritsos, L., Furman, R., Flinn, I.W., Foreno-Torres, A. , Flynn, J. M., Stromatt, S. C., Byrd, J. C. 2009, 'A Phase 1 Trial of TRU-016, An Anti-CD37 Small Modular Immunopharmaceutical (SMIP™) Protein in Relapsed and Refractory CLL: Early Promising Clinical Activity [abstract 3017].', *J Clin Oncol.*, vol. 27.

Badoux, X.C. et al. 2011, 'Lenalidomide as initial therapy of elderly patients with chronic lymphocytic leukemia', *Blood*.

Bello, C. & Sotomayor, E.M. 2007, 'Monoclonal antibodies for B-cell lymphomas: rituximab and beyond', *Hematology Am Soc Hematol Educ Program*, pp. 233-42.

Byrd J, C.J., Flinn I, et al. 2008, ' Lumiliximab in combination with FCR for the treatment of relapsed chronic lymphocytic leukemia (CLL): results from a phase I/II multicenter study', *Ann Oncol* vol. 19(suppl 4):iv130 (Abstract 145).

Byrd, J.C. et al. 2007a, 'Flavopiridol administered using a pharmacologically derived schedule is associated with marked clinical efficacy in refractory, genetically high-risk chronic lymphocytic leukemia', *Blood*, vol. 109, no. 2, pp. 399-404.

Byrd, J.C. et al. 2007b, 'Phase 1 study of lumiliximab with detailed pharmacokinetic and pharmacodynamic measurements in patients with relapsed or refractory chronic lymphocytic leukemia', *Clin Cancer Res*, vol. 13, no. 15 Pt 1, pp. 4448-55.

Byrd, J.C. et al. 2003, 'Randomized phase 2 study of fludarabine with concurrent versus sequential treatment with rituximab in symptomatic, untreated patients with B-cell chronic lymphocytic leukemia: results from Cancer and Leukemia Group B 9712 (CALGB 9712)', *Blood*, vol. 101, no. 1, pp. 6-14.

Byrd, J.C. et al. 2005, 'Addition of rituximab to fludarabine may prolong progression-free survival and overall survival in patients with previously untreated chronic lymphocytic leukemia: an updated retrospective comparative analysis of CALGB 9712 and CALGB 9011', *Blood*, vol. 105, no. 1, pp. 49-53.

Carnahan, J. et al. 2007, 'Epratuzumab, a CD22-targeting recombinant humanized antibody with a different mode of action from rituximab', *Mol Immunol*, vol. 44, no. 6, pp. 1331-41.

Carnahan, J. et al. 2003, 'Epratuzumab, a humanized monoclonal antibody targeting CD22: characterization of in vitro properties', *Clin Cancer Res*, vol. 9, no. 10 Pt 2, pp. 3982S-90S.

Catovsky, D. et al. 1988, 'The UK Medical Research Council CLL trials 1 and 2', *Nouv Rev Fr Hematol*, vol. 30, no. 5-6, pp. 423-7.

Catovsky, D. et al. 2007, 'Assessment of fludarabine plus cyclophosphamide for patients with chronic lymphocytic leukaemia (the LRF CLL4 Trial): a randomised controlled trial', *Lancet*, vol. 370, no. 9583, pp. 230-9.

Chanan-Khan, A. et al. 2006, 'Clinical efficacy of lenalidomide in patients with relapsed or refractory chronic lymphocytic leukemia: results of a phase II study', *J Clin Oncol*, vol. 24, no. 34, pp. 5343-9.

Cheson, B.D. 2006, 'Monoclonal antibody therapy of chronic lymphocytic leukemia', *Cancer Immunol Immunother*, vol. 55, no. 2, pp. 188-96.

Coiffier, B. et al. 2008, 'Safety and efficacy of ofatumumab, a fully human monoclonal anti-CD20 antibody, in patients with relapsed or refractory B-cell chronic lymphocytic leukemia: a phase 1-2 study', *Blood*, vol. 111, no. 3, pp. 1094-100.

Di Gaetano, N. et al. 2003, 'Complement activation determines the therapeutic activity of rituximab in vivo', *J Immunol*, vol. 171, no. 3, pp. 1581-7.

Diehl, L.F. et al. 1999, 'The American College of Surgeons Commission on Cancer and the American Cancer Society. The National Cancer Data Base report on age, gender, treatment, and outcomes of patients with chronic lymphocytic leukemia', *Cancer*, vol. 86, no. 12, pp. 2684-92.

Dighiero, G. et al. 1998, 'Chlorambucil in indolent chronic lymphocytic leukemia. French Cooperative Group on Chronic Lymphocytic Leukemia', *N Engl J Med*, vol. 338, no. 21, pp. 1506-14.

Elter, T. et al. 2005, 'Fludarabine in combination with alemtuzumab is effective and feasible in patients with relapsed or refractory B-cell chronic lymphocytic leukemia: results of a phase II trial', *J Clin Oncol*, vol. 23, no. 28, pp. 7024-31.

Faderl, S. et al. 2003, 'Experience with alemtuzumab plus rituximab in patients with relapsed and refractory lymphoid malignancies', *Blood*, vol. 101, no. 9, pp. 3413-5.

Ferrajoli, A. et al. 2008, 'Lenalidomide induces complete and partial remissions in patients with relapsed and refractory chronic lymphocytic leukemia', *Blood*, vol. 111, no. 11, pp. 5291-7.

Fischer, K., Cramer, P., Stilgenbauer, S., Busch, R., Balleisen, L., Kilp, J., Fink, A-M., Boettcher, S., Ritgen, M., Kneba,M.,Staib, P., Döhner, H., Schulte, S., Eichhorst, B.F., Hallek, M., Wendtner, C-M., and the German CLL Study Group (GCLLSG) 2009, ' Bendamustine Combined with Rituximab (BR) in First-Line Therapy of Advanced CLL: A Multicenter Phase II Trial of the German CLL Study Group (GCLLSG)', *Blood*, vol. (ASH Annual Meeting Abstracts) 114: 205.

Fischer, K., Stilgenbauer, S., Schweighofer, C.D. , Busch, R., Renschler, J., Kiehl, M., Balleisen, L., Eckart, M.J., Fink, A-M., Kilp,J., Ritgen, M., Böttcher, S., Kneba, M., Döhner, H., Eichhorst, B.F., Hallek, M., Wendtner, C-M., and The German CLL Study Group 2008, 'Bendamustine in combination with rituximab (BR) for patients with relapsed chronic lymphocytic leukemia (CLL): A multicentre phase II trial of the German CLL Study Group (GCLLSG).', *Blood*, vol. 112, p. 128.

Fournier, S. et al. 1992, 'CD23 antigen regulation and signaling in chronic lymphocytic leukemia', *J Clin Invest*, vol. 89, no. 4, pp. 1312-21.

Golay, J. et al. 2000, 'Biologic response of B lymphoma cells to anti-CD20 monoclonal antibody rituximab in vitro: CD55 and CD59 regulate complement-mediated cell lysis', *Blood*, vol. 95, no. 12, pp. 3900-8.

Goldenberg, D.M. et al. 2010, 'Veltuzumab (humanized anti-CD20 monoclonal antibody): characterization, current clinical results, and future prospects', *Leuk Lymphoma*, vol. 51, no. 5, pp. 747-55.

Goldenberg, D.M. et al. 2009, 'Properties and structure-function relationships of veltuzumab (hA20), a humanized anti-CD20 monoclonal antibody', *Blood*, vol. 113, no. 5, pp. 1062-70.

Gopal, A.K. & Press, O.W. 1999, 'Clinical applications of anti-CD20 antibodies', *J Lab Clin Med*, vol. 134, no. 5, pp. 445-50.

Grillo-Lopez, A.J. et al. 1999, 'Overview of the clinical development of rituximab: first monoclonal antibody approved for the treatment of lymphoma', *Semin Oncol*, vol. 26, no. 5 Suppl 14, pp. 66-73.

Group., C.T.C. 1999, 'Chemotherapeutic options in chronic lymphocytic leukemia: a meta-analysis of the randomized trials', *J Natl Cancer Inst.*, vol. 91:861-868.

Hagenbeek, A. et al. 2008, 'First clinical use of ofatumumab, a novel fully human anti-CD20 monoclonal antibody in relapsed or refractory follicular lymphoma: results of a phase 1/2 trial', *Blood*, vol. 111, no. 12, pp. 5486-95.

Hale, G. et al. 1990, 'The CAMPATH-1 antigen (CDw52)', *Tissue Antigens*, vol. 35, no. 3, pp. 118-27.

Hallaert, D.Y. et al. 2007, 'Crosstalk among Bcl-2 family members in B-CLL: seliciclib acts via the Mcl-1/Noxa axis and gradual exhaustion of Bcl-2 protection', *Cell Death Differ*, vol. 14, no. 11, pp. 1958-67.

Hallek, M., Fingerle-Rowson, G., Fink, A.M., et al. 2008, ' Immunochemotherapy with fludarabine (F), cyclophosphamide (C), and rituximab (R) (FCR) versus fludarabine and cyclophosphamide (FC) improves response rates and progression-free survival (PFS) of previously untreated patients (pts) with advanced chronic lymphocytic leukemia (CLL) [abstract]', *Blood*, vol. 112(11):125 Abstract 325.

Hallek, M. et al., 'Addition of rituximab to fludarabine and cyclophosphamide in patients with chronic lymphocytic leukaemia: a randomised, open-label, phase 3 trial', *Lancet*, vol. 376, no. 9747, pp. 1164-74.

Hanada, M. et al. 1993, 'bcl-2 gene hypomethylation and high-level expression in B-cell chronic lymphocytic leukemia', *Blood*, vol. 82, no. 6, pp. 1820-8.

Hansen, M.M. et al. 1988, 'CHOP versus prednisolone + chlorambucil in chronic lymphocytic leukemia (CLL): preliminary results of a randomized multicenter study', *Nouv Rev Fr Hematol*, vol. 30, no. 5-6, pp. 433-6.

Hillmen, P. et al. 2007, 'Alemtuzumab compared with chlorambucil as first-line therapy for chronic lymphocytic leukemia', *J Clin Oncol*, vol. 25, no. 35, pp. 5616-23.

Huhn, D. et al. 2001, 'Rituximab therapy of patients with B-cell chronic lymphocytic leukemia', *Blood*, vol. 98, no. 5, pp. 1326-31.

Iannitto, E. et al. 2011, 'Bendamustine with or without rituximab in the treatment of relapsed chronic lymphocytic leukaemia: an Italian retrospective study', *Br J Haematol*, vol. 153, no. 3, pp. 351-7.

Itala, M. et al. 2002, 'Standard-dose anti-CD20 antibody rituximab has efficacy in chronic lymphocytic leukaemia: results from a Nordic multicentre study', *Eur J Haematol*, vol. 69, no. 3, pp. 129-34.

Jaksic, B. et al. 1997, 'High dose chlorambucil versus Binet's modified cyclophosphamide, doxorubicin, vincristine, and prednisone regimen in the treatment of patients with advanced B-cell chronic lymphocytic leukemia. Results of an international multicenter randomized trial. International Society for Chemo-Immunotherapy, Vienna', *Cancer*, vol. 79, no. 11, pp. 2107-14.

Johnson, S. et al. 1996, 'Multicentre prospective randomised trial of fludarabine versus cyclophosphamide, doxorubicin, and prednisone (CAP) for treatment of advanced-stage chronic lymphocytic leukaemia. The French Cooperative Group on CLL', *Lancet*, vol. 347, no. 9013, pp. 1432-8.

Kay, N.E. et al. 2007, 'Combination chemoimmunotherapy with pentostatin, cyclophosphamide, and rituximab shows significant clinical activity with low accompanying toxicity in previously untreated B chronic lymphocytic leukemia', *Blood*, vol. 109, no. 2, pp. 405-11.

Keating, M.J. et al. 2005, 'Early results of a chemoimmunotherapy regimen of fludarabine, cyclophosphamide, and rituximab as initial therapy for chronic lymphocytic leukemia', *J Clin Oncol*, vol. 23, no. 18, pp. 4079-88.

Kipps, T.J., Wierda, W.G., Jones, J.A., Swinnen, L.J., Yang, J., Cui, Y., Busman, T., Krivoshik, A., Enschede, S., and Humerickhouse, R. 2010, 'Navitoclax (ABT-263) Plus Fludarabine/Cyclophosphamide/Rituximab (FCR) or Bendamustine/Rituximab (BR): A Phase 1 Study In Patients with Relapsed/Refractory Chronic Lymphocytic Leukemia (CLL) ', vol. ASH Annual Meeting Abstracts 2010; Abstract 2455.

Knauf, W.U. et al. 2009, 'Phase III randomized study of bendamustine compared with chlorambucil in previously untreated patients with chronic lymphocytic leukemia', *J Clin Oncol*, vol. 27, no. 26, pp. 4378-84.

Konopleva, M. et al. 2008, 'Mechanisms of antileukemic activity of the novel Bcl-2 homology domain-3 mimetic GX15-070 (obatoclax)', *Cancer Res*, vol. 68, no. 9, pp. 3413-20.

Leonard, J.P. et al. 2005, 'Combination antibody therapy with epratuzumab and rituximab in relapsed or refractory non-Hodgkin's lymphoma', *J Clin Oncol*, vol. 23, no. 22, pp. 5044-51.

Leonard, J.P. et al. 2003, 'Phase I/II trial of epratuzumab (humanized anti-CD22 antibody) in indolent non-Hodgkin's lymphoma', *J Clin Oncol*, vol. 21, no. 16, pp. 3051-9.

Leonard, J.P. et al. 2004, 'Epratuzumab, a humanized anti-CD22 antibody, in aggressive non-Hodgkin's lymphoma: phase I/II clinical trial results', *Clin Cancer Res*, vol. 10, no. 16, pp. 5327-34.

Leonard, J.P. & Goldenberg, D.M. 2007, 'Preclinical and clinical evaluation of epratuzumab (anti-CD22 IgG) in B-cell malignancies', *Oncogene*, vol. 26, no. 25, pp. 3704-13.

Leonard, J.P. et al. 2008, 'Durable complete responses from therapy with combined epratuzumab and rituximab: final results from an international multicenter, phase 2 study in recurrent, indolent, non-Hodgkin lymphoma', *Cancer*, vol. 113, no. 10, pp. 2714-23.

Leporrier, M. et al. 2001, 'Randomized comparison of fludarabine, CAP, and ChOP in 938 previously untreated stage B and C chronic lymphocytic leukemia patients', *Blood*, vol. 98, no. 8, pp. 2319-25.

Lepretre, S., Aurran, T., Mahe, B., et al. 2009, ' Immunochemotherapy with Fludarabine (F), Cyclophosphamide (C), and Rituximab (R) (FCR) Versus Fludarabine (F), Cyclophosphamide (C) and MabCampath (Cam) (FCCam) in Previously Untreated Patients (pts) with Advanced B-Chronic Lymphocytic Leukemia (BCLL): Experience On Safety and Efficacy within a Randomised Multicenter Phase III Trial of the french Cooperative Group On CLL and WM (FCGCLL/MW) and the "Groupe Ouest-Est d'Etudes Des Leucemies Aigues Et Autres Maladies Du sang" (GOELAMS) : CLL2007FMP (for fit medically patients).', *ASH Annual Meeting Abstracts. 2009;114(22):538-.*

Lin, T.S. et al. 2009, 'Phase II study of flavopiridol in relapsed chronic lymphocytic leukemia demonstrating high response rates in genetically high-risk disease', *J Clin Oncol*, vol. 27, no. 35, pp. 6012-8.

Lozanski, G. et al. 2004, 'Alemtuzumab is an effective therapy for chronic lymphocytic leukemia with p53 mutations and deletions', *Blood*, vol. 103, no. 9, pp. 3278-81.

Manches, O. et al. 2003, 'In vitro mechanisms of action of rituximab on primary non-Hodgkin lymphomas', *Blood*, vol. 101, no. 3, pp. 949-54.

Marvromatis, B., Rai, K., Wallace, P.K., et al. 2006, 'Impact of prognostic markers on outcomes in patients with advanced chronic lymphocytic leukemia treated with the regimen of fludarabine/rituximab plus oblimersen (Bcl-2 Antisense) ', *[abstract 6609] ASCO Annual Meeting Proceedings; 2006. p.24.*

Mason, K.D. et al. 2009, 'The BH3 mimetic compound, ABT-737, synergizes with a range of cytotoxic chemotherapy agents in chronic lymphocytic leukemia', *Leukemia*, vol. 23, no. 11, pp. 2034-41.

Mavromatis, B., Rai, K.R., Wallace, P.K., et al. 2005, 'Efficacy and Safety of the Combination of Genasense™ (Oblimersen Sodium, Bcl-2 Antisense Oligonucleotide), Fludarabine and Rituximab in Previously Treated and Untreated Subjects with Chronic Lymphocytic Leukemia', *ASH Annual Meeting Abstracts 2005;106:2129.*

McLaughlin, P. et al. 1998, 'Rituximab chimeric anti-CD20 monoclonal antibody therapy for relapsed indolent lymphoma: half of patients respond to a four-dose treatment program', *J Clin Oncol*, vol. 16, no. 8, pp. 2825-33.

Micallef, I.N. et al. 2006, 'A pilot study of epratuzumab and rituximab in combination with cyclophosphamide, doxorubicin, vincristine, and prednisone chemotherapy in patients with previously untreated, diffuse large B-cell lymphoma', *Cancer*, vol. 107, no. 12, pp. 2826-32.

Mone, A.P. et al. 2006, 'Alemtuzumab induces caspase-independent cell death in human chronic lymphocytic leukemia cells through a lipid raft-dependent mechanism', *Leukemia*, vol. 20, no. 2, pp. 272-9.

Montserrat, E. et al. 1996, 'Fludarabine in resistant or relapsing B-cell chronic lymphocytic leukemia: the Spanish Group experience', *Leuk Lymphoma*, vol. 21, no. 5-6, pp. 467-72.

Morschhauser, F., Cartron, G., Lamy, T., et al. 2009, 'Phase I study of RO5072759 (GA101) in relapsed/refractory chronic lymphocytic leukemia [abstract]. ASH Annual Meeting Abstracts. 2009;114:884.'.

Morschhauser, F. et al. 2009, 'Humanized anti-CD20 antibody, veltuzumab, in refractory/recurrent non-Hodgkin's lymphoma: phase I/II results', *J Clin Oncol*, vol. 27, no. 20, pp. 3346-53.

O'Brien, S. et al. 2007, 'Randomized phase III trial of fludarabine plus cyclophosphamide with or without oblimersen sodium (Bcl-2 antisense) in patients with relapsed or refractory chronic lymphocytic leukemia', *J Clin Oncol*, vol. 25, no. 9, pp. 1114-20.

O'Brien, S.M. et al. 2009, 'Phase I study of obatoclax mesylate (GX15-070), a small molecule pan-Bcl-2 family antagonist, in patients with advanced chronic lymphocytic leukemia', *Blood*, vol. 113, no. 2, pp. 299-305.

O'Brien, S.M. et al. 2005, 'Phase I to II multicenter study of oblimersen sodium, a Bcl-2 antisense oligonucleotide, in patients with advanced chronic lymphocytic leukemia', *J Clin Oncol*, vol. 23, no. 30, pp. 7697-702.

Patz M, F.N., Muller B, et al. 2009, 'Depletion of chronic lymphocytic leukemia cells from whole blood. Samples mediated by the anti-CD20 antibodies rituximab and GA101 [abstract]', vol. ASH Annual Meeting Abstracts 114, p. 2365.

Pepper, C. et al. 1997, 'Bcl-2/Bax ratios in chronic lymphocytic leukaemia and their correlation with in vitro apoptosis and clinical resistance', *Br J Cancer*, vol. 76, no. 7, pp. 935-8.

Phelps, M.A. et al. 2009, 'Clinical response and pharmacokinetics from a phase 1 study of an active dosing schedule of flavopiridol in relapsed chronic lymphocytic leukemia', *Blood*, vol. 113, no. 12, pp. 2637-45.

Plunkett, W. et al. 1993, 'Fludarabine: pharmacokinetics, mechanisms of action, and rationales for combination therapies', *Semin Oncol*, vol. 20, no. 5 Suppl 7, pp. 2-12.

Rai, K.R. et al. 2000, 'Fludarabine compared with chlorambucil as primary therapy for chronic lymphocytic leukemia', *N Engl J Med*, vol. 343, no. 24, pp. 1750-7.

Raphael, B. et al. 1991, 'Comparison of chlorambucil and prednisone versus cyclophosphamide, vincristine, and prednisone as initial treatment for chronic lymphocytic leukemia: long-term follow-up of an Eastern Cooperative Oncology Group randomized clinical trial', *J Clin Oncol*, vol. 9, no. 5, pp. 770-6.

Robak, T., Moiseev, S., Dmoszynska, A., et al. 2008, 'Rituximab, fludarabine, and cyclophosphamide (R-FC) prolongs progression free survival in relapsed or refractory chronic lymphocytic leukemia (CLL) compared with FC alone: final results from the international randomized phase III REACH trial', *Blood*, vol. 112(11):LBA-1 Abstract 157420.

Robertson, L.E. et al. 1996, 'Bcl-2 expression in chronic lymphocytic leukemia and its correlation with the induction of apoptosis and clinical outcome', *Leukemia*, vol. 10, no. 3, pp. 456-9.

Salles, G., Morschhauser, F., Lamy, T., et al. 2009, 'Phase I study of RO5072759 (GA101) in patients with relapsed/refractory CD20 non-Hodgkin lymphoma (NHL) [abstract] ASH Annual Meeting Abstracts. 2009;114:1704.'.

Schulz, H. et al. 2002, 'Phase 2 study of a combined immunochemotherapy using rituximab and fludarabine in patients with chronic lymphocytic leukemia', *Blood*, vol. 100, no. 9, pp. 3115-20.

Shustik, C. et al. 1988, 'Treatment of early chronic lymphocytic leukemia: intermittent chlorambucil versus observation', *Hematol Oncol*, vol. 6, no. 1, pp. 7-12.

Steurer, M. et al. 2006, 'Single-agent purine analogues for the treatment of chronic lymphocytic leukaemia: a systematic review and meta-analysis', *Cancer Treat Rev*, vol. 32, no. 5, pp. 377-89.

Stilgenbauer, S. & Dohner, H. 2002, 'Campath-1H-induced complete remission of chronic lymphocytic leukemia despite p53 gene mutation and resistance to chemotherapy', *N Engl J Med*, vol. 347, no. 6, pp. 452-3.

Tam, C.S. et al. 2008, 'Long-term results of the fludarabine, cyclophosphamide, and rituximab regimen as initial therapy of chronic lymphocytic leukemia', *Blood*, vol. 112, no. 4, pp. 975-80.

Tam, C.S. et al. 2006, 'Fludarabine, cyclophosphamide, and rituximab for the treatment of patients with chronic lymphocytic leukemia or indolent non-Hodgkin lymphoma', *Cancer*, vol. 106, no. 11, pp. 2412-20.

Teeling, J.L. et al. 2004, 'Characterization of new human CD20 monoclonal antibodies with potent cytolytic activity against non-Hodgkin lymphomas', *Blood*, vol. 104, no. 6, pp. 1793-800.

Umana, P., Moessner, E., Bruenker, P., et al. 2007, ' GA101, a novel humanized type II CD20 antibody with glycoengineered Fc and anhanced cell death induction, exhibits superior anti-tumor efficacy and superior tissue B cell depletion in vivo. Blood 2007;110: 694a (Abstract 2348). '.

Umana, P., Moessner, E., Bruenker, P., Unsin, G., Puentener, U., Suter, T., et al. 2006, 'Novel third-generation humanized Type II CD20 antibody with glycoengineered Fc and modified elbow hinge for enhanced ADCC and superior apoptosis induction', *Blood*, vol. 108 ; (abstract #229).

Wierda G, K.T., Mayer J, et al. 2009, 'High activity of single-agent ofatumumab, a novel CD20 monoclonal antibody in fludarabine- and alemtuzumab-refractory or bulky fludarabine - refractory chronic lymphocytic leukemia, regardless of prior rituximab exposure [abstract].EHA Annual Meeting 2009;0919.'.

Wierda, W. et al. 2005, 'Chemoimmunotherapy with fludarabine, cyclophosphamide, and rituximab for relapsed and refractory chronic lymphocytic leukemia', *J Clin Oncol*, vol. 23, no. 18, pp. 4070-8.

Wierda, W.G. et al. 2010, 'Chemoimmunotherapy with O-FC in previously untreated patients with chronic lymphocytic leukemia', *Blood*, vol. 117, no. 24, pp. 6450-8.

Zenzl, T., Volden, M., Mast, T., et al. 2009, 'In vitro activity of the type II anti-CD20 antibody GA101 in refractory, genetic high-risk CLL [abstract]', vol. ASH Annual Meeting Abstracts 2009;114:2379.

# 9

# Present and Future Application of Nanoparticle Based Therapies in B-Chronic Lymphocytic Leukemia (B-CLL)

Eduardo Mansilla[1,2], Gustavo H. Marin[2], Luis Núñez[3],
Gustavo Larsen[4], Nelly Mezzaroba[5] and Paolo Macor[5]
[1]*National University of La Rioja, UNLAR, La Rioja,*
[2]*CUCAIBA, Ministry of Health, La Plata, Buenos Aires*
[3]*University of Chicago, Chicago, Illinois, USA and Bio-Target, Chicago, Illinois,*
[4]*LNK Chemsolutions, Lincoln Nebraska, USA and Bio-Target, Chicago,*
[5]*Department of Life Science, University of Trieste,*
[1,2]*Argentina*
[3,4]*USA*
[5]*Italy*

## 1. Introduction

We describe a variety of polymer biodegradable nanoparticles (BNPs) that can be created in an attempt to find an effective and durable treatment for B-Chronic Lymphocytic Leukemia (B-CLL). Many different drugs including those like Chlorambucil (CLB) that has been the gold standard B-CLL´s chemotherapeutic treatment preference for years (1), or even those not traditionally considered or used as antineoplastic agents like Hydroxychloroquine (HCQ) (2), can safely be encapsulated inside nanoparticles and specifically be targeted to the selected tumor cells by the coating of monoclonal antibodies in their surface (3,4). In this way all these drugs could be released in a steady manner exclusively into the desired neoplastic cells. This would give several advantages in relation to traditional drug delivery methods as a significant less toxicity is produced in non cancer cells while very high concentrations of the therapeutic compounds with great apoptotic effect are reached only at the targeted selected B-CLL cells level.

Therapeutic systems of this kind are relatively easy to produce in the large scale, are probably very safe, and will elicit a negligible immune response (3). BNPs like the ones we have developed, will offer a great promise as non-viral biocompatible and biodegradable vectors and carriers of drugs, peptides or other substances, with targeting capacities to specific cell sites by surface receptors of monoclonal antibodies (mAbs). Our data indicate that these nanoparticles with surface mAbs are suitable as a selective drug delivery method to treat B-CLL, other lymphomas and probably autoimmune disease such as Rheumathoid Arthritis and Lupus Erythematosus between many others. When loaded with the lysosomotropic agent HCQ alone, or combined with CLB, they elicited a strong apoptotic effect (3) (4). Additional data revealed that these BNPs were non-toxic for healthy animals, and had prolonged an outstanding survival in mice models of human lymphoma and B-CLL. There is a real need to comprehend and define all the basic processes needed in order to commercially produce viable products of this kind. This includes the present knowledge that has been acquired in the development and use of nanoparticles for the cure of B-CLL as well as all the possibilities that have been opened by their introduction, such as regulatory/safety, environmental, health and societal implications of these new treatments (5).

## 2. B-CLL and the need for new therapeutic approaches: An opportunity for nanoparticle systems

B-CLL is the most common form of leukemia in the western world. It results from a relentless accumulation of small mature monoclonal lymphocytes. Following a recent demonstration of a significant increase in the proliferative pool of CLL cells in vivo, the gradual accumulation of malignant B-CLL cells seems to be primarily the consequence of their selective survival advantages relative to their normal B-cell counterparts (6). As the disease is mainly caused by defective apoptosis it is thus a good candidate for treatment by pro-apoptotic agents. Even though a large amount of research has been done during the last past years, the prognosis has not changed (7). A major problem with treating patients with cancer and B-CLL by traditional chemotherapeutic regimes is that their tumors often develop a multidrug resistant (MDR) phenotype and subsequently become insensitive to a range of different chemotoxic drugs. One cause of MDR is overexpression of the drug-effluxing protein, P-glycoprotein. It is now apparent that P-glycoprotein may also possess a more generic antiapoptotic function that protects P-glycoprotein–expressing cancer cells and normal cells from death (8). B-CLL cells with unfavorable cytogenetic alterations such as deletion of chromosome 17p with loss of p53 are often resistant to fludarabine and cyclophosphamide (9,10). Similarly, CLL cells from patients with advanced disease stages or having a history of prior chemotherapy, exhibit elevated oxidative stress (11) and thus may have a greater potential to acquire additional mutations and genetic abnormalities, leading to drug resistance and disease progression.

## 3. The history of the first biodegradable nanoparticle system for the treatment of B-CLL and lymphomas that could also work for autoimmune disease

By the end of 2007 Dr. Luis Núñez, a biochemist that founded with Dr. Gustavo Larsen, Bio-Target, a Chicago, USA, start-up nanotechnology company, with a new interesting intellectual property in the production of biodegradable nanoparticles that could be loaded with many drugs and coated with monoclonal antibodies, contacted Dr. Eduardo Mansilla in La Plata, Argentina, and agreed to develop together ideas and products in this direction. By that time Dr. Mansilla was very involved in B-CLL research, and for many years looked for a system that could deliver HCQ in enough concentrations inside tumor B-CLL cells. In this situation the technology offered by Bio-Target seemed to him the wright one to use. In less than six months the research group in Argentina of which Dr. Gustavo H. Marin was also intensively participating, had the particles ready and the in vitro testing done with superior results, having the anti-CD20 antibody Rituximab coated in the surface of the BNPs. The nanoparticles were specifically attaching to the B-CLL cells and as they were penetrating them, an outstanding apoptotic process was seen with more than 95% killing effect in less than 48 hrs. In this way, we produced and tested in vitro in an amazing fast time the first biodegradable nanoparticle system in the history of medicine with a non-traditional antineoplastic old drug such as HCQ and a monoclonal antibody approved by the FDA, Rituximab, for the treatment of B-cell malignancies, with very good efficacy. We did some further testing with particles coated with the anti-CD19 mAb and its combination with the anti-CD20, as well as mixtures of HCQ and CLB. Then, we offered our technology to the Italian group, from Trieste, conducted by Dr. Paolo Macor in order to do more in vitro testing and a large animal study in a mouse model of Burkkit´s lymphoma. The results were reproduced in the same manner with similar results in vitro. The animal study was a great surprise, as almost all animals treated with the nanoparticle system were alive after more than 120 days, while the control group was all dead by that time. After that, we started conversations with United States and European research groups to introduce this technology into further more animal studies not only for B-CLL and Lymphoma but also for autoimmune disease, specially SLE and Reumathoid Arthritis, as well as a human clinical trial for B-CLL patients. At this time, it is clear that the developmental steps of this new technology was successful and done in just a few months, later on, the industrialization and approval by regulatory agencies, as well as the commercialization and final benefit of the patients is taking an unacceptable but predictable long time and delay. These new therapeutic strategies are really urgently needed, especially because they could easily switch on new apoptotic responses and restore sensitivity to drugs in B-CLL cells. In this way, nanoparticle-based "smart" therapeutics will generate both evolutionary as well as revolutionary products in the near future for B-CLL. There is enough evidence now, in order to think that these systems will profoundly impact the next generation of treatments for this disease and probably others. If this is to happen, there will be a few key biological requirements for such technologies to be introduced and routinely used by the onco- hematology community. All these aspects, specially related to their design, delivery capacity and their tremendous selectivity in their targeting to specific B-CLL cell sites, is urgently needed to be addressed.

## 4. Old drugs re-discovered to be used inside BNPs for B-CLL

CLB, which belongs to a family of drugs known as alkylating agents, has been in use for decades to treat hematological malignancies including B-CLL (12). This drug is given orally, which is normally an advantage but in this case, causes problems because the rate at which the drug is absorbed into the bloodstream can vary tremendously from patient to patient (13). Drug developers have tried a variety of techniques to offer new forms of delivery of this interesting old drug, but each of these methods has proven less than optimal (14). Now, however, we have created these BNPs that appear to could solve these issues and hold the promise of improving the utility of CLB not only in B-CLL but in many other cancer therapies. This could also be true for many other old onco-hematologic chemo-therapeutic agents with a fairly interesting efficacy and safety profile that could be re-discovered for their use in B-CLL and other leukemias and lymphomas by delivering them in nanoparticles. This could be the case of doxorubicin or tamoxifene (15,16), or even bendamustine. This last drug has been used for more than 30 years in the treatment of lymphoma, but little is known about the optimal dosing schedule in relapsed or refractory B-cell chronic lymphocytic leukemia (CLL). Various dose and treatment schedules have been used empirically, and several studies have shown impressive efficacy specially in heavily pre-treated and treatment-refractory patients (17,18).

## 5. Non-classical drugs for the treatment of B-CLL: HCQ, magnolol, honokiol, parthenolide, phenylethyl-isothio-cyanate (PEITC) and others delivered in BNPs

Many compounds non-traditionally used as anti-neoplastic agents have been shown to put cancer cells into pro-apoptotic programs and could be very useful for B-CLL treatment. A great diversity of still undefined compounds with anti-cancer properties can be obtained from botanical species. The pharmaceutical industry has been substantially but slowly scaling-up research efforts and partnering up with research universities for finding natural herbal and natural alternatives to fight cancer instead of the conventional expensive and tedious large scale process of screening thousands of synthetic compounds to find a final cure or solution to cancer. Scientists have given proof of the valuable anti-inflammatory, antioxidant, and cholesterol-lowering benefits of resveratrol, curcumin, and green polyphenols, natural compounds between many other that are found in red wine, curry, and green tea extracts respectively (17,18). Some of these natural products could be effective in B-CLL by activating different cell death pathways. The active principles of a group of very well known herbs like tanacetum parthenium, magnolia grandiflora, cruciferous vegetables, turmeric, and many others, have been previously described as components of different Japanese, Latin American or Chinese traditional medicine having recognized anti-angiogenic and/or anti-tumor properties (19). Many of the difficulties found in human application of these drugs have been related mainly to bioavailibility and toxicological issues. In this way and considering that these drugs are usually very cheap and can be obtained from botanical species in unlimited amounts it is very interesting to speculate in its use in B-CLL by its administration inside nanoparticles. It is an interesting issue that many of these herbs contain parthenolide (PTL) as one of their major active components (20). This last substance is a sesquiterpene lactone, a novel natural NF-kappa B inhibitor with antineoplastic properties (21). In general, parthenolide is well tolerated by humans, making it a good candidate for further clinical testing as an anti B-CLL agent. Obtained mainly from Tanacetum parthenium , Magnolia grandiflora and other plants, it has recently demonstrated an interesting anti-tumoral activity against CLL, some solid tumors and acute myeloid leukemia (21,22), but it was only tried in B-CLL in a study done by our group (23). We showed for the first time that PTL has a potent apoptotic effect on B-CLL cells without a great impact on normal PBMC (24). PTL displayed potent cytotoxic and apoptotic effects on B-CLL cells in vitro. B-CLL cells treated with PTL resulted in a dose and time dependent cytotoxicity. PTL mediated cytotoxicity occurred at a concentration of 1 µ M and above. A significant decrease in the cell viability of B-CLL cells obtained from 5 patients was seen after one day of culture (38.1± 6.37%) and at 72 h (90± 5.19%) with a PTL concentration of 8 µ M. (Fig. 1). All these responses were dose and time dependent for PTL values from 1 to 10 uM. By contrast, this compound had little apoptotic or cytotoxic effect in PBMCs of healthy donors even at higher concentrations. These results provided clues for interesting pathways involving different aspects of B-CLL cell apoptosis that could be exploited in therapies with this product. It could be speculated that parthenolide increased the amount of the NF-kappa B inhibitory protein, I kappa B-alpha, and decreased NF-kappa B DNA binding activity. All this evidence suggests that parthenolide may provide an anti-B-CLL effect and could be a potentially effective repertoire for chronic lymphocytic leukemia treatment specially if given in combination with other drugs in nanoparticle systems. Even though all our patients were Rai II and CD38-, compromising mainly a potentially less aggressive category of disease, the results obtained in this work were more than satisfactory and probably could also be transfered to patients with a poor prognosis. As this compound had little cytotoxic in vitro impact on normal human PBMCs, side effects in the clinical setting could probably be minimized, especially if given inside a nanoparticle system, and this of course, will be a very important aspect to be considered in a chronic disease like B-CLL. It is also possible that a formulation combining parthenolide with some other natural molecules like honokiol or magnolol, obtained indeed from the Magnoliaceae family of plants, or the classical treatments, might have a synergistically beneficial effect in B-CLL, being a potential promising strategy for the treatment of this hematological malignancy.

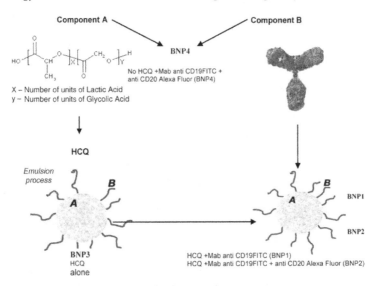

Fig. 1. Targeted biodegradable nanoparticle desing scheme.

Magnolia Grandiflora mainly contains Honokiol, Magnolol and Parthenolide (23) Honokiol and Magnolol are the major active constituents extracted from the bark of different Magnoliaceae species like Magnolia officinalis and Magnolia Grandiflora. They have a variety of pharmacological effects, such as anti-inflammatory, (21) antithrombotic, (25) anti-arrhythmic, (26)antioxidant (27)and anxiolytic effects, (28)and more recently, cytotoxic activity by inducing cell apoptosis in some cell lines (29). Magnolol and Honokiol-triggered apoptotic process is accompanied with down-modulation of Bcl-XL molecules (30) or through Caspase cascades activation (31) We have also shown that an aqueous Magnolia extract displayed a strong apoptotic effect on untreated as well as in heavily CLB treated B-CLL cells in vitro. We have published that Magnolia's extracts have efficacy in apoptosis and cytotoxicity induction and that these properties are exhibited mainly in tumors and not in normal cells, suggesting that an increase in NF-kappa B inhibitory protein and a decrease in NF-kappa B DNA binding activity or EGFR/PI3K/Akt signaling pathway or inhibition of telomerase activity might be involved in apoptosis induction (32). Phenylethyl-isothio-cyanate (PEITC) is abundant in cruciferous vegetables, has potent preventing antineoplastic properties as well as pro-apoptotic activities against a large variety of cancers, it is also a ROS-generating agent capable to kill B-CLL cells in vitro and probably in vivo.

## 6. Hydroxychloroquine for CLL

Concerning HCQ, it could be say that it is an anti malarial and a Disease-Modifying Antirheumatic Drug (DMARD), very active against rheumatoid arthritis and lupus erythematosus which operates by inhibiting lymphocyte proliferation, antigen presentation in dendritic cells, release of enzymes from lysosomes, release of reactive oxygen species from macrophages, and production of IL-1 (33). Also it has demonstrated to be active as an antiviral agent, since it impedes the completion of the viral life cycle by inhibiting some processes occurring within intracellular organelles and requiring a low pH. For HIV-1, chloroquine and hydroxychloroquine also inhibit the glycosylation of the viral envelope glycoprotein gp120, which occurs within the Golgi apparatus (34). For all of this HCQ, that has been used in the clinic for decades with good results and a very safe profile (35) is a very interesting option to be loaded in nanoparticles with the intention to treat B-CLL and autoimmune diseases and maybe also some viral infections like HIV. Recently HCQ by itself has demonstrated an interesting pro-apoptotic effect and has been selected by the NIH as an anti-cancer drug that deserves further testing. Its antineoplastic properties in vitro depend on its concentration but this cannot routinely be obtained in vivo by the usual oral route of administration (3). HQC, induces a decrease in B-CLL cell viability in a dose- and time-dependent manner when tested in vitro. The mean LC50 calculated for the cells of 20 patients was 32 +/- 7 microg/ml (range, 10-75 microg/ml). A large increase in apoptotic cell numbers after 24 h of incubation with 50 microg/ml HCQ (55 +/- 6 vs. 23 +/- 3% in medium alone, p < 0.001). Indeed, HCQ in leukemic cells induced the features of apoptosis (cell shrinkage, decrease in mitochondrial transmembrane potential, phosphatidylserine externalization, chromatin condensation and DNA fragmentation). HCQ had marked selective cytotoxicity when compared with normal blood mononuclear cells, in which the LC50 was >100 microg/ml at 24 h. HCQ induced the proteolytic cleavage of poly(ADP(adenosine 5'-diphosphate)ribose) polymerase (PARP) and increased the activity of caspase-3. The expression of bcl-2 and bax proteins was significantly modified after incubation with the drug and HCQ activity against CLL cells occurred independently of the presence of IL-4, sCD40L and bone marrow stromal cells (36). The mechanisms behind the effects of HCQ on cancer are currently being investigated. The best- known effects (investigated in clinical and pre-clinical studies) include radiosensitizing effects through lysosome permeabilization, and chemosensitizing effects through inhibition of drug efflux pumps (ATP-binding cassette transporters) or other mechanisms like those of a lysosomotropic agent, meaning that it accumulates preferentially in the lysosomes of cells and in this way promotes apoptosis (37)

## 7. New treatments

### 7.1 Monoclonal antibodies

At present, there are mainly two antibodies with great clinical value for patients with CLL. The first is rituximab (Rituximab, Mabthera) that targets the CD20 antigen(38). This CD20 molecule is expressed on almost all B-cells of patients with B-CLL, but the intensity of expression appears to be lower than in patients with non Hodgkin lymphoma (NHL) (39,40). The second approved mAb is alemtuzumab (Campath-1H), a humanized therapeutic mAb that recognizes the CD52 antigen expressed on normal and neoplastic lymphoid cells. Alemtuzumab is an effective drug in CLL patients with poor risk cytogenetics, such as deletions in 17p. However, alemtuzumab is ineffective in patients with bulky nodal disease (>5 cm) (41-43). Both these "gaps" of these two mAbs, low CD20 expression and bulky nodal disease, could be overcome by nanoparticles technology. Ofatumumab (HuMax-CD20; Arzerra), is a second-generation, fully human, anti-CD20, IgG1 mAb. Ofatumumab recognizes a different CD20 epitope to rituximab (44,45). Compared with rituximab, ofatumumab has similar antibody- dependent cellular cytotoxicity (ADCC) but stronger complement-dependent cytotoxicity (CDC) and does not induce cell death by apoptosis. Ofatumumab potentially represents an active treatment option with clinical benefit for patients with very poor prognosis who have exhausted standard treatment options but also is a very interesting option for the construction of our particles. Lumiliximab is a genetically primatized, macaque human chimeric anti-CD23 IgG1; mAb investigated for the treatment of relapsed CLL. It induces ADCC and CDC, and enhances apoptosis when combined with current or emerging CLL therapies including CLB, fludarabine, alemtuzumab and rituximab. TRU-016 is an intravenously administered anti-CD37 IgG fusion protein for the potential treatment of B-cell malignancies, including CLL and non-Hodgkin's lymphoma. In addition, several other mAbs directed against lymphoid cells have been recently developed and investigated in preclinical studies and clinical trials. These treatments include epratuzumab, galiximab and anti-CD40 mAbs (46).

### 7.2 Phenethyl isothiocyanate-PEITC

Epidemiological studies support the evidence that the consumption of cruciferous vegetables has long been associated with a reduced risk in the occurrence of cancer at various sites, including the prostate, lung, breast, and colon (47).1 The anticarcinogenic effect of cruciferous vegetables is attributed to organic isothiocyanates (ITCs), which are present in a variety of edible cruciferous vegetables such as broccoli, watercress, cabbage, and so on (47). Phenethyl isothiocyanate (PEITC) is one of the ITC family of compounds that has attracted a great deal of attention owing to its remarkable cancer chemopreventive activity (48). In one study samples tested for genetic abnormalities, with deletion of 17p., and exhibiting resistance to F-ara-A ($IC_{50} > 10$ μM), consistent with the crucial effect of p53 on sensitivity to fludarabine remained sensitive to PEITC. The loss of p53 is known to promote genetic instability and mitochondrial dysfunction (49), which not only confers drug resistance but may also promote ROS production (50). In this way it is conceivable that the p53-null CLL cells may have elevated ROS generation and would be highly sensitive to PEITC. Since the loss of p53 is prevalent in cancer and associated with resistance to many standard therapeutic agents (51), the novel ROS-mediated strategy using agents such as PEITC may have potentially broad clinical implications. The increase in ROS generation in CLL cells may render them highly sensitive to PEITC, whereas normal lymphocytes with low ROS output are less vulnerable to this compound. CLL cells from patients in advanced stages refractory to fludarabine-based therapy still remain highly sensitive to PEITC due to their increased ROS generation (52).

To improve their efficacy, HDACi have been paired with other antitumor agents. There are several combination therapies, such as ROS-generating agents, that together may provide a therapeutic advantage over single-agent vorinostat (53).

This last combination of Vorinostat and a ROS generating agent like, Phenylethyl-isothiocyanate (PEITC), has already been tested by us in nanoparticles systems with very good results, and so, it would be a best to associate them in this way for the production of the next generation of BNPs.

## 7.3 Histone deacetylase inhibitors (HDACi)

Histone acetylation is another recent alternative for CLL treatment that consists in a posttranslational modification that plays a role in regulating gene expression.

More recently, other non-histone proteins have been identified to be acetylated which can regulate their function, stability, localization, or interaction with other molecules. Modulating acetylation with histone deacetylase inhibitors (HDACi) has been validated to have anticancer effects in preclinical and clinical cancer models. This has led to development and approval of the first HDACi, Vorinostat, for the treatment of cutaneous T cell lymphoma. The impressive anticancer activity observed in both in vitro and in vivo cancer models, together with their preferential effect on cancer cells, have led to a huge effort into the identification and development of HDACi with different characteristics. To date, several clinical trials of HDACi conducted in solid tumors and hematological malignancies have shown a preferential clinical efficacy of these drugs in hematological malignancies and in particular in cutaneous T-cell lymphoma (CTCL), peripheral T-cell lymphoma (PTCL), Hodgkin lymphoma (HL) and myeloid malignancies. Several agents are also beginning to be tested in combination therapies, either as chemo-sensitizing agents in association with standard chemotherapy drugs or in combination with DNA methyltransferase inhibitors (DNMTi) in the context of the so-called "epigenetic therapies", aimed to revert epigenetic alterations found in cancer cells. Vorinostat has demostrated also efficacy in Hodgkin and Non-Hodgkin Lymphomas (53-56). However, to date, targeting acetylation with HDACi as a monotherapy has shown modest activity against     other cancers including B-CLL.

## 7.4 New biodegradable nanoparticle systems for the treatment of B-chronic lymphocytic leukemia and lymphomas

The pharmaceutical industry as well as the scientific community has been dedicating a big effort as well as a large financial investment in the generation of promising targeted new therapeutic approaches for the treatment of all types of cancers including B-CLL and other Non-Hodgkin lymphomas. These attempts have been design mainly to overcome the challenges associated with the development of drug resistance. Also novel strategies are urgently needed to by-pass the adverse side effects of standard and new chemo and biologic therapeutic agents given by oral, IV or IM routes. In this way, we and others, have proposed to use monoclonal coated and drug loaded biodegradable nanoparticles (BNPs) specially to promote cell epitope specific delivery, and an increased sensitivity to anti-neoplastic drugs. Nanoparticle-based systems are already a real possibility to treat B-CLL. This innovative strategy will generate a pipeline of products in the near future, which will change the way we will treat these patients as well as others with different but also complex and severe diseases. There will probably be no big differences between products of this kind but this little varieties will also not be trivial. The best available products such as those non-traditional pro-apoptotic compounds or its combinations, will be the substances to be selected and loaded in these particles, and this will be one of the clues for these particles to work. HCQ is one of the best candidates as seen in all our research studies. It will be important for the hematologist to completely understand the mechanisms of action of this substance when delivered inside BNPs. Many drugs as well as other biologic agents have poor cellular bioavailability (56). At low or suboptimal concentrations these compounds are not pro-apoptotic at all or their effects could be very different to those we are looking for. Consistent with this, HCQ in clinical trials for B-CLL given orally like for malaria or rheumatic disease, might not be provoking the desired effects or even some, that could be not good at all for the patients, specially considering that its apoptotic effects are only reach at very high concentrations that are impossible to obtained by the oral route. Combining HCQ with CLB will probably be synergistic especially for those patients with already resistant disease or with bad prognosis gene mutations (57). Also PEITC associated with Vorinostat as well as Parthenolide with Honokiol/Magnolol seem to be interesting combinations to try. In relation to the monoclonal antibodies that will coat the first generation of BNPs for B-CLL treatment, those that target the anti-CD20 receptor alone or in combination with the anti-CD19 antibody are surely the best candidates to begin. Then the anti-CD52 and anti-CD23 would also be good possibilities to be used. There are some biological needs for these treatments to succed: (i) they must exhibit "stealth" qualities to evade macrophage attack and the immune response; (ii) be nontoxic, traceable and biodegradable following systemic administration through any route; (iii) display effective pharmacokinetic properties; (iv) the polymer must protect the embedded therapeutics; and (v) they must be selective in their targeting to specific tissue sites. All these qualities are fulfilled by our BNPs. Regulatory changes are needed also at the FDA. FDA must provide clear regulatory/safety guidelines for therapeutic nanoparticles including those related to environmental and health issues, but must help to accelerate the introduction of these technologies as soon as possible in the market.

## 8. Production and characterization of the first generation of biodegradable nanoparticles and its use in the treatment of B-CLL

We have already described that almost all FDA approved antineoplastic drugs in clinical use today are not selective to cancer cells and can produce very toxic side effects (58). In order to obtain better results and tolerability other therapeutic strategies should be developed, specially those that could carry drugs in new delivery systems designed to specifically target cell receptors or epitopes an introduce the desired therapeutic agents loaded in a carrier such as a nanoparticle. These systems are a new technology for cancer therapy (59). Receptor-targeted nanoparticles like the ones presented here (200~300 nm) are good drug carriers and can transport large amounts of drugs, while having a prolonged circulation time (specially when surface PEGylated), as well as a very selective tumor penetration when coated with monoclonal antibodies such as the anti-CD20 Rituximab. These nanoparticles can release enough amounts of drugs inside the cancer cells and in this way overcome multidrug resistance (MDR) mechanisms which are over-expressed in many B-CLL cells (60). Other nanoparticles (e.g., liposomes, micelles, polymers, dendrimers) have demonstrated efficacy both in vitro and in vivo (61). Nanoparticles systems have emerged as important tools to modify the release profile for a large number of drugs including inhibitors, protein and peptide molecules. They are produced from biocompatible and biodegradable FDA approved materials, making them a promising therapeutic strategy for drug targeting and delivery, and surmounting the inherent limitations of regulation acceptance. Additional advantages include reduction of drug toxicity and increase of drug bioavailability . Several previous studies have already demonstrated the goal, and it is well known that when used to deliver chemotherapeutics to cancer models, nanoparticles have a higher maximum tolerated dose than free drug. Nanoparticles for example provide a promising carrier for cisplatin administration avoiding its side effects without a reduction of the efficacy, which was consistent with a higher activation of apoptosis than free-drug. Moreover, this simple strategy can promote co-assembly of drugs, imaging agents and targeting moieties into multifunctional nano-pharmaceutics. Most current anticancer agents do not greatly differentiate between cancerous and normal cells, leading to systemic toxicity and adverse effects. This lack of differentiation greatly limits the maximum drug allowable dose, but the overexpression of receptors or antigens in human cancers lends itself to efficient uptake by receptor mediated endocytosis. There is some previous but limited published experience with nanoparticles in lymphomas, including in vivo studies in lympho-proliferative diseases. We have already published (3) the possibility of using these pharmaceutical new systems to overcome drug resistance of B-Chronic Lymphocytic Leukemia cells. We used for this purpose, PEG-PLGA polymers based BNPs specially designed to be loaded with HCQ and coated with specific monoclonal antibodies. These BNPs induced apoptosis of malignant B-CLL cells at low concentrations. HCQ-BNPs with mAbs induced a decrease in cell viability in a dose and time-dependent manner. In leukemic cells, the nanoparticles reduced cell viability in doses and times significantly lower than in normal lymphocytes. In vitro treatment of drug-resistant B-CLL cells with these HCQ-loaded BNPs was shown to be significantly more effective (P<0.001) than BNPs without drug, indicating that treatment with empty BNPs had little impact on cell viability. BNPs encapsulated with HCQ, but without mAbs, had significantly less impact on in vitro cell viability (P<0.001). Anti-CD19 and anti-CD20 antibodies suspended in PBS with 10% BSA in AIM V medium alone without BNPs produced no significant apoptoticeffect in B-CLL or normal lymphocytes. Active targeting is based on specific interactions with receptors on target cells that may promote enhanced internalization of nanoparticles through receptor mediated endocytosis. In addition, a common method for reducing the recognition of nanoparticles by the RES is to coat their surfaces with polyethylene glycol (PEG). In addition to specific interactions between the ligands on the surface of nanoparticles and receptors expressed on the tumor cells, this may trigger receptor mediated endocytosis. Furthermore, active targeting has shown the potential to suppress multidrug resistance (MDR) via bypassing of P-glycoprotein-mediated drug efflux. The targeting ligands may not play a role until the targeted nanoparticles find the tumor sites. This is very easy for our particles as the targeted cells reside mainly inside the vascular compartment or in tissues with high accessibility to the vasculature, such as in the case of B-CLL. In this situation, targeting occurs relatively quickly and easily. When BNPs were coated with human anti-CD19 and anti-CD20 antibodies the apoptotic effect was more pronounced and enhanced. Confirming the idea that nano-constructs such as these ones targeting B-CLL cells should serve as customizable, targeted drug delivery vehicles capable of ferrying large doses of chemotherapeutic agents into malignant cells while sparing healthy ones. Our nanoparticles beside the original idea of loading them with an anti-malarial immune modifying drug such as HCQ, have the advantage of their special production process in which nano core shells of a median diameter of 250 nm can be obtained by a non-emulsion-polymerization method, and in which several different drugs or petides can be easily encapsulated while one or more monoclonal antibodies can be coated in their surface. We also tried a similar kind of nanoparticles, both, in-vitro and in-vivo, in a mice living model of human lymphoma, but

HCQ was combined this time with CLB in order to potentiate its effects, and Rituximab, the first anti-human CD20 monoclonal antibody approved by the FDA for the treatment of lymphomas (62), was attached to the surface of the BNPs. We have developed a special type of biodegradable targeted nanoparticles with demonstrated efficacy in vitro and in vivo in animal studies for B-CLL, lymphomas and autoinmune diseases. The rational design of these nanoparticles considered the possibility of delivering high concentrations of HCQ and its combination with CLB loaded in biodegradable (PLGA) nanoparticles and coated with the mentioned antibody. Ordinarily, CLB-resistant B-CLL lymphocytes are 5- to 6-fold more resistant in vitro, using the MTT assay, as compared to sensitive lymphocytes (IC50 CLB of _61.0 mmol=L can be considered sensitive). This is why delivering CLB in nanoparticle systems seems to be a good idea indeed in resistant phenotypes. Loss of viability in human CLL cells correlated with the early induction of apoptosis.

## 9. Encapsulation of CLB and HCQ sulfate in BNPs containing anti-human-CD20 monoclonal antibody rituximab functional groups on their outer shells

BNPs with an average diameter in the range of 250 nm (measured by Dyamic Light Scattering) were produced by a non-emulsion-polymerization proprietary technology (Bio-Target Inc. USA). The particles had a -0.05 mV surface potential, measure by its zeta potential. The nano- capsules used in this study included a shell region and a core region. The shell was made of three biocompatible biodegradable polymers: PEG-PLA (polyethylene-glycol-poly-lactic-acid) and PCL (polycaprolactone). The monoclonal antibody Rituximab was coated in their surface.

The core included two therapeutic agents: HCQ and CLB. In this way a capsule including two encapsulated anti-neoplastic agents were produced by this methodology. One specific aspect of these BNPs, was an anti human CD20 functional group (Rituximab) dispersed on the outer surface of the shell region. Three different kinds of BNPs were specially designed. BNP0: only polymer-BNPs (PEG-PLA-PCL) at a concentration of 1.66 mg/ml. BNP1: Polymer (PEG-PLA- PCL) at a concentration of 1.66mg/ml coated with the anti human-CD20 monoclonal antibody, Rituximab, at a concentration of 8.824 ug/ml, combined with a cyanine 5.5 (CY5.5) dye, a fluorescent molecular beacon that emits photons in the near-IR, at 0.465 ug/ml. BNP2: antihuman- CD20-BNPs + (HCQ + CLB) with polymer (PEGPLA- PCL) at 1.66mg/ml, Rituximab at 8.824 ug/ml, CY5.5 dye at 0.465 ug/ml, and CLB at 5mg/ml-HCQ at 5mg/ml. The particles were produced under class 100 clean room conditions and the CY5.5 dye was chemically attached after preparation of the base BNPs as described below. B-CLL Cells and Cell Culture with BNPs Heparinized blood was obtained after informed consent from 3 B-CLL (median age 64.4 years old) Rai-IV, p-53 mutated, patients. The mononuclear cell fractions were isolated by centrifugation on Ficoll-Hypaque gradients. Primary tumor B cells positive for CD5, CD19, CD23, CD20, CD38 and ZAP70, with unmutated Ig genes and p53 mutations were isolated from the B-CLL patient's mononuclear cell fractions respectively using a B-Cell Isolation Kit. Briefly, 2 x 105 freshly isolated cells, from the CLL patients, were incubated in triplicate for all experiments at 37°C and 5% CO2 at various concentrations of BNPs in RPMI 1640 serum-free medium. All BNPs were suspended at the time of use in PBS with 10% Bovine Serum Albumin (BSA) at a final total mass concentration of 900 ug/ml. Aliquots of 0.2, 0.5, 1, and 2 ul from these solutions were used for experiments. After 24 and 48 hours of incubation at 37°C, the number of residual viable cells was estimated in each BNPs system using Ethidium Bromide/Acridine Orange staining and immune-fluorescent microscopy counting as well as measurement of cell apoptosis using annexin-V and propidium-iodide by FACS analysis. Direct Tumor Cell Cytotoxicity Assays using BJAB and MEC-1 cells were also done. The procedure was modified from Macor et al. (63) in order to evaluate the effect of BNPs on BJAB cells, a human Burkitts lymphoma cell line already used to characterize Rituximab activity and on MEC-1, a cell line derived from a patient with chronic lymphocytic leukemia. 2x105 cells of each class were incubated in triplicate in RPMI 1640 serum-free medium (Sigma-Aldrich Italy) with various amounts of BNPs. All BNPs were suspended at the time of use in PBS with 10% Bovine Serum Albumin (BSA) at a final total mass concentration of 900 ug/ml. Aliquots of 0.2, 0.5, 1, and 2 ul from these solutions were used for experiments. After 48 hours of ncubation at 37°C, the number of residual viable cells was estimated using the MTT assay and percentage of dead cells was calculated. For toxicology Studies, 4 groups of 4 C57/Bl mice each were treated intraperitoneally with different amounts of BNP2 in order to evaluate their effects on healthy animals: Group 1 received 10 ul of BNP2 for 4 times (50 ug HCQ + 50 ug CLB). Group 2 received 20 ul BNP2 for 4 times (100 ug HCQ + 100 ug CLB) and Group 3 received 40 ul BNP2 for 4 times(200 ug HCQ+ 200 ug CLB). Group 4: 80 ul BNP2 for 4times(400 ug HCQ + 400 ug CLB). Each animal was treated on days 0, 2, 4 and 7 and followed up to day 21. Therapeutical tudies using a Human/Mouse Model of Burkitt's Lymphoma were performed. Female severe combined immunodeficiency (SCID) mice (4-6 weeks of age) were purchased from Charles River and maintained under pathogen- free conditions. A SCID xenograft model of Human Lymphoma specially developed to investigate the in vivo distribution and therapeutic effects of monoclonals antibodies was used to analyze the effects of BNPs after the toxicology studies. BJAB cells were expanded in vitro and then implanted intraperitoneally (2x106 cells/mouse) in 15 SCID mice (day 0). Ten of these mice were used as controls and the other 5 mice were treated i.p. with 80 ul BNP2 (400 ug HCQ + 400 ug CLB) at days 4, 7, 10, 13. We analyzed survival of controls and treated mice for more than 120 days (end of experiment). Histological and immunohistochemicals analysis were done. Tumor peritoneal masses and liver were collected from sacrificed mice (for ethic reasons) and maintained in buffered- formaline for 16 hours. Samples were first washed in EtOH 70% for 2 hours and then in EtOH 100%. Histological and immunohistochemicals analysis were performed. Results obtained from the prior assays shown that BNPs2 formulated with the human anti-CD20 monoclonal antibody Rituximab, and drugs (HCQ and CLB) efficiently induced apoptosis of malignant human B-CLL cells in vitro. At 0.5 ul concentration, and 24 hs of cuture, these BNPs2 induced 4-fold more apoptosis in malignant B-CLL cells compared to BNPs0 and BNPs1, reaching at 48 hs of culture almost a 95% cell killing effect. Reductions of living B-CLL cells were observed in vitro at 24 and 48 hours for injections of all concentrations of BNPs2. Loss of viability correlated with early induction of apoptosis as confirmed by monitoring the B-CLL cells after Annexin V/propidium iodide staining. BNPs2 with Rituximab and drugs induced a decrease in cell viability in a dose and time dependent manner. In vitro treatment of these B-CLL cells with BNPs2 showed to be more effective than BNPs without drugs (BNP0) indicating that treatment with empty BNPs had little impact on cell viability. BNPs1 encapsulated with HCQ and CLB but without monoclonal antibody had almost no impact on in vitro cell viability. The killing effect of the different BNPs on the B-CLL derived cell line MEC-1 was also analysed. BNPs0 and BNPs1 had 0% cell killing effect after 48 hs in culture, while BNPs2 had 94% killing effect using 0,5 ul. One or 2ul concentrations added little killing effect in the assays. The same experiments performed with BNPs and the Burkitt´s lymphoma cell line (BJAB) showed similar results, obtaining levels of 94% cell killing with 1 ul of BNPs2. In vivo studies start analyzing BNP2 toxicity in healthy mice. C57/Bl mice were treated intraperitoneally with different amounts of BNP2 (10 ul, 20 ul, 40 ul or 80 ul) for 4 injection on days 0, 2, 4 and 7 and followed up to day 21 in order to see possible adverse effects. No side effects have been detected in all the study period in any of the animals injected with BNPs. Histological and immunochemical studies performed on survival animals do not produce information about the distribution of the BNPs because the analysis was performed several weeks after BNPs injections. The in vivo therapeutic effect study was concluded 120 days after the administration of the tumor cells to the animals. Control mice died within day 63 after tumor cell injection. Three treated mice died between day 72 and 98 and tumor mass and liver were collect from these animals. At day 120 only 2 treated mice appeared healthy even at the end of the study. Histological studies were performed on samples derived from tumor masses developed in the peritoneum of treated and untreated mice. The peritoneal masses observed in all untreated animals were mainly composed of sheets of homogeneous round- shaped, medium-sized malignant lymphoid elements showing cohesive growth. However, necrotic areas were seen in peritoneal histological masses derived from all BNPs2-treated mice.

## 10. Final discussion

We have studied and described a new kind of therapeutic BNPs with a functional specific group attached to their outer shell, the first human anti-CD20, FDA approved for Lymphoma treatment, monoclonal antibody Rituximab. We have also combined in these BNPs an antimalarial agent, Hydroxychloroquine, known to have pro-apoptotic properties, with the old anti-leukemic drug Chlorambucil. This last agent has been the gold standard treatment for B- CLL for many decades until the general acceptance of Fludarabine as first line choice treatment (64). Both drugs have been used alone or in combination with Rituximab and other agents for the treatment of many B cell malignancies (65). After initial good responses, these hematological neoplasias usually mutate, and become resistant to all modalities of standard treatments. B-CLL and Lymphomas seem to be different sides of the same coin. Their malignant cells have the same potential to kill the patients, but also the same potential to dye by apoptosis under similar targeted therapies, like the one we propose here. With the use of these BNPs we were able to specifically target a variety of B malignant cells such as those from B-CLL patients, as well as BJAB and MEC-1 cell lines, with outstanding cell killing efficiency by apoptotic mechanisms. These BNPs induced high levels of responses beside having some of those cells, like the ones from CLL patients, bad prognostic markers such as mutation of the p- 53 gen. Then, a BNP coated with Rituximab and loaded with HCQ and CLB could be an interesting therapeutic strategy in which the antimalarial drug with pro-apoptotic activity seems to have a synergistic effect when associated with a cytotoxic agent. Those mechanisms of drug resistance usually found in Lymphomas after several treatment modalities could be overcome by the use of these BNPs and this drug combination. We did not see any adverse effect related to the use of BNPs when tested in living mice models. This could be a good evidence of the safety of this kind of treatment. The survival advantage of those animals implanted with human lymphoma cells when treated with BNPs is provocative, but in some way it was expected after the good results obtained in our in vitro assays. This prolonged overall survival of the treated animals probably correlates well with some of the histological findings, in which cell apoptosis and necrosis were seen only in B cell tumor areas after injecting the mice models with BNP2. For all of this, it seems reasonable to do more animal studies of the same kind in order to accelerate a possible introduction of this promising technology into a first human clinical trial. Maybe changing at last, the high mortality associated with B-CLL and other indolent lymphomas.

## 11. References

[1] Raphael B, Andersen JW, Silber R, et al. Comparison of chlorambucil and prednisone versus cyclophosphamide, vincristine, and prednisone as initial treatment for chronic lymphocytic leukemia: long-term follow-up of an Eastern Cooperative Oncology Group randomized clinical trial. J Clin Oncol. 1991;9(5):770-6.

[2] Lagneaux L, Delforge A, Carlier S, Massy M, Bernier M, Bron D. Early induction of apoptosis in B-chronic lymphocytic leukaemia cells by hydroxychloroquine: activation of caspase-3 and no protection by survival factors.Br J Haematol.2001;112(2):344-52.

[3] Mansilla E, Marin GH, Nuñez L, et al. The lysosomotropic agent, hydroxychloroquine,delivered in a biodegradable nanoparticle system, overcomes drug resistance of B-chronic lymphocytic leukemia cells in vitro. Cancer Biother Radiopharm. 2010Feb;25(1):97-103.

[4] Marin GH, Mansilla E, Mezzaroba N. Exploratory study on the effects of biodegradablenanoparticles with drugs on malignant B cells and on a human/mouse model ofBurkitt lymphoma. Curr Clin Pharmacol. 2010;5(4):246-50.

[5] Bawa R. Nanoparticle-based Therapeutics in Humans: A Survey. Nanotechnology Law & Business. 2008; 5,2:135-155.

[6] Deglesne PA, Chevallier N, Letestu R. et al. Survival response to B-cell receptor ligation is restricted to progressive chronic lymphocytic leukemia cells irrespective of Zap70 expression. Cancer Res. 2006;66(14):7158-66.

[7] Zucchetto A, Bomben R, Dal Bo M et al. A scoring system based on the expression of sixsurface molecules allows the identification of three prognostic risk groups in B-cell chronic lymphocytic leukemia. J Cell Physiol. 2006;207(2):354-63.

[8] Ricky W. Johnstone, Erika Cretney, and Mark J. Smyth. P-Glycoprotein ProtectsLeukemia Cells Against Caspase-Dependent, but not Caspase-Independent, Cell Death. Blood 1999; 93,3: 1075-1085.

[9] Turgut B, Vural O, Pala FS, et al. 17p Deletion is associated with resistance of B-cell chronic lym- phocytic leukemia cells to in vitro fludarabine- induced apoptosis. Leuk Lymphoma. 2007;48: 311-220.

[10] Grever MR, Lucas DM, Dewald GW, et al. Com- prehensive assessment of genetic and molecular features predicting outcome in patients with chronic lymphocytic leukemia: results from the US Intergroup Phase III Trial E2997. J Clin Oncol. 2007; 25:799-804.

[11] Zhou Y, Hileman EO, Plunkett W, Keating MJ, Huang P. Free radical stress in chronic lympho- cytic leukemia cells and its role in cellular sensitivity to ROS-generating anticancer agents. Blood 2003;101:4098-4104.

[12] Kalil N, Cheson BD. Management of chronic lymphocytic leukaemia. Drugs Aging. 2000;16(1):9-27

[13] Silvennoinen R, Malminiemi K, Malminiemi O, Seppälä E, Vilpo J. Pharmacokinetics of chlorambucil in patients with chronic lymphocytic leukaemia: comparison of different days, cycles and doses.Pharmacol Toxicol. 2000;87(5):223-8.

[14] Tam KY, Leung KC, Wang YX. Chemoembolization agents for cancer treatment. Eur J Pharm Sci. 2011;44(1-2):1-10.

[15] Ren D, Kratz F, Wang SW. Protein nanocapsules containing doxorubicin as a pH-responsive delivery system. Small. 2011;7(8):1051-60

[16] Bergmann MA, Goebeler ME, Herold M, et al. Efficacy of bendamustine in patients with relapsed or refractory chronic lymphocytic leukemia: results of a phase I/II study of the German CLL Study Group. Haematologica. 2005;90(10):1357-64.

[17] Fischer K, Cramer P, Busch R. Bendamustine Combined With Rituximab in Patients With Relapsed and/or Refractory Chronic lymphocytic Leukemia: A Multicenter Phase II Trial of the German Chronic Lymphocytic Leukemia Study Group. J Clin Oncol. 2011 ; 8(1):38-47 .

[18] Cavalli R, Bisazza A, Bussano R. Poly(amidoamine)-Cholesterol Conjugate Nanoparticles Obtained by Electrospraying as Novel Tamoxifen Delivery System. J Drug Deliv. 2011;2011:587604.

[19] Magrone T, Jirillo E. Potential application of dietary polyphenols from red wine to attaining healthy ageing. Curr Top Med Chem. 2011;11(14):1780-96.

[20] Chow HH, Hakim IA. Pharmacokinetic and chemoprevention studies on tea in humans. Pharmacol Res. 2011 Aug;64(2):105-12.

[21] Song WZ, Cui JF, Zhang GD. Studies on the medicinal plants of the Magnoliaceae tuhoupo of Manglietia. J Chin Herbs 1989;24:295-9.

[22] Ross JJ, Arnason JT, Birnboim HC. Low concentrations of the fever few component parthenolide inhibit in vitro growth of tumor lines in a cytostatic fashion. Planta Med 1999;65:126-9.

[23] Yip-Schneider MT, Nakshatri H, Sweeney CJ, Marshall MS, Wiebke EA, Schmidt CM. Parthenolide and sulindac cooperate to mediate growth suppression and inhibit the nuclear factor-kappa B pathway in pancreatic carcinoma cells. Mol Cancer Ther 2005;4:587-94.

[24] Sweeney CJ, Mehrotra S, Sadaria MR, Kumar S, Shortle NH, Roman Y, et al. The sesquiterpene lactone parthenolide in combination with docetaxel reduces metastasis and improves survival in a xenograft model of breast cancer. Mol Cancer Ther 2005;4:1004-12.

[25] Marin GH, Mansilla E. Apoptosis induced by Magnolia Grandiflora extract in chlorambucil-resistant B-chronic lymphocytic leukemia cells.J Cancer Res Ther. 2010; 6(4):463-5.

[26] Marin G.H., Mansilla E. Parthenolide has apoptotic and cytotoxic selective effect on B-chronic lymphocytic leukemia cells. J. Appl. Biomed.2006; 4: 135–139.

[27] Yang SE, Hsieh MT, Tsai TH, Hsu SL. Inhibitory effect of magnolol and honokiol from Magnolia obovata on human fibrosarcoma HT-1080. Invasiveness in vitro. Planta Med 2001;67:705- 8.

[28] Sweeney CJ, Mehrotra S, Sadaria MR, Kumar S, Shortle NH, Roman Y, et al. The sesquiterpene lactone parthenolide in combination with docetaxel reduces

metastasis and improves survival in a xenograft model of breast cancer. Mol Cancer Ther 2005;4:1004-12.

[29] Battle TE, Castro-Malaspina H, Gribben JG, Frank DA. Sustained complete remission of CLL associated with the use of a Chinese herbal extract: Case report and mechanistic analysis. Leuk Res 2003;27:859-63.

[30] Wiedhopf RM, Young M, Bianchi E, Cole JR. Tumor inhibitory agent from Magnolia grandiflora (Magnoliaceae). I. Parthenolide. J Pharm Sci 1973;62:345.

[31] Clark AM, El-Feraly FS, Li WS. Antimicrobial activityof phenolic constituents of Magnolia grandiflora L. J Pharm Sci 1981;70:951-2.

[32] Yang SE, Hsieh MT, Tsai TH, Hsu SL. Down-modulation of BCl-XL, release ofcytochrome c and sequential activation of caspases during honokiol-inducedapoptosis in human squamous lung cancer CH27 cells. Biochem Pharmacol 2002; 63:1641-51.

[33] Ross JJ, Arnason JT, Birnboim HC. Low concentrations of the feverfew component parthenolide inhibit in vitro growth of tumor lines in a cytostatic fashion. Planta Med 1999;65:126-9.

[34] Kanno S, Kitajima Y, Kakuta M, Osanai Y, Kurauchi K, Ujibe M, et al. Costunolide-induced apoptosis is caused by receptor-mediated pathway and inhibition of telomerase activity in NALM-6 cells. Biol Pharm Bull 2008;31:1024-8

[35] Amaravadi RK, Lippincott-Schwartz J, Yin XM et al.Principles and current strategies for targeting autophagy for cancer treatment. Clin Cancer Res. 2011 Feb 15;17(4):654-66.

[36] Aguirre-Cruz L, Torres KJ, Jung-Cook H, Fortuny C, Sánchez E, Soda-Mehry A, Sotelo J, Reyes-Terán G Preferential concentration of hydroxychloroquine in adenoid tissue of HIV-infected subjects. AIDS Res Hum Retroviruses. 2010;26(3):339-42.

[37] Das SK, Pareek A, Mathur DS, Efficacy and safety of hydroxychloroquine sulphate in rheumatoid arthritis: a randomized, double-blind, placebo controlled clinical trial--an Indian experience. Curr Med Res Opin. 2007 Sep;23(9):2227-34.

[38] Lagneaux L, Delforge A, Dejeneffe M, Massy M, Bernier M, Bron D Leuk Hydroxychloroquine-induced apoptosis of chronic lymphocytic leukemia involves activation of caspase-3 and modulation of Bcl-2/bax/ratio.Lymphoma. 2002;43(5):1087-95.

[39] Rahim R, Strobl JS. Hydroxychloroquine, chloroquine, and all-trans retinoic acid regulate growth, survival, and histone acetylation in breast cancer cells. Anticancer Drugs. 2009;20(8):736-45.

[40] Robak T. Monoclonal antibodies in the treatment of chronic lymphoid leukemias. Leuk. Lymphoma.2004;45:205–19.

[41] Onrust SV, Lamb HM, Balfour JA. Rituximab. Drugs. 1999;58:79–88.

[42] O'Brien SM, Kantarjian H, Thomas DA, et al. Rituximab dose-escalation trial in chronic lymphocytic leukemia. J. Clin. Oncol. 2001;19:2165–70.

[43] Robak T. Alemtuzumab for B-cell chronic lymphocytic leukemia. Expert Rev. Anticancer Ther. 2008;8:1033–51

[44] Robak T. Novel monoclonal antibodies for the treatment of chronic lymphocytic leukemia. Curr Cancer Drug Targets. 2008;8:156–71.

[45] Coiffier B, Lepretre S, Pedersen LM, et al. Safety and efficacy ofofatumumab, a fully human monoclonal anti-CD20 antibody, in patients with relapsed or refractory B-cell chronic lymphocytic leukemia. A phase I–II study. Blood. 2008;11:1094–1100

[46] Robak T. Novel drugs for chronic lymphoid leukemias: mechanism of action and therapeutic activity.Curr Med Chem. 2009;16:2212–34.

[47] Conaway CC, Yang YM, Chung FL. Isothiocyanates as cancer chemo-preventive agents: their biological activities and metabolism in rodents and humans. Curr Drug Metab. 2002;3:233–255.

[48] Stoner GD, Morrissey DT, Heur YH, Daniel EM, Galati AJ, Wagner SA. Inhibitory effects of phenethyl isothiocyanate on N-nitrosobenzylmethylamine carcinogenesis in the rat esophagus. Cancer Res. 1991; 51:2063–2068.

[49] Matoba S, Kang JG, Patino WD, et al. p53 regulates mitochondrial respiration. Science 2006;312:1650-1653.

[50] Achanta G, Sasaki R, Feng L, et al. Novel role of p53 in maintaining mitochondrial genetic stability through interaction with DNA Pol gamma. EMBO J 2005;24: 3482-3492.

[51] Gasco M, Crook T. p53 family members and chemoresistance in cancer: what we know and what we need to know. Drug Resist Updat 2003;6:323-328.

[52] Trachootham D, Zhang H , Zhang W, Feng L, Du M, Zhou Y, Chen Z, Pelicano H, Plunkett W, Wierda W, Keating M, and Huang P. Effective elimination of fludarabine-resistant CLL cells by PEITC through a redox-mediated mechanism. Blood 2008; 112, 5: 1912-1922.

[53] Kirschbaum M, Frankel P, Popplewell L et al. Phase II study of vorinostat for treatment of relapsed or refractory indolent non-Hodgkin's lymphoma and mantle cell lymphoma. J Clin Oncol. 2011;29(9):1198-203.

[54] Miller CP, Singh MM, Rivera-Del Valle N, Manton CA, Chandra J. Therapeutic strategies to enhance the anticancer efficacy of histonedeacetylase inhibitors. J Biomed Biotechnol. 2011;20:5142-61.

[55] Robak T. Application of New Drugs in Chronic Lymphocytic Leukemia. Mediterr J Hematol Infect Dis.2010; 2(2): e2010011.

[56] Mercurio C, Minucci S, Pelicci PG. Histone deacetylases and epigenetic therapies of hematological malignancies.Pharmacol Res. 2010 ;62(1):18-34.

[57] Krystof V, Uldrijan S. Cyclin-dependent kinase inhibitors as anticancer drugs. Curr Drug Targets. 2010;11(3):291-302.

[58] Meng-Dan Z, Fu-Qiang H, Yong-Zhong D. Coadministration of glycolipid-like micelles loading cytotoxic drug with different action site for efficient cancer chemotherapy .Nanotechnology 2009; 20,5: 55-9. Jønsson V, Gemmell CG, Wiik A. Emerging concepts in the management of the malignant haematological disorders. Expert Opin Pharmacother. 2000;1(4):713-35.

[59] Islam T, Josephson L.Current state and future applications of active targeting in malignancies using superparamagnetic iron oxide nanoparticles. Cancer Biomark. 2009;5(2):99-107.

[60] Rao DA, Forrest ML, Alani AW, Kwon GS, Robinson JR. Biodegradable PLGA based nanoparticles for sustained regional lymphatic drug delivery. J Pharm Sci. 2010; 99(4):2018-31.

[61] Luo G, Yu X, Jin C, Yang F, et al LyP-1-conjugated nanoparticles for targeting drug delivery to lymphatic metastatic tumors. Int J Pharm. 2010; 385(1-2):150-6.

[62] Schulz H, Rehwald U, Morschhauser F et al. Rituximab in relapsed lymphocyte-predominant Hodgkin lymphoma: long-term results of a phase 2 trial by the German Hodgkin Lymphoma Study Group (GHSG). Blood. 2008;111(1):109-11.

[63] Macor P, Tripodo C, Zorzet S, et al. In vivo targeting of human neutralizing antibodiesagainst CD55 and CD59 to lymphoma cells increases the antitumor activity ofrituximab. Cancer Res 2007; 67(21): 10556-63.

[64] Rai K, Peterson BL, Appelbaum FR. Fludarabine compared with chlorambucil as primary therapy for chronic CLL. N. Engl. J Med 2000; 343: 1750-8.

[65] Huhn D., von Schilling C., Wilhelm M. Rituximab therapy of patients with B-cell CLLL. Blood 2001; 5: 1326-31

# Permissions

The contributors of this book come from diverse backgrounds, making this book a truly international effort. This book will bring forth new frontiers with its revolutionizing research information and detailed analysis of the nascent developments around the world.

We would like to thank Pablo Oppezzo, PhD, for lending his expertise to make the book truly unique. He has played a crucial role in the development of this book. Without his invaluable contribution this book wouldn't have been possible. He has made vital efforts to compile up to date information on the varied aspects of this subject to make this book a valuable addition to the collection of many professionals and students.

This book was conceptualized with the vision of imparting up-to-date information and advanced data in this field. To ensure the same, a matchless editorial board was set up. Every individual on the board went through rigorous rounds of assessment to prove their worth. After which they invested a large part of their time researching and compiling the most relevant data for our readers. Conferences and sessions were held from time to time between the editorial board and the contributing authors to present the data in the most comprehensible form. The editorial team has worked tirelessly to provide valuable and valid information to help people across the globe.

Every chapter published in this book has been scrutinized by our experts. Their significance has been extensively debated. The topics covered herein carry significant findings which will fuel the growth of the discipline. They may even be implemented as practical applications or may be referred to as a beginning point for another development. Chapters in this book were first published by InTech; hereby published with permission under the Creative Commons Attribution License or equivalent.

The editorial board has been involved in producing this book since its inception. They have spent rigorous hours researching and exploring the diverse topics which have resulted in the successful publishing of this book. They have passed on their knowledge of decades through this book. To expedite this challenging task, the publisher supported the team at every step. A small team of assistant editors was also appointed to further simplify the editing procedure and attain best results for the readers.

Our editorial team has been hand-picked from every corner of the world. Their multi-ethnicity adds dynamic inputs to the discussions which result in innovative outcomes. These outcomes are then further discussed with the researchers and contributors who give their valuable feedback and opinion regarding the same. The feedback is then collaborated with the researches and they are edited in a comprehensive manner to aid the understanding of the subject.

Apart from the editorial board, the designing team has also invested a significant amount of their time in understanding the subject and creating the most relevant covers. They scrutinized every image to scout for the most suitable representation of the subject and create an appropriate cover for the book.

The publishing team has been involved in this book since its early stages. They were actively engaged in every process, be it collecting the data, connecting with the contributors or procuring relevant information. The team has been an ardent support to the editorial, designing and production team. Their endless efforts to recruit the best for this project, has resulted in the accomplishment of this book. They are a veteran in the field of academics and their pool of knowledge is as vast as their experience in printing. Their expertise and guidance has proved useful at every step. Their uncompromising quality standards have made this book an exceptional effort. Their encouragement from time to time has been an inspiration for everyone.

The publisher and the editorial board hope that this book will prove to be a valuable piece of knowledge for researchers, students, practitioners and scholars across the globe.

# List of Contributors

L. Michaux
Center for Human Genetics, Catholic University of Leuven, Leuven, Belgium

N. Put, I. Wlodarska and P. Vandenberghe
Department of Hematology, University Hospital UCL Saint-Luc, Brussels, Belgium

José-Ángel Hernández
Hospital Universitario Infanta Leonor, Madrid, Spain

Marcos González and Jesús-María Hernández
Hospital Clínico Universitario, Salamanca, Spain

Leticia Huergo-Zapico, Azahara Fernández-Guizán, Andrea Acebes Huerta, Alejandro López-Soto and Segundo Gonzalez
Functional Biology Department, Instituto Universitario Oncologico del Principado de Asturias (IUOPA), University of Oviedo, Oviedo, Spain

Ana P. Gonzalez-Rodríguez
Hematology Department, Hospital Universitario Central de Asturias, Oviedo, Spain

Juan Contesti
Hematology Department, Hospital Cabueñe, Gijón, Spain

Jovana Bogojeski, Biljana Petrović and Živadin D. Bugarčić
University of Kragujevac, Faculty of Science, Department of Chemistry, Serbia

Farhad Abbasi
Bushehr University of Medical Sciences, Iran

Günter Krause, Mirjam Kuckertz, Susan Kerwien, Michaela Patz and Michael Hallek
Department I of Internal Medicine, University of Cologne, Center of Integrated Oncology Köln Bonn, Germany

Nina C. Dempsey-Hibbert, Christine Hoyle and John H.H. Williams
Chester Centre for Stress Research, University of Chester, United Kingdom

Reslan Lina and Dumontet Charles
Université Lyon 1, Lyon, France

Eduardo Mansilla
National University of La Rioja, UNLAR, La Rioja, Argentina

**Gustavo H. Marin**
CUCAIBA, Ministry of Health, La Plata, Buenos Aires, Argentina

**Luis Núñez**
University of Chicago, Chicago, Illinois, USA and Bio-Target, Chicago, Illinois, USA

**Gustavo Larsen**
LNK Chemsolutions, Lincoln Nebraska, USA and Bio-Target, Chicago, USA

**Nelly Mezzaroba and Paolo Macor**
Department of Life Science, University of Trieste, Italy

Printed in the USA
CPSIA information can be obtained
at www.ICGtesting.com
JSHW011404221024
72173JS00003B/423